Lazaretto

*How Philadelphia Used an Unpopular Quarantine
Based on Disputed Science to Accommodate Immigrants and
Prevent Epidemics*

David Barnes

Johns Hopkins University Press
Baltimore

© 2023 Johns Hopkins University Press
All rights reserved. Published 2023
Printed in the United States of America on acid-free paper
9   8   7   6   5   4   3   2   1

Johns Hopkins University Press
2715 North Charles Street
Baltimore, Maryland 21218
www.press.jhu.edu

Library of Congress Cataloging-in-Publication Data is available.

ISBN 978-1-4214-4644-8 (hardcover)
ISBN 978-1-4214-4645-5 (ebook)

A catalog record for this book is available from the British Library.

Special discounts are available for bulk purchases of this book. For more information, please contact Special Sales at specialsales@jh.edu.

To Dan and Nick, with pride and joy

Contents

Illustrations

Lazaretto

Grace under Pressure, 1879

If this book has a hero, it is William T. Robinson.

As resident physician at the Lazaretto, Philadelphia's quarantine station on Tinicum Island, Robinson used his medical and leadership skills from 1878 through 1883 to save the lives of people suffering from a deadly disease—all while placating business interests anxious to keep commerce flowing. He had the imperturbable confidence needed to keep everyone calm during yellow fever outbreaks as he faced down politicians' threats. And he had the wisdom to focus on providing the best medical advice and attention he could, letting any controversy swirl past him.

In one of the few surviving photographs of him, there is a soft, knowing twinkle in Dr. Robinson's eye that hints at a depth of character and a humanistic outlook on life not found in every medical man or public servant of his era. This he knew: if nothing bad happened during his tenure, praise was unlikely, but blame would surely find him if disaster occurred on his watch. Public service was a calling he took seriously. Equanimity and political savvy served him well.

Seventy-eight years after the Lazaretto's opening in 1801, the quarantine station and the area around it had changed dramatically. Nearby Chester, a thriving shipbuilding city, was growing rapidly, as was the industrial behemoth of Philadelphia. Both cities' populations were slowly creeping outward toward the Tinicum Island site, which had been chosen for its remoteness. The Philadelphia, Wilmington, and Baltimore Railroad stopped at the Lazaretto. Federal officers stationed at the breakwater protecting the mouth of the Delaware Bay could warn the quarantine station via telegraph whenever a vessel was headed its way, and even whether illness was aboard.[1] The telegraph also allowed instant communication between the Lazaretto and the Board of Health in the city, a far cry from the twice-daily mail runs, which had delayed decisions on many critical occasions.

Robinson embraced progress at the Lazaretto and continually sought to reassure Philadelphia's merchants that there was no inherent conflict between protecting public health and preserving the free flow of commerce.[2] He also considered himself a progressive man of science, and his tenure on Tinicum Island coincided with the most dramatic developments in the bacteriological revolution.

Equanimity certainly came in handy in July 1879, when the filthy brig *Shasta* limped up the Delaware River to Tinicum Island. A soft breeze carried the brig to the Lazaretto, but to Dr. Robinson it carried the ominous, unmistakable stench of yellow fever, an odor described in the textbooks of the day as a blend of human cadavers and putrid fish. Sure enough, as soon as he boarded, he saw something close to a worst-case scenario: nine haggard men, famished and out of provisions, seven of them sick with yellow fever. Even with all nine working together, they were too weak to heave the anchor over the side. The *Shasta*'s 46-year-old captain, Albert Batson, lay prostrate with a severe case.[3]

Anyone in Robinson's position would have detained the *Shasta* for quarantine at the Lazaretto; it was an easy call. But it was the last easy decision he would face during what turned into a seven-week ordeal of public fear, rumor, outrage, defiance, and recriminations.

Anchored at "a safe distance" from the Lazaretto, the brig was taking on water and needed three men at the pumps to keep it afloat. Robinson brought the captain and the five seamen sickest with yellow fever ashore, where they were bathed, dressed in clean clothing, and admitted to the hospital. The two healthy sailors and the one with the mildest symptoms remained aboard the leaky vessel, where the Lazaretto steward provided them with vegetables, bread, and meat. The Lazaretto gates were closed, and placards surrounding it proclaimed "No Admittance." Dr. Robinson refused an invitation from the Board of Health to send his wife and four children away from the station for their safety; if his family left, he reasoned, the station would be demoralized, and staff might leave their posts in panic. "I think I can prevent the station from becoming infected, and feel perfectly capable of managing everything to the satisfaction of the Board of Health," Robinson told the board.[4]

The *Shasta*'s cargo of logwood from the northern coast of Haiti was destined for the Sharpless Dye Works just outside Chester, 3 miles west of the Lazaretto, where a newspaper reported that the sickly brig's arrival "naturally excited much anxiety." Before the day was out, rumors were already circulating in Chester that Dr. Robinson was presiding over an open-door policy at the Lazaretto, "riding around the community himself" and allowing others to come and go as they pleased.[5]

Back at the station, Robinson did not have time at first to respond to the criticism in the press. He ordered the *Shasta* patients' old clothing to be fumigated in a shed with sulfuric acid mixed into chlorinated lime. As soon as the three seamen remaining on board were fed and rested, the bargemen used the same mixture to fumigate the enclosed spaces of the brig itself. Robinson privately despaired of Captain Batson's recovery, but he nevertheless managed to maintain a placid demeanor.

By July 21, though, Robinson felt compelled to write to the board denying reports that he had visited Chester after the brig's arrival. He had not left the Lazaretto even for a minute, he insisted. Savvy political observer that he was, the doctor knew that the anxious rumors emerged from a populace still reeling from the Lazaretto's darkest hour, in 1870, when its previous physician, William Thompson, had botched the quarantine of the brig *Home* and paid for it with his life. The filthy vessel from Jamaica had spread yellow fever throughout the Lazaretto site and even to neighboring houses on Tinicum Island, killing eighteen people, including the quarantine master, matron, and head nurse, in addition to Thompson. The disease spread to the neighborhood around Swanson Street in Philadelphia, where thirteen more died. Two Chester physicians, led by J. F. M. Forwood, had treated some of the Lazaretto staff and neighbors during that terrible outbreak, while the Chester doctors and Philadelphia's Board of Health traded accusations of meddling and incompetence.

Forwood was left embittered by the events of 1870, believing not only that the Lazaretto was poorly managed but that it posed a threat to its neighbors. By 1879 that feeling had grown along with the county's population. By then, too, Forwood's brother, Dr. Jonathan L. Forwood, had been elected mayor of Chester.[6] As a Democrat, he operated from a baseline level of distrust toward Republican appointees like W. T. Robinson and the political machine that dominated Philadelphia's municipal government.

When the *New York Tribune* picked up the rumors emanating from Chester and reported that the doctor and other Lazaretto employees came and went "at their pleasure," the Board of Health issued a strenuous denial, but the stakes had been raised for Dr. Robinson, who felt the need to carry out a "thorough investigation" of the charges. The board promptly released the report on the investigation's outcome to the press. In it, Robinson "explicitly and positively" denied the charges that any Lazaretto officer or employee, "except the mail boy and one other whose duty it is to obtain supplies," had left the station for any purpose and called the charges "false and malicious."[7]

While the doctor was being attacked in the press, his patients thrived under his regimen of quinine, beef broth, lemonade, and nursing care. All six were released from the hospital as cured thirteen days after their miserable arrival. Even Captain Batson walked out of the Lazaretto healthy. The fate of the *Shasta* and its cargo of logwood, however, remained unresolved.

With the *Shasta*'s owners pressing for permission to unload the brig so it could be disinfected and readied for its next voyage, Mayor Forwood refused to allow the brig or its cargo anywhere inside the Chester city limits. While the board's Lazaretto Committee expressed concern about the logwood being unloaded at the wharf next to the quarantine station, the board, in a testament to the trust and esteem that Robinson enjoyed among his nominal superiors, voted to defer to Dr. Robinson's judgment in the matter.[8]

What would Robinson do? He would remain vigilant, arguing that the brig and its cargo should stay put for the time being, and that when the logwood was unloaded, it should be unloaded in the stream of the river, onto small cargo barges called *lighters*. His priority: keep the vessel and its cargo as far as possible from populated areas. The owners' agent ridiculed the notion that yellow fever could be transmitted through logwood, noted that the *Shasta*'s rigging was "rotting rapidly," and complained that each day of continued quarantine was costing the owners more than fifty dollars. The board, unmoved, backed Robinson's recommendation.[9]

Meanwhile, Captain Batson was not satisfied with simply being alive. He wanted to be paid, and that would happen only when the logwood was delivered to the consignee on the wharf in Chester. Seemingly oblivious to the battle playing out around his brig and its cargo, Batson went to Chester to arrange the delivery. In a face-to-face confrontation with Mayor Forwood, who expressed indignation that Batson had ignored Chester's official decisions on the matter, Batson shot back with his own contemptuous surprise that a small-time local official would presume to dictate to him what he could and could not do with his own ship, which had already been cleaned to his satisfaction. Forwood seized the opportunity to appear defiant and pugnacious in public, sent Batson packing, and went straight to the press, vowing in one reporter's telling that "if the *Shasta* attempted to tie up at the wharf here, he would blow her out of the water with Gatling guns."[10]

Although the *Shasta* had been fumigated, the mayor insisted that the logwood remained "alive with germs of yellow fever" and confidently predicted that half of the population of his city would die of yellow fever if the cargo was unloaded there. He promised that he would mount cannons on Chester's old ramparts before he allowed such a calamity.[11]

With the Lazaretto physician Robinson and the doctor-mayor Forwood each standing firm, the next move belonged to the Board of Health. On August 14, four weeks to the day after the *Shasta*'s arrival, the board permitted the brig's owners to unload the cargo onto lighters so that the vessel and cargo could be thoroughly fumigated. Because the board's ruling did not rescind the quarantine (which in principle covered both vessel and cargo), it brought the logwood no closer to either Chester or Philadelphia. But it did ratchet tensions up a notch. Mayor Forwood stationed a corps of heavily armed policemen along the Chester riverfront, then rushed to see Dr. Robinson at the Lazaretto. Forwood demanded to know whether the board's decision included permission for the lighters to take the logwood to the Chester wharves. The doctor calmly replied, "I do not so understand it."[12]

Five days after the board's resolution, the owners had done nothing. They did not have a fixed date for delivering the logwood, and they rightly judged the prospect of paying forty dollars a day to rent lighters for an indefinite period to be an unattractive business proposition. Miffed at the owners' inaction, Robinson told the board that until the logwood was unloaded, he could not properly fumigate it or the *Shasta*, and that until they were fumigated, he could not release either cargo or brig from quarantine. Although he did not commit himself, he sent a signal to the owners by telling the board that if the logwood was properly fumigated, "it might be safe" to deliver the cargo in Chester.[13]

August turned to September, and the stalemate dragged on. The *Shasta* had been anchored off the Lazaretto for more than six weeks. Maybe its owners finally understood what Dr. Robinson was conveying in his message and decided to unload the vessel for fumigation, hastening its release from detention. Maybe Mayor Forwood decided that he had already reaped all the political advantage to be had from his bellicose bluster and let it be known that Chester's wharves were open for any and all deliveries. Maybe the owners of the Sharpless Dye Works tired of waiting for their raw material and pressured the mayor into softening his posture. Or maybe Robinson somehow persuaded the various parties that the danger had passed, and that the time had come to settle the matter of the quarantined brig and its cargo.

No police, no cannons, and no Gatling guns greeted the lighters as they approached Chester on September 2 to unload the logwood. Robinson confirmed to the board two days later that the *Shasta* had been emptied of her cargo and was "in an extremely filthy condition in her hold." He ordered the owners to send in a gang of cleaners, as soon as he performed a preliminary fumigation to make it safe for them, to scrub with brooms and thoroughly whitewash every surface. When they were done, a more thorough fumigation and final inspection followed. On September 6, 1879, Lazaretto physician W. T. Robinson discharged the brig from quarantine.[14]

Shortly after dawn on July 17, when Robinson had first set eyes on the *Shasta* and its desperate crew, he must have considered the range of likely outcomes. The deaths of most of the starving, feverish seamen would not have been surprising. The outbreak of 1870 pointed to the possibility of yellow fever spreading at or near the station, but in 1879, with thicker settlement nearby, who knew how much damage the brig might do? An outcome in which everyone survived physically and politically unscathed must have seemed, on July 17, most unlikely.

Yet that is exactly what happened. All six sailors stricken with yellow fever recovered under the doctor's care. No illness broke out at the station, in its environs, or among those who unloaded or cleaned the *Shasta* or handled its cargo. In the eye of the political storm, beset by personal attacks, Robinson stayed vigilant while steering a course of imperturbable confidence. He took action that made the difference between life and death: he got food to people who were starving and provided clean beds for people who needed rest. With the board's support, he muddled through while projecting a sense of security and control to skittish politicians and a fearful populace alike. With little fanfare, but with strategic intervention in the press when needed, he navigated around catastrophe.

During the twenty-first-century COVID-19 pandemic, Americans looked desperately to public health experts for strong leadership amid a maelstrom of denial, ignorance, rumors, and government mendacity. A few officials, including National Institutes of Health infectious-disease director Anthony Fauci, were hailed as heroes at the time for their fearless, plain-spoken transparency under extreme pressure.[15] Had they known about W. T. Robinson, Fauci and the others might have drawn some measure of inspiration and comfort from his example. Viewed from nearly a century and a half's hindsight, Robinson's understated calm and determination seem courageous, and even heroic, in an old-fashioned way.

The events recounted in this book took place from the 1790s to the 1890s, in the city of Philadelphia and its Lazaretto quarantine station on Tinicum Island. Philadelphians in this era knew epidemics and quarantine well—too well. As epidemic followed epidemic, one of the few defenses the city could mount was to quarantine anyone and anything suspected of harboring disease. The Lazaretto was built in response to yellow fever, and typhus was the most commonly treated disease at the Lazaretto hospital, but the officers there and the city's Board of Health were trying to prevent *any* disease that might become epidemic from entering Philadelphia. Their perspective and their weapons—like medicine itself for most of its history—were not disease specific.

When epidemic disease was circulating, politicians sparred over whether preserving commerce or the public's health was more important, while doctors disagreed among themselves over cause, containment, and treatment. Nineteenth-century theories about yellow fever—none of which involved viruses or mosquitoes, and all of which have long since been rejected as fundamentally erroneous—actually provided perfectly adequate and plausible explanations of the disease's observed incidence. The seasonal pattern was obvious: yellow fever epidemics happened exclusively in the warmer months. In most years the epidemic season (and the quarantine season) began on May 1 or June 1 and ended on October 1, this being the period of greatest danger from yellow fever. To those who held that yellow fever was imported, one obvious route for disease to enter the city was evident, too: ships from foreign lands. If they proceeded directly to the city dock, these ships and their goods and passengers could seed a disease that might quickly grow to epidemic proportions.

Cured. That simple word appears more often than any other in the Lazaretto hospital register from the mid to late nineteenth century. It is hard not to be astonished by the carpet of "cured" appearing down the "Result" column on page after page. Eighty-eight percent of patients treated at the Lazaretto between 1847 and 1893 were listed as "cured." Yellow fever—cured. Typhus—cured. Smallpox—cured. Cholera—cured. At first, I read these records with extreme skepticism. These doctors, I thought, were lucky not to *kill* most of their patients with their strange treatments, and here they were, arrogant enough to assume (like the rooster whose crowing makes the sun rise) that they had *cured* them? It took a deeper reading of nineteenth-century medical treatises, textbooks, and dictionaries for me to understand what treatment was about, and what *cure* meant at the Lazaretto.

In the nineteenth century, *cure* often referred to a patient's restoration to health, with or without a doctor's active intervention. By the mid-nineteenth century most physicians acknowledged that their role in curing the sick was important but limited. Nature healed; the doctor helped.[16] What makes it hard for us to take seriously the "cure" rate at the Lazaretto is not their arrogance, but ours. Medicine prior to penicillin, we hear, was nothing but folly and delusion—worthless at best, harmful at worst, or "placebos that did nothing and poisons that made you sicker." One historian thinks that "if we define medicine as the ability to cure diseases, then there was very little medicine before 1865." Another says that it was not until sometime after 1910 that an average patient seeing an average doctor for a random disease had a better than even chance of benefiting from medical care.[17] First the germ theory of disease and then the discovery of antibiotics fostered the expectation that each disease has (or ought to have) its cure: a specific treatment that targets the germ or other specific cause of the disease.

But Philadelphia's Lazaretto physicians fought yellow fever and other diseases with no recognizably scientific understanding of their causes or means of transmission. Their methods were crude: detention of ships, cargo, passengers, and crew; isolation of and care for patients; and fumigation and ventilation of vessels and goods. Medical treatment in the Lazaretto hospital was based on principles that were 2,000 years old.

And yet it worked. Somehow it worked. The ruthlessly murderous yellow fever epidemics that had devastated Philadelphia four times in the 1790s became less frequent and less deadly. Nine in ten patients treated in the hospital recovered. The city thrived. And the institution of quarantine itself—frequently denounced, occasionally mocked, and almost universally resented—managed to survive even into the age of germ theory and laboratory medicine.

This is the story of how quarantine worked, and how America's growth as a nation was made possible in part by this 600-year-old tradition-bound institution. The long history of quarantine has never *not* been controversial. It has been marked by xenophobia, arbitrariness, uneven enforcement, and deprivation, but also at times by earnestness, flexibility, competence, and humanity.[18] *These contradictions are our history*; they fill these pages, and they will surely color our future, too.

Lazaretto tells the dramatic and often tragic stories of diseases spreading insidiously from house to house and neighborhood to neighborhood, of destitute immigrants risking their lives on notorious "coffin ships" to find a better life in a new place, and of doctors and policymakers wrestling with scientific uncertainty and public pressure as they tried to keep epidemics at bay without crippling the city's economy. Like policymakers today fighting pandemics or terrorism or climate change, they needed to scare the public just enough to motivate them to take preventive action, but not so much as to cause panic. They needed to provide people with arenas in which to demonstrate their collective will to fight back against these often invisible threats—even when the specific preventive measures undertaken might not actually be effective. Places like the Lazaretto contain the stories that made us who we are today.

PART I / Struggling for Survival, 1793–1803

Chapter One

The Nation's Capital at Rock Bottom, 1793–1798

P resident John Adams and the Congress had made up their minds: they would escape Philadelphia before another summer plague overtook the city. At the first sign of warm weather, in March 1798, they returned to their homes in Massachusetts and elsewhere, away from the nation's capital. Secretary of State Timothy Pickering and Secretary of War James McHenry, along with many diplomats and military strategists, were still needed in the city, however, because trouble was brewing between the United States and France. Federalist politicians were spouting bellicose anti-French sentiments, the French government refused to meet with a delegation of American envoys, and McHenry was mobilizing officers from various states in case hostilities broke out.

Then yellow fever returned. By early August 1798, less than two weeks after the first reports of a malignant fever in the crowded streets near the river, Philadelphia was in full panic. All federal government offices shut down in a hurry and moved to Trenton, New Jersey, 35 miles away. "The fever is more malignant than in any former year," Pickering reported to Rufus King, the US ambassador in London. "The poor are the principal sufferers. Most of those who have the means have left, and are leaving, the city."[1] Pickering and McHenry were among them.

Memories of the great epidemic of 1793 and its aftershock outbreak in 1797 were so fresh and so dreadful that even many of those who had stayed in Philadelphia and survived the earlier ordeals considered it prudent to leave town in 1798. Among doctors, the experience of previous epidemics had led to nearly universal agreement on one point and one point alone: the surest way to avoid yellow fever was to "leave quickly, go far away, and return late."[2] Doctors faced with plague epidemics had been delivering this advice for centuries.

People began fleeing around August 7, and the pace accelerated over the next two weeks. By mid-September, about 40,000 of the city's 55,000 or 60,000 residents had left. Per capita, this was the largest urban exodus in American history.[3]

When William Penn and his surveyor Thomas Holme first laid out the plans for the city in 1682, they envisioned a "greene countrie towne," with large lots separated by abundant open space. Within a few decades, what had sprung up instead was a chaotic free-for-all of subdivided lots and improvised settlements densely clustered along the river.[4]

By 1798, Philadelphia was a bustling and crowded city. Nearly all of its population lived and worked within six blocks of the Delaware River, in an area of less than half of a square mile. One could easily walk from the northwest corner of the populated part of the city to the southeast corner in a half hour. Add the immediately adjacent sections of the Northern Liberties and Southwark Township (administratively separate from the city but directly tied into its economy), and between 50,000 and 60,000 people lived within only about fifty city blocks (figures 1 and 2).

The heart of the city—the place where its lifegiving pulse could be seen, heard, and felt most clearly—was not the High Street Market, nor the New Market on Second Street near Lombard, and certainly not the State House (today known as Independence Hall) on Chestnut Street between Fifth and Sixth Streets, where the new nation's blueprints had been so recently sketched. No, the heart of the city was the river itself, and the cacophonous wharfside blocks that adjoined it.

A stroll along a two-block stretch of Front Street, on either side of High (Market) Street, would have given visitors an immediate taste of how compact, busy, and crowded the American capital city was in 1798. A profusion of trades and goods of all kinds jostled for space and customers' attention. Their eyes would certainly have been drawn to the fashionable bonnets for ladies and colored hats for men and boys just in from London and Liverpool at Baker & Comegys, by the Irish linens at Murland & Bowden, and by the assortment of fine glassware, china, "queen's ware" (a cream-colored style of ceramic ware developed by Josiah Wedgwood), and "Japanned ware" (articles finished with a Japanese-inspired black varnish) at the store of James Gallagher, China merchant. Ships periodically arrived in port carrying exotic goods from China and Batavia (today Jakarta, Indonesia) to tempt luxury-minded Philadelphians, alongside the more familiar goods arriving frequently from the West Indies, the British Isles, and northern Europe.[5]

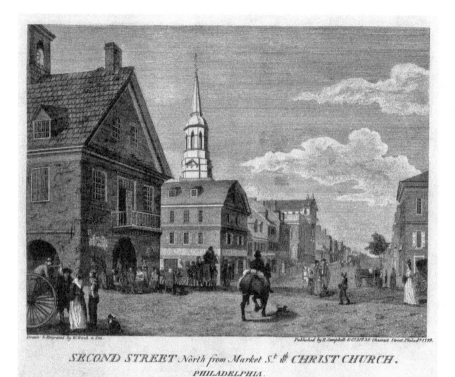

SECOND STREET. North from Market S.t ⚓ CHRIST CHURCH.
PHILADELPHIA.

Figure 1. Northward view along Second Street from Market Street, 1800, by William R. Birch. William R. Birch, *The City of Philadelphia,* [. . .] *as It Appeared in the Year 1800* ([Philadelphia], 1800).

Visitors' ears would be ringing with the clanging of tools and the cries of shop-keepers. The sounds of gold- and silversmith Abner Reeder, coppersmith Robert Orr, and ironmongers Peirce & Smith struck up an industrious music with those of chairmaker William Cox, upholsterer Thomas Jaquett, and clockmakers Jacob Carver and Ephraim Clark. (Often, one would struggle to hear anything over the din of the riverside wharves just a hundred feet or so to the east.) The smell of leather filled the air from the shops of saddler Thomas Moore, cordwainer William Young, and not one but four shoemakers. The grassy, faintly sweet aroma of cured tobacco wafted out from tobacconist William Miller's shop. Visitors' appetites would be whetted by the offerings of grocers Elizabeth Thomson and Joseph McClurg (who also sold liquor), baker Henry Dankle, fruit sellers Robert Taylor and Mrs. Cranchel, and tavernkeepers Philip Redmond and Richard Thorne.[6]

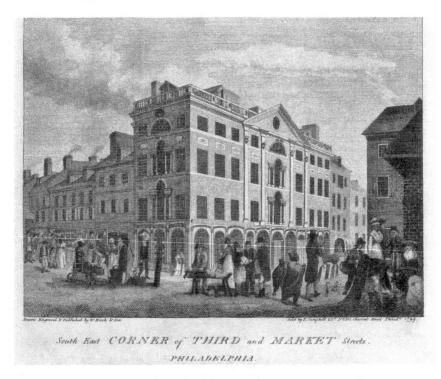

Figure 2. Southeast corner of Third and Market Streets, 1800, by William R. Birch. William R. Birch, *The City of Philadelphia*, [. . .] *as It Appeared in the Year 1800* ([Philadelphia], 1800).

All these and five hatters, a pocketbook maker, a druggist, and eighty-nine more tradesmen, shopkeepers, and merchants competed for the attention and business of customers along just two blocks of Front Street, on either side of High Street. Every time yellow fever returned to desolate Philadelphia, it found its home and headquarters in places like this, the riverfront heart of this busy seaport city.

After the August 1798 exodus, an eerie emptiness settled on the city, disturbed only by the "frequent and loud" "howlings and cries" of abandoned dogs and cats— sounds that so disturbed the prominent Black minister Richard Allen and his remaining neighbors that he placed a newspaper advertisement in which he took "the liberty of hinting to the owners of such animals as remain in this state of con- finement and starvation, the propriety of empowering some friend in town to liberate them as speedily as possible." While many Philadelphians of means fled

Yellow Fever

Symptoms: Sudden and intense headache, body aches, chills, fever, followed by remission; in severe cases, jaundice, internal bleeding, vomiting.

Mortality: In the nineteenth century, an estimated 20 to 50 percent of severe cases were fatal.

Pathogen: Arbovirus of the *Flavivirus* genus, first identified in 1927.

Vector: *Aedes aegypti* mosquito; its role in transmission was first demonstrated in 1900.

Treatment: As of this writing, no specific medication exists for treatment of yellow fever infection. Treatment consists primarily of easing symptoms.

Sources: Lauren E. Blake and Mariano A. Garcia-Blanco, "Human Genetic Variation and Yellow Fever Mortality during 19th-Century U.S. Epidemics," *mBio* 5, no. 3 (2014): e01253-14; Thomas P. Monath, "Yellow Fever Vaccine," *Expert Review of Vaccines* 4, no. 4 (2005): 553–74; Thomas P. Monath, "Yellow Fever: An Update," *Lancet Infectious Diseases* 1, no. 1 (2001): 11–20; Donald B. Cooper and Kenneth F. Kiple, "Yellow Fever," in *The Cambridge World History of Human Disease*, ed. Kenneth F. Kiple (Cambridge: Cambridge University Press, 1993), 1100–1107.

the city for the safety of country estates, Allen organized a volunteer corps of nurses to tend to the indigent sick.[7]

This was nothing new for Richard Allen. Born enslaved in Delaware, he purchased his freedom as a young man, became a Methodist minister, and moved to Philadelphia. With another formerly enslaved preacher, Absalom Jones, Allen formed the Free African Society to advocate for the interests of Philadelphia's free Black population and broke from the white-dominated Methodist church. Allen and Jones each established a new Black-run church in the city. When yellow fever struck with sudden ferocity in 1793, Dr. Benjamin Rush (believing erroneously that people of African descent were immune to yellow fever) called for free Black people to volunteer to provide nursing care, to transport patients to Bush Hill hospital, and to help bury the dead. Rush, one of the nation's founding fathers and its most famous physician, was a quintessential man of the Enlightenment and played a leading role in the abolitionist movement, as well as many other reform causes. Seeing the desperate need—as well as an opportunity to advance the status of their community—Allen and Jones agreed and organized an extensive corps of volunteers. For their tireless efforts, when the epidemic ended, they were met with scurrilous published accusations of profiteering and even stealing from patients and their families.[8]

Quaker architect and philanthropist Edward Garrigues also remained behind in 1798 when so many others fled. He too organized relief efforts with heroic dedication. Garrigues volunteered to help organize the campaign to bring shelter, food, and medical care to the sick, poor, and homeless who remained in the city. A huge tent encampment was set up on the east bank of the Schuylkill River near Walnut Street. Merchants, farmers, and others dropped off donations of straw for bedding, food, and even cash at the site. Volunteers like those organized by Allen provided rudimentary care to the sick. At least 1,200 Philadelphians sought shelter at the encampment.[9]

On August 18, Garrigues wrote in his diary that the epidemic was widespread and that "none really affected therewith recover." When it finally began to abate more than two months later, he attributed the relief entirely to "Divine Providence," adding that "all human endeavors have not been adequate to the Cause." He did not, however, see a deadly epidemic as an outcome to be avoided at all costs. When mass flight put a stop to the everyday "worldly business" of the city, he expressed the hope that the suspension of commercial pursuits would have a "weaning effect" on the "avidity" with which his fellow citizens pursued success in business. He reserved his harshest condemnation for himself, for he considered himself to be more preoccupied with "temporals than Spirituals."[10]

Throwing himself into poor relief and attending the sick gave Garrigues "peculiar satisfaction" and combated his preoccupation with the material and the mundane. "I have been glad to feel my heart tendered on seeing the accumulated distress which I have witnessed," he wrote on August 31. Yellow fever was a great ordeal, a trial of biblical proportions. "We of this City are in nearly equal jeopardy with the Israelites of Old," he observed with relish in early September. Even when he became sick with the fever at the end of that month, he declared himself "glad to be here . . . in preference to having removed [from the city] to try to avoid this bodily suffering." Each encounter with misery and distress was another occasion to cultivate humility, each death a chance to witness a soul "released to enjoy the peace prepared for the Righteous."[11] The epidemic was a spiritual opportunity not to be squandered.

Opportunities of a different kind were to be had too, of course. The Bank of Pennsylvania was robbed of $162,821.61 in cash and notes on September 2, after which that bank, the Bank of North America, and the Bank of the United States took the pragmatic step of moving their offices to Germantown for a time. A city-wide dragnet eventually caught a carpenter named Isaac Davis. Davis was arrested, and nearly all the money was recovered.

Earlier, on August 18, a group of prisoners had tried to take advantage of upheaval at the Walnut Street Jail, whose warden had deserted his post when the fever penetrated the walls. During a medical visit, these prisoners grabbed the cellblock keys, knocked two guards to the ground, and called out to prisoners in the yard to join them. The guards and Mayor Robert Wharton (who, along with citizen volunteer Peter Helm, had stepped in to assist the short-handed jailers) reestablished order only after fatally shooting two of the would-be escapees. Two months later, in the waning days of the epidemic, seven convicts dug a tunnel under the east wall of the jail and escaped; only two of them were ever caught.[12]

By the time cold weather set in and the epidemic had run its course, survivors had begun to assess the human damage. The Board of Health calculated the death toll at 3,645; others had it at over 4,000, including those infected in the city who fled and died in the country. Of the city's population of about 60,000, 40,000 had fled in panic. Of every ten Philadelphians who had stayed, two succumbed to the fever.[13]

When the last body was finally buried, it was time to reflect on the lessons of the epidemic and to plan for the future. Benjamin Stoddert, secretary of the navy, wrote to President Adams in November, asking him to work with Congress to create a plan for "the removal of the offices of government for the summer and autumn months." Waiting until the last minute and leaving in haste, he complained, had caused severe disruptions in government operations and the loss of important papers.[14] The president took no action on the matter.

Nor did the latest epidemic manage to budge the medical professionals. Some doctors believed that yellow fever was contagious and was imported from the West Indies aboard ships, while others insisted it was not contagious and was generated locally in hot weather by decaying organic matter and other kinds of filth. Their contagion dispute had become so intense during the 1797 epidemic that a faction of the College of Physicians of Philadelphia, the nation's first professional medical society, split away and formed a rival society, the Academy of Medicine. Led by Benjamin Rush of the University of Pennsylvania, the academy promoted the localist view that yellow fever originated locally in accumulated filth and could not spread from person to person.

Rush's primary antagonist, Dr. William Currie, and the College of Physicians of Philadelphia were certain that yellow fever had been imported from the West Indies and had spread from person to person by contact. Like Rush, Currie was a son of the Enlightenment and believed that the United States represented the vanguard of democracy in the world. Like Rush, he praised Philadelphia as a mecca of "learning, manufactures, and human improvements of every kind"—an ideal capital for an enlightened age. But where Rush was fervent and mercurial, Currie was calm and measured. Less quick to take offense than Rush, Currie nevertheless did not shrink from medical polemics and skirmishes in print. He blamed Philadelphia's yellow fever outbreaks on an inadequate quarantine at the pesthouse on State Island, located at the confluence of the Schuylkill and Delaware Rivers, and lax enforcement of the health law. Rush and the Academy of Medicine likewise stood their ground: yellow fever had arisen domestically, through foul air generated under particular atmospheric conditions by "filthy matter . . . highly concentrated" on the docks and in gutters, cellars, and yards. It could not spread from person to person, they insisted, and quarantine was a pointless waste of money and an unnecessary burden on trade and prosperity.[15]

The high-stakes struggles among the doctors over the source of yellow fever and how to respond to it were as vehement as they were fruitless. What was different in 1798 from 1793 and 1797 was a dawning recognition of the most terrifying prospect of all: that what had originally been seen as a single shocking catastrophe was beginning to seem like a recurring affliction. And this third time, Philadelphians' patience with the quarreling doctors was wearing thin.[16] Their city, after all, was the leading medical and scientific center in the United States. The experts who were so quick to proclaim their authority had had ample opportunity to study yellow fever, but by 1798 it was becoming clear that none of the vaunted treatments was uniformly effective on large numbers of patients. Some recovered and some did not, regardless of medication. Moreover, neither of the theories about the causes of the disease fully explained why it did not strike in every city every year. It often appeared in hot, wet weather, but some especially hot and wet years remained healthy. In some instances it seemed to strike everyone in a family, block, or neighborhood one after the other, and in others it struck hit or miss—as if at random. No preventive policy recommended by the doctors seemed to have any appreciable effect on the likelihood or severity of an outbreak. The physicians' self-assured rhetoric had produced meager results.

After the devastating epidemic of 1798, Philadelphia's fortunes were at a low ebb. Death, flight, and loss of trade threatened to depopulate the nation's capital and largest city. If what had seemed in 1793 a once-in-a-lifetime calamity had truly become a nearly annual visitation, then surely the city would not recover. Vice President Thomas Jefferson, who saw cities as inherently corrupting and incompatible with democratic values, predicted a year later that the recurring calamity of yellow fever in Philadelphia would not only cause Philadelphians to abandon their city but also inhibit the development of large cities throughout the nation.

Jefferson saw the "yeoman farmer," who owned the land he worked, as the paragon of American democracy. He touted the virtues of agrarian self-reliance and deplored the elitism of the urban merchant class. But his letters hint that his antipathy to cities went further than that. During the yellow fever epidemics, Jefferson urged his Philadelphia associates to flee. He asked one friend about "the effects of these visitations on that place." "It will naturally deter, but will it not also drive off some of the present inhabitants . . . [and if so] of what descriptions?" Depopulation alone would be salutary, he implied, but especially if those who abandoned the city were the "lower sorts"—the free Blacks and poor whites who had no steady source of employment or income. He even seemed to greet reports of yellow fever's shocking death tolls with grim satisfaction. They promised both direct and indirect depopulation of the city. During the outbreak in 1799, he confided to Benjamin Rush that he expected the calamity would "prevent the growth of cities beyond a very moderate size," before adding drily, "Perhaps manners will not be the worse for that." As a remedy for the evils of urban life, yellow fever was harsh but perhaps necessary, in Jefferson's view.[17]

Most outside observers had more tact than Jefferson, but everyone knew that the prospects of this leading American metropolis were dire.

At noon on December 7, 1798, Pennsylvania governor Thomas Mifflin stood before both houses of the state legislature in the Pennsylvania State House (now known as Independence Hall) to give his annual address. In the very building where the nation's independence and Constitution had been debated in the previous two decades, the former president of the Continental Congress, quartermaster general, and brigadier-general of the Continental Army beseeched the lawmakers to rescue and defend what many surely considered a lost cause: Philadelphia. The crisis of recurring epidemics went well beyond local concerns, he told them: "It is natural that I should wish to secure, for the last acts of my administration, the pride and the solace of contributing to rescue our country from the greatest physical evil, to which it has ever been exposed."[18] Just one month after the last reported case of yellow fever, Mifflin put into words what many people were feeling in the pit of their stomachs.

As a politician, Mifflin had a straightforward goal: outline the priorities of state government and convince the legislature to pay for them. But as a statesman and former military leader, he grasped the scale of the undertaking that he was proposing, and he understood that extraordinary ventures required extraordinary motivation. He laid out a vision of a people and a government united by bonds of humanity, solidarity, and trust, guided by the Enlightenment principles on which the young nation had been founded. He began with a solemn evocation of the scale of the 1798 disaster—how many dead, how many dispersed—and remarked that for years to come, "a numerous train of widows and orphans" would act as a constant reminder of the tragedy.

Compounding the human tragedy, Mifflin added, was the "incalculable loss" to the "opulence of [the] metropolis." So important was Philadelphia's economic health to that of the rest of the state that none in the chamber could feel sheltered from the epidemic's impact: "The general prosperity of the state will be imminently endangered," Mifflin insisted, "unless the resources of public wealth and wisdom, as well as the exertions of private industry and virtue, shall be sedulously applied, not merely to repair the injuries that have been already suffered, but to avert, as far as human agency can avail, the recurrence of so awful a visitation." Prompt action was a matter of economic self-interest as well as simple human decency.[19]

In a careful rhetorical pivot, Mifflin then lamented the neglect of "precautions which experience, policy, and humanity dictate." He reminded the legislators that earlier plans to prevent pestilence had faltered in their chambers. (Blame was left implicit.) Without pressing the point, the governor quickly went on to proclaim himself "confident that the liberal sentiments of our constituents, in perfect unison with your own, have prepared you to adopt and enforce, among the earliest acts of legislation, every measure" designed to protect the capital's health. "Wasted and depressed" citizens of Philadelphia needed immediate relief, Mifflin said, and "the honor of the state" demanded "an adequate appropriation of the public wealth, and an energetic reformation of the public police." Only a vigorous government response would "effectually redeem the reputation of our climate, and rescue our metropolis from the desolation which . . . unhappily obscures the splendor of its prospects." "To an appeal thus made," Mifflin noted, "no generous mind will allow the suggestions of a parsimonious policy to reply."[20]

He left them no choice.

Claiming (though he knew full well it was not true) that the doctors' views had "subsided into a unanimous sentiment" that yellow fever could "equally" be generated locally or imported, the governor called for specific health reforms carried out in solidarity and cooperation. They included drawing from Wissahickon Creek and the Schuylkill River to ensure an adequate, clean water supply for the city. This would go a long way toward meeting one of the central demands of the localists, who would use the water to cleanse persistent deposits of filth from the streets and alleyways.[21]

But the centerpiece of Mifflin's extravagantly optimistic agenda was what he called a "radically new" quarantine system. The Board of Health would be empowered to appoint several officers, who would be permanent employees with expanded powers. A new quarantine station would be built at a greater distance from the city than the existing one on State Island, with ample accommodations for the sick, the convalescent, and the "suspected." It would include storehouses for cargo and stoves for fumigating any goods that might be subject to contamination. While a full summertime embargo of West Indian ports would be "injurious to the mercantile interests of the state," the new regime would keep all such traffic at arm's length from the city, at the new quarantine station. All vessels arriving from infected ports, no matter what the season, would be "carefully cleansed and aired," as well as detained for a period fixed by law. Finally, "every transgression of these regulations should be denounced as highly criminal, subject to the severest penalties, which should never, in any instance, be mitigated or remitted."[22]

Mifflin's closing words were sanguine but conditional. The country's continued existence as a "united and happy" people, and as a "free, independent and powerful" republic, he said, depended on the willingness of "every public agent" to rise above partisan invective and seize the "present fair and favorable opportunity" to take drastic measures. Success was likely as long as "the principles of a mutual and merited confidence shall be seasonably disseminated between the government and the people."[23] Among Mifflin's most important lingering messages was this: neither

Chapter Two

Righteousness and Desperation, 1799

B etween 1793 and 1800, most of the mid-Atlantic and northeastern seaport cities in the young nation experienced at least one epidemic of yellow fever.[1] The epidemic of 1793 was not the first yellow fever outbreak in Philadelphia, but there had been nothing like it before. This cataclysmic epidemic left the city deeply traumatized. Nearly 5,000 Philadelphians in a population of 50,000 died in less than three months. That was bad enough, but it kept coming back. In 1797 and 1798, yellow fever again took thousands of lives.

After the 1793 epidemic, devastated Philadelphians had established a twelve-member Board of Health to oversee the city's cleanliness and to administer the Marine Hospital on State Island (formerly Province Island), which served as the port's quarantine inspection station.[2] (The Marine Hospital was also re-ferred to on occasion as a "pesthouse" and as "the Lazaretto.") When yellow fever visited the city in 1797 and again in 1798, however, it was clear that the system was not working: passengers and cargo were routinely landed from detained ves-sels at the State Island quarantine ground, which was located only 7 miles from the city by water, and less than 5 by road. Goods and passengers could easily make their way to the city, and it was just as easy for city residents to board ships at State Island, in flagrant violation of the law (and despite the Board of Health's regular legal proceedings against accused quarantine scofflaws).

A year later, another epidemic season was upon the city. It was time for a new system.

Wanting to increase the influence of physicians on decisions affecting the public's health, the College of Physicians lobbied Governor Thomas Mifflin in 1799 to shrink the size of the Board of Health from twelve to five members, two of whom would be physicians. "The professional knowledge of the medical characters," the college argued, "will be necessary to direct the measures of the board." The members of the current board saw things differently, proposing that the board remain at twelve members and not necessarily include doctors: "The collision of medical theories, instead of illuminating, may envelop the true origin of the calamity still deeper in the clouds of controversy; the tenacity of science, and illusion of theory, are not likely to produce that harmony of sentiment and action, without which no Board of Health can discharge with promptitude the duties of their office to the public advantage." In other words, too much learning could be a dangerous thing. What the public needed was not theory or even science—which had shown itself to be paralyzing—but decisive action. When the new health law was passed in April 1799, the board was given expanded powers, but its membership remained at twelve, with no provision for medical representation (although in practice, the board never had fewer than two physicians).[3]

During the previous summer's epidemic, Edward Garrigues had volunteered to oversee emergency relief to thousands of Philadelphians.[4] This time, however, as reports of sudden illnesses and deaths near the wharves of Lombard Street and Southwark began to circulate, Garrigues held a position that made him responsible for preventing another epidemic, as well as for organizing the city's response if the disease did return: he had been appointed president of the Board of Health. It was an impossible position, requiring medical acumen, humanitarian compassion, and political savvy in equal measure. Yellow fever was saturated with controversy: physicians were bitterly divided over its causes and treatment, and seemingly every Philadelphian with access to a printing press had a definitive plan to prevent it and a thoroughly developed critique of others' erroneous plans. All agreed that the survivors of previous epidemics and their families still urgently needed assistance, but public coffers were depleted. Another epidemic would surely strain even Philadelphia's much-touted charity beyond its limits.[5] The viciously partisan political atmosphere of the early republic guaranteed that every public utterance would be met with an immediate denunciation in the press. And to make matters worse, rival port cities like New York stood ready to trumpet even the slightest rumor of illness in Philadelphia to divert business toward their own wharves and warehouses.

Garrigues, 43, was neither a physician nor a politician. He was a "master builder"—essentially, an architect and building contractor—and a member of Philadelphia's economic elite. He owned considerable property, participated actively in civic life, and gave generously of his money and time when his fellow citizens were in need. Doubtless his civic mindedness and philanthropy owed much to his Quaker faith. His diary portrays him as either the most pious or the most impious man in America. In every entry, he proclaimed his desire to forsake worldly concerns and give himself over entirely to God's will, and in every entry he lamented his inability to do so. He found himself pulled in several directions—by his private pursuit of wealth, his public commitment to the poor and suffering, and his spiritual quest for self-abandonment.

What Edward Garrigues chose to do was leave the board's expanded powers sitting on the shelf, unused. As the summer of 1799 arrived, and the rest of the city began to see every low-grade fever or upset stomach as the first sign of the coming plague, Garrigues greeted the hot weather without high anxiety. He did not worry that an epidemic was coming; he expected that it was. He only worried about how he would measure up when it did. After all, if an epidemic was the ultimate in suffering, if all suffering was a divine trial, and if withstanding trials was the path to salvation, then why would he run from yellow fever, or even fear it? On the contrary, he should embrace it, as he had the previous year. The only problem was that this time, he was president of the Board of Health, not the supervisor of spiritual purity.

In April he had noted in his diary that "the public mind" was "agitated" about another epidemic and wanted "all human means of mitigating . . . the impending scourge" to be implemented. "My fears have been excited," he added, "that we are depending too much on the arm of flesh"—the "human endeavors" that had not been "adequate to the Cause" the previous year. As the first reports of yellow fever cases began to circulate in late June, Garrigues looked on the bright side: "May it please Divine Providence if [it be] in His Wisdom to permit this scourge to visit this once highly favored city, again grant that it may be means of turning many to righteousness."[6]

The president of the Board of Health wanted to save Philadelphia—but not from yellow fever.

The first three reported cases came unusually early in the year, and the signs were ominous. On June 15, a Mr. Thomas arrived at the wharves in Southwark on a ship from the island of Curaçao off the coast of Venezuela. The next day, an unnamed young woman who lived nearby on Front Street suddenly took sick. On the seventeenth, both Thomas and a Mr. Ashmead, another neighbor on Front Street, fell ill.[7] The three illnesses followed an all-too-familiar pattern: in each case, an otherwise healthy adult was struck suddenly by a splitting headache right behind the eyes, shooting from temple to temple.[8] It came with alternating chills and high fever, severe lethargy, and an intense thirst for cold drinks.

The symptoms disappeared within a day or two, but the remission was short lived. The thirst increased and was accompanied by constant nausea and violent projectile vomiting. The patients seemed indifferent or resigned; they may have slipped into unconsciousness interrupted by more vomiting. Thomas and the young woman seem to have begun to recover at this point, but Ashmead's copious vomit turned chocolate colored or black—the classic, indisputable sign of yellow fever. He uncontrollably passed bloody, tar-like stools, which smelled like rotting corpses. Jaundice yellowed his skin and turned his eyes a ghostly bloodshot yellow. Vivid, painful dreams made his sleep as frightening as his waking moments. He hiccupped constantly and had difficulty swallowing; what he did swallow, he could not keep down. His speech became halting and incoherent, his vision dimmed, and delirium gradually set in. On June 23, six days after his first symptoms, Ashmead fell into a cold, clammy sweat, made a rattling sound in his throat, and died in violent convulsions.[9] The doctors called it "malignant fever" (meaning that it was extremely severe and potentially fatal), "bilious fever" (marked by vomiting), "remitting fever" (in which the temperature periodically rises and falls), or "malignant bilious remitting fever." Ordinary people just called it "the yellow fever."

Philadelphians were anxious. These first three cases and a few more were clustered in the area of the city where disease was most liable to spread: the wharfside district along the Delaware River. On the other hand, some cases were not necessarily yellow fever, because the patients' vomit was not black. And the handful of initial cases was followed by a lull lasting a few weeks.[10] Maybe it was just the ordinary seasonal "bilious fever," and not the beginning of an epidemic. It was June, after all, and yellow fever did not typically strike the city until August and September. But then again, that people could speak knowledgeably of what "typically" happened in a yellow fever outbreak showed just how much had changed in the past six years.

When Garrigues and the board looked to the medical community for guidance, they found only the same old discord and acrimony. On July 1, William Currie and the College of Physicians urged the board to immediately order the removal of all ships docked or at anchor between Pine and South Streets and the evacuation of the infected district, with no contact to be permitted between residents of that neighborhood and other Philadelphians.[11]

Meanwhile, Rush and the Academy of Medicine urged the Board of Health to hire inspectors to remove from the city's streets, gutters, and ponds all matter that was subject to putrefaction in warm weather, to use water pumped from the Schuylkill River to cleanse "the impure parts of the city," and to take other steps to prevent the accumulation of filth in yards, cellars, and alleyways. Rush was tired of seeing this advice fall on deaf ears year after year, and he was tired of the ridicule and accusations that were his only recompense for trying to save his city from panic and ruin. In a pamphlet published just after the first fever cases of 1799, he complained that for six years, he had tried "to persuade the citizens of Philadelphia that the yellow fever is of domestic origin." He eventually decided to give up on "all further attempts to produce conviction upon this subject," he wrote, but later changed his mind. He would try one more time: "A retrospect of the scenes of distress which I have witnessed from that terrible disease, and the dread of seeing them speedily renewed, with aggravated circumstances, have induced me to make one more effort to prevent them, by pointing out their causes and remedies."[12]

Rush was well aware of the likely consequences of speaking out yet again:

> I anticipate from it a renewal of the calumnies to which my opinion of the origin of our annual calamity has exposed me; but these will be less difficult to bear, than the suppression of truths which involve in their consequences the prosperity of our city, and the lives of many thousand people, whom poverty and despair will finally compel to become the unwilling victims of the fever, should it again prevail in our city.

It was not too late, Rush insisted with righteous indignation, for the proud citizens of Philadelphia to "admit the unwelcome truth . . . that the yellow fever is engendered in her own bowels" and to take action accordingly: "May heaven forbid this catastrophe to the present capital of the United States! and in mercy command the destroying angel of pestilence to sheath his uplifted sword!"[13]

The reports of suspicious illnesses in June revived rumors and fanned anxiety in the city. The college demanded immediate action: remove the ships and evacuate the neighborhood. The academy demanded immediate action: remove the filth and cleanse the streets. Caught in the middle, Garrigues was pressured to act, and he held the fate of the city in his hands.

He decided to do nothing.

On July 2, the board declined to order an evacuation of ships or residents from the riverside district between Pine and South Streets. "A public notification would perhaps create a terror that might add to the predisposing cause of the sickness," the board announced. Its members were "convinced of the necessity of early precaution, but they also dread[ed] to give an alarm which must injuriously affect the welfare of the city and which may perhaps eventually be unnecessary." They even took the step of warning the College of Physicians against feeding panic by making public statements regarding the situation.[14]

For more than a week, no new cases were reported. An unnamed member of the college—either Currie or a colleague parroting his arguments—wrote the board to caution against further delay. In each of the previous three epidemics, the letter claimed, a modest and highly localized initial cluster of cases had been followed by a marked pause before the fever spread out over the entire city. This lull in the first week of July would prove to be that pause and nothing more. Now was precisely the time for decisive action, before it was too late. The letter went on to recommend early identification of cases; when cases were detected, every patient and the patient's entire household with all of its belongings must be evacuated to "a safe distance from the city," followed by the cleansing of all affected residences.[15]

Garrigues, however, remained preoccupied with the other kind of cleansing. On July 4, he complained in his diary that "the minds of many are abundantly engrossed in festivity" in celebration of Independence Day, "notwithstanding the dread of another scourge." Amid the revelry, he joined with the few "secret mourners" who turned toward "the Divine Countenance" rather than "celebrating any anniversary of outward things." Signs of widespread fear and excessive concern with earthly survival disheartened him, while any indication that people were "disposed to acquiesce with Divine appointment in their trial" gave him cheer.[16]

Meanwhile, in response to an inquiry from Baltimore authorities, the Board of Health flatly denied reports of an epidemic in Philadelphia. Cases had been isolated and unrelated, it insisted, and ten days had passed without any new ones: "The alarm has entirely subsided." Currie reacted caustically to the board's denial. "No one is willing to believe the destroyer is at work," he grumbled, "lest business should be suspended and the interest of the city suffer." He had seen it all before: "Everyone endeavors to persuade himself and his neighbor that it is not come, till he discovers it at his own door. Everyone is offended with him who pronounces the disagreeable truth." Physicians often served as the scapegoats of choice, he added sourly.[17]

In 1799, as in previous years, quarantine rules were routinely flouted—especially at night, when there was no guard on duty at State Island. Passengers who were quarantined aboard detained vessels regularly came up to the city—some by swimming to shore—and returned to quarantine before daybreak. Philadelphians had no trouble boarding vessels to visit, bring supplies, or conduct business. Some vessels brazenly ignored the law in order to avoid quarantine. One evening, Captain Carson of the sloop *Dependence* from La Guaira, Venezuela, disembarked and rowed ashore at State Island to summon the resident physician for inspection, but Joseph Bressell, the pilot responsible for guiding the sloop upriver, simply proceeded up to the port without stopping.[18] The pilot apparently feared the delay entailed by a possible quarantine more than he feared local law enforcement.

The Board of Health dutifully pursued every alleged violation of the health law, and prosecuted the violators and witnesses—if they could be located. Seven city residents were caught later in the summer attempting to board vessels detained in quarantine, and the board had them confined on State Island for fifteen days. Many defendants pleaded ignorance of the health law, however, and were acquitted or pardoned. Joseph Bressell's brazen crime happened early in the quarantine season, and the board was eager to make an example of him. Bressell was convicted and appealed to the governor for clemency, pleading ignorance of the law even though Captain Carson had expressly ordered him to stop, and even though all Delaware River pilots had been informed of the law a month beforehand. When Governor Mifflin pardoned Bressell, the Board of Health again found itself enforcing a law with no teeth.[19] Philadelphia's quarantine was leaking badly, and everyone knew it.

On July 12, several new suspicious illnesses were reported in the southern wharfside neighborhoods. July 15 saw more headaches, chills, vomiting, and fever, over a wider area. On the seventeenth, there were nineteen funerals in the city, and new cases continued to appear over the following week. The pause was over, and the murmurs of alarm grew louder. Garrigues fretted that his fellow citizens were more "agitated" about how to flee the yellow fever than they were "prepared to meet the Great Judge of the Quick and the Dead by a Godly and circumspect life."[20]

When Boston imposed a quarantine on all vessels from Philadelphia, Garrigues fired off an angry letter of protest to the Boston Board of Health. He insisted that Boston's "injurious" decision had been based only on "reports which credulity has diffused, and to which fear has given a gigantic stature." Denial was becoming harder to sustain, but when the beginning of August brought another slowdown in new cases, Garrigues and the board stuck to their position: there was no epidemic. The new lull was short lived, however, and the fever surged in the middle of the month, steadily encroaching on previously untouched parts of the city.[21]

On August 21, the College of Physicians again called upon the Board of Health to act decisively, reiterating its claim that the same "malignant contagious fever" that had so desolated the city in recent summers "prevails amongst us at this time to a very alarming degree." The board barely budged. Garrigues released a statement the next day admitting only that "a number of persons" had taken ill during the previous six days in Philadelphia and in the township of Southwark, "many of whom have died," and that there were "still a considerable number sick." "At present there is not sufficient ground for the great alarm which pervades the city," he insisted, expressing optimism that most of the sick were on the road to recovery and that recent cool weather would block the disease's progress. Less than a week later, Pickering's State Department, McHenry's War Department, and the rest of the federal government offices were again forced to relocate to Trenton, as they had the year before.[22]

Although the board's daily meetings kept Garrigues very busy, he continued to visit the homes of the poor and the sick, offering what relief he could. He saw the misery firsthand, and he recorded his sorrow in his diary. But he continued to hope that the epidemic would be "the means of turning many to righteousness." When his visits took him to the home of a neighbor dying of yellow fever, he stayed with him until the end, writing in his diary that his "mind felt a peaceful quiet" at the moment of the neighbor's death.[23]

Garrigues may have felt pressure from his friends in Philadelphia's merchant class to deny the existence of an epidemic. But his deep determination to treat suffering as a purifying trial gave him an even more powerful motive to persist in minimizing the danger. Furthermore, no matter how much yellow fever he saw in his daily charitable rounds, he was suspicious of everything the doctors told him. He did not trust Currie and the contagionist College of Physicians, and he did not trust Rush and the localist Academy of Medicine. Garrigues wrote in his diary that residents were "much alarmed by some of the Doctors reporting this to be a contagious disease, while others among them with equal earnestness declare it is not—plainly evincing to the mind of the beholders that they [the doctors] know nothing about this fatal disease."[24]

Yellow fever epidemics in Philadelphia tended to gradually wane over the early fall, until the first hard frost snuffed out any lingering embers. In fact, the only thing that all parties agreed on was that weather—the only variable not subject to human control—determined the conditions in which the disease flourished then disappeared. In 1799, the fever eventually spread throughout all but the westernmost districts of Philadelphia. By September 1, much of the city was deserted. New cases and deaths continued until the second half of October, when a few consecutive nights of severe frost brought the epidemic to an end. The death toll from yellow fever in 1799 was significantly lower than that of the previous year—probably just over 1,000.[25] "Only" 1,000 deaths, with the expectation of more to come the next year, still represented a serious blow to the city's pride, reputation, and commerce. Moreover, no policy or intervention could be credited with mitigating yellow fever's severity, for the simple reason that no action had been taken. The only lesson learned from 1799 was that the current system of prevention was conclusively not working.

In hindsight, it is clear that Garrigues was the right man to lead Philadelphia's relief operations during the 1798 epidemic and exactly the wrong man to preside over the Board of Health in 1799. When fearlessness, solidarity with the downtrodden, and the ability to mobilize resources on short notice were needed, he was there. When his city looked to its health authorities for strong leadership in preventing or mitigating a grave danger, he could not provide it, because he saw the danger as a trial sent by God—a good and necessary thing—rather than a preventable tragedy.

But most Philadelphians, including other members of the Board of Health, did not share Garrigues's fatalism. While the fires of yellow fever began burning in the city for the fourth time in six years, the Board of Health announced in June 1799 that in response to the continuing threat, a new quarantine station would be built.

In the fifteenth century, Italians used the word *lazaretto* to designate a pesthouse; the word is derived from the biblical figure Lazarus, patron saint of lepers. Four centuries later, Philadelphians deemed it an appropriate name for their new quarantine station, which would be situated on Tinicum Island. The main building of the station was to be constructed of Flemish bond brickwork, a trademark of stately architectural ambition. The brickwork, the long colonnaded portico, and the elegant cupola of the main building would announce the grand vision of the Lazaretto's founding without revealing the trauma that had made it necessary. Along the riverfront, four smaller outbuildings, handsome but not extravagant, would complement the imposing main building, flanking it in symmetrical harmony. They would house the Lazaretto physician, the quarantine master, and the laborers who transported personnel and cargo between the ships and the station. The serene mile-wide expanse of the Delaware flowed past Tinicum Island and the Lazaretto on its way from Philadelphia through the Delaware Bay and

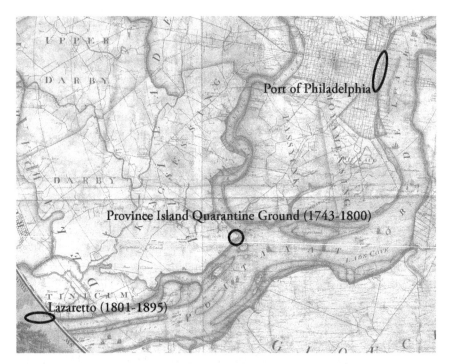

Figure 3. Map showing Philadelphia's quarantine stations at State Island (formerly Province Island), Tinicum Island, and the Port of Philadelphia. Underlying map from John Hills, *A Plan of the City of Philadelphia and Environs Surveyed by John Hills* (Philadelphia, 1808). Courtesy of Eli Zebooker Collection, Athenaeum of Philadelphia.

out to the Atlantic Ocean. Facing the Lazaretto was Little Tinicum Island, a ribbon of green wilderness that divided the river into the relatively calm inner channel in front of the station and the broader, deeper main shipping channel on the New Jersey side.

It was along those shipping lanes that both prosperity and the threat of epidemics sailed from the Atlantic toward Philadelphia. The new Lazaretto, though, would stand sentry for Philadelphians against the recurrent threat of disease. If they could get quarantine right, they could keep disease away from their city.

In choosing Tinicum Island as the site of the new quarantine station, the Board of Health aimed to project a sense of control and authority in a time of fear and desperation. The island's remoteness was its greatest asset: located 13 miles downriver from the city, it would provide a much more effective buffer than State Island. The facilities there were abandoned when the new station opened (figure 3).

"We expect that expedition, utility, economy and beauty will recognize each other in these public buildings." In other words, we will build this new Lazaretto quickly; it will be effective; we will not waste your money; and you will be proud of it. So proclaimed a notice that appeared in Philadelphia newspapers in late June 1799 above the pseudonym "Citizens," which was almost certainly a press release issued by the Board of Health to announce the site that it had chosen for a new quarantine station. The location was remote enough to prevent unauthorized comings and goings, but close enough to the city that mail and other supplies could be regularly delivered, and anyone having business at the Lazaretto could make the round trip in a morning or in an afternoon. The board glossed over the fact that nearly all of Tinicum Island consisted of low-lying wetlands, which were notorious breeding grounds for disease. The announcement insisted that the site was uniquely healthy, with soil "capable of absorbing any quantity of moisture," exposed to salutary southerly breezes but protected from the stormy northwesterly and northeasterly winds. The "variegated scenery" and views were, according to the board, "not surpassed by any on the river Delaware." "Expedition, utility, economy and beauty": this combination gave the board reason to hope that "under God, by the faithful execution of the health law, Philadelphia will be secure from the yellow fever by importation."[26]

Construction of the Lazaretto would begin immediately. It was an act of desperation, but also of defiance and resolve.

Chapter Three

A New Lazaretto, 1800–1801

W hile the new Lazaretto was under construction on Tinicum Island, yellow fever spared Philadelphia for the first time in four years. Even so, that last quarantine season of 1800 at the old State Island Lazaretto did not lack for drama. What stirred the city's emotions that summer was the human cargo conveyed aboard two American schooners. It took nearly a month, the indignation of the press and prominent citizens, and a federal judge's intervention to determine the fate of the vessels and their cargo.

On August 4, the American schooner *Phoebe* tied up at State Island. When resident physician James Hall and quarantine master Thomas Egger boarded the vessel for inspection, they found it controlled not by its own sailors but by a prize crew from the US naval warship *Ganges*. The cargo, they discovered, consisted of thirty casks of water, two and a half barrels of bread, a half barrel of beef, a half barrel of port, and 118 human beings from Africa, naked and "in a very wretched condition."[1]

Patrolling off the coast of Cuba to protect American merchant vessels against the depredations of French privateers, the *Ganges* had also been on alert for violations of the 1794 Slave Trade Act, which prohibited US-outfitted ships from participating in the slave trade. After capturing the *Phoebe* on July 21 near Havana, Captain John Mullowny of the *Ganges* decided to put his prize crew at the helm of the slaving schooner and send it to Philadelphia, the capital of the early abolitionist movement in America. Mullowny chose this destination over one of the closer southern US ports, where the prize crew might have shared in the proceeds after the sale of the Africans. As soon as Hall and Egger saw the *Phoebe*'s cargo, they set about to "land and encamp" the Africans, many of whom were seriously ill.[2]

Philadelphians learned about the unusual arrival in the next morning's newspapers, where the Board of Health had published a notice pleading for immediate clothing donations:

HUMANITY.

Arrived at the Lazaretto yesterday, one hundred and eighteen Black People, without the least cloathing, being taken on board the schr. Phoebe, prize to the United States ship Ganges—the humane citizens are requested to send to the Health Office at the State House, any kind of linen cloaths for their accommodation, as well as to prevent the shock their decency will be exposed to by so many of both sexes being thus exposed naked.

To right-minded Philadelphians, slavery and the brutal reality of the Middle Passage were horrors. Exposing people naked was a further indignity—one Philadelphians could do something about. The machinery of the city's collective charity quickly sprang into action. "I look'd upon this as a call on humanity indeed," boasted Elizabeth Drinker in her diary, "and set about making up a bundle . . . of good and suitable things for the poor naked creatures." Drinker's women friends called on her that same day to ask for clothing donations and were pleased to find that she had already answered the call. Like horror, pity—and public piety—moved fast.[3]

Two days after the *Phoebe*, the American schooner *Prudent* arrived at State Island with a prize crew from the *Ganges* and sixteen more Africans aboard. According to newspaper accounts, a husband and his pregnant wife had been forcibly separated by the slavers in West Africa, with one placed aboard the *Phoebe* and the other on the *Prudent*. When the Africans from the *Prudent* were landed at the Lazaretto, the couple was suddenly and unexpectedly reunited. "Lost for a moment in an ecstasy of surprise," the *Gazette of the United States* reported, "they exhibited a scene of tenderness which would have softened even the savage hearts of those who had occasioned their separation." Overcome by the emotional reunion, the woman spontaneously miscarried.[4]

One day after the *Prudent* arrived, the Pennsylvania Abolition Society called an emergency meeting. Officially named the Pennsylvania Society for Promoting the Abolition of Slavery, the Relief of Free Negroes Unlawfully Held in Bondage, and the Improvement of the African Race, the group counted many prominent Philadelphians among its members, including Benjamin Rush, who served as its president for the last ten years of his life. At its meeting the society appointed a committee to look out for the welfare of the newly arrived Africans and to advocate on their behalf before the state and federal governments. One of the committee's members was the Quaker abolitionist Edward Garrigues—the philanthropist who had organized the relief effort during the 1798 yellow fever epidemic and had done nothing to prevent the 1799 outbreak. As president of Philadelphia's Board of Health he knew the State Island Lazaretto well.[5]

US District Court judge Richard Peters, a member of the Abolition Society, declared the 134 Africans from the two schooners free, and the society assumed custody of them while they recovered at the Lazaretto. Either the judge or the society determined that all the Africans would be given the surname Ganges. As many as 48 of those originally enslaved had died aboard the *Phoebe* and the *Prudent* during the Middle Passage. Six more died while under care at the hospital on State Island.[6]

The 128 survivors were gradually indentured to employers and families (many of them Quakers) in Philadelphia and the surrounding area. The Abolition Society attempted to preserve family connections and to place the Ganges Africans in clusters where they could provide a semblance of community for one another. The indentures provided for a kind of involuntary apprenticeship; girls were bound until age 18, boys until age 21, and adults for four years. Strict terms prescribed rules of conduct for the apprentices and enjoined masters to provide shelter, food and drink, clothing, washing, and education. The employers appear to have chosen first names for their charges: names like John, Peter, and Sarah as well as Furry, Abana, and Tamby. Girls and women were to learn "the Art and Mystery of Housewifery," while boys and men were to be taught their master's trade—in most cases farming. Captain Mullowny of the *Ganges* took on Thomas Ganges as an apprentice sailor.[7]

One 9-year-old girl given the name Mary Ann was destined to stay in quarantine for nine years. She was indentured to former sea captain Thomas Egger, the last quarantine master at the State Island Lazaretto and the first quarantine master at the new Lazaretto on Tinicum Island. Like her shipmates, she arrived in a strange new world as it entered a new century. Her life had been turned upside down, and the country that liberated and indentured her after enslaving her was about to undergo dramatic transformations of its own. After a 6,000-mile voyage from West Africa to Cuba and then to Philadelphia, Mary Ann's 7-mile journey from State Island to Tinicum Island paralleled a city's transition to a new era of vigilance against disease, and a nation's journey into a new era of economic expansion and immigration.

Giving thanks for a year's exemption from their summertime scourge, Philadelphians began to turn their attention downriver toward the stage on which the next century's drama of danger, vigilance, and purification would be played out. They knew that disease was almost certainly on its way up the Delaware River aboard arriving ships, whether the Lazaretto quarantine station was ready or not.

And so, as the weather turned warm in April 1801, the city's Board of Health declared the mostly completed Lazaretto open for business. Eight of the board's twelve members were newly appointed, and they surely understood that their decisions would be put under the microscope of public scrutiny. A flagpole tall enough to be visible for miles was erected at the foot of the Lazaretto pier, and to mark the opening of the first of what would turn out to be ninety-five quarantine seasons on Tinicum Island, the international symbol of quarantine was hoisted up the pole: a yellow flag with a black letter Q, which signaled to all arriving captains and pilots that they must anchor in the river and await inspection.

Philadelphians knew from intimate experience how yellow fever, typhus, and other diseases threatened their loved ones and their livelihoods. They fervently hoped the Lazaretto would seal the city's porous disease defenses. Those in charge of the Lazaretto faced an impossible task: keep the commerce of the port flowing freely, but do not allow in anyone or anything that might start another epidemic— even though it was not at all clear what category of person or thing carried or spread epidemic diseases. Also, they were to remain supremely vigilant at all times, but treat all with compassion and charity. Considering what had happened in the 1790s—quarantine laws widely flouted, four deadly summers, more than 10,000 yellow fever deaths in a city of 50,000 people—there was every reason to be pessimistic.

To face those impossible tasks, the new station's steward in residence would have to be someone who could be trusted to dependably oversee day-to-day operations, maintain the physical plant, make sure the facility was always well supplied, and keep sick patients adequately fed, clothed, and sheltered. For this weighty job, the 1801 Board of Health chose Edward Garrigues—a surprising choice, considering that he had proved himself incapable of decisive action under pressure during the 1799 yellow fever crisis, when his delay and denial failed to prevent that year's epidemic.

Garrigues's troubles would continue at the Tinicum Island Lazaretto. Shortly after assuming his new duties there, he was accused in the press of selling substandard bread to desperate passengers and sailors aboard quarantined ships, of charging more than triple the Philadelphia market price for it, and of responding like a bully when confronted with the allegations.[8] The allegations must have stung, given how hard he had worked to establish his reputation as a dedicated philanthropist and humanitarian. Whether or not the charges were true, the Board of Health had clearly decided that an organized, pious man who greeted disease outbreaks as opportunities to exercise his faith and charity would make an excellent steward for the new Lazaretto.

Ship inspections, medical treatment, and quarantine decisions fell to the Lazaretto physician. The board made another controversial choice for that position in selecting Dr. James Hall. Hall, a founding member of the College of Physicians, had in recent years seen trouble in his position as port physician. He had been accused of being inattentive to his duty and of lying publicly about whether anyone in the city had yellow fever.[9] Nevertheless, he was an experienced and respected medical man who had apprenticed in the hospitals of London and participated in various philanthropic ventures. Neither political attacks in the press nor shiploads of people ill with typhus were likely to shake his stolid demeanor.

Garrigues and Hall were an unlikely pair to lead the city's defense at the Lazaretto—and yet they created an outpost that did what the city needed. It acted, in effect, as a massive harbor sluice at the city's gates that could be opened up or shut off by degrees, allowing people and goods in while keeping disease out. But it was a clumsy operation even in the best of times, never perfect and always unpopular.

The steward, the physician, and Thomas Egger, the quarantine master (who was charged with cargo inspection and disinfection), scrambled to inspect and accommodate each arriving ship.[10] Cargo had to be unloaded and each sickly vessel disinfected. Laundry had to be done, food provided, patients treated, and bodies buried. Everybody waited while cargo and cargo holds were thoroughly ventilated. Everybody waited to see if patients recovered, and if healthy passengers and sailors remained so. Time was money, then as now, and merchants, sailors, and passengers abhorred quarantine-caused delays. Even doctors questioned quarantine's purpose, bemoaned its inefficiency, and denounced its uneven enforcement.

The officers responsible for enforcing quarantine regarded their work as, at best, an unpleasant necessity. As soon as the masts of an arriving vessel came into view on the southwestern horizon, the watchman rang the bell to summon the physician, the quarantine master, and the bargemen. Six bargemen rowed Hall and Egger out to board the schooner from Havana or the brig from Jamaica or the bark from Liverpool, which anchored in the channel between the Lazaretto and the narrow forested strip of Little Tinicum Island.

Egger inspected the vessel's hold and cargo for signs of rot or other disease-causing foulness, while Dr. Hall interrogated the captain under oath. What port did you sail from? When did you depart? What was the prevailing state of health of that city at the time? What is your cargo? How many passengers were aboard at the start of the voyage? Were there any illnesses or deaths aboard during the voyage? Hall's list of questions was long, and the penalties for lying or concealing evidence were harsh: a $500 fine and a sentence of hard labor lasting one to five years.

The physician also visually inspected all seamen and passengers for signs of illness. Anyone found to be sick was brought to the Lazaretto hospital (in the wings of the main building), where they were clothed, fed, and treated until death or recovery. After weighing the evidence, Hall had to decide the ship's fate as well: at his discretion (subject to Board of Health approval), the vessel, the cargo, the passengers—or all three—could be detained for days, weeks, or even months. When the physician ordered a thorough "cleansing and purification," even healthy passengers were landed, to be provided by steward Garrigues with necessary supplies and sheltered overnight if necessary. Meanwhile, the crew and the bargemen unloaded all cargo that the quarantine master decreed had to be aired. The vessel was whitewashed, and the hold fumigated and ventilated.

Garrigues and Hall had expected that ships bringing yellow fever would arrive from the West Indies soon after the new Lazaretto opened. Instead, an entirely different threat entered the station from Europe and the British Isles: typhus, also known as "famine fever" or "ship fever." Whenever large numbers of poor people were crowded together aboard ships with inadequate food supplies, typhus outbreaks were sure to follow. No disease was encountered more frequently at the Lazaretto.[11]

When the brig *Venture Again* arrived on July 31 carrying destitute immigrants ill with typhus, the brand-new station was overwhelmed. One hundred and two Welsh immigrants who planned to work off the cost of their passage and start new lives in the United States had boarded the vessel in Liverpool, but only 49 survived the voyage, and every one of them arrived at the Lazaretto seriously ill, along with all but one of the crew.[12] With no advance warning, Hall had to treat the Welsh

Epidemic Typhus

Symptoms: Fever, headache, body aches, rash, extreme exhaustion, delirium, stupor.

Mortality: 10 to 40 percent of cases not treated with antibiotics are fatal.

Pathogen: *Rickettsia prowazekii* bacterium, first identified in 1916.

Vector: Human body louse (*Pediculus humanus corporis*); its role in transmission was first demonstrated in 1909.

Treatment: Since the 1940s, typhus has been treatable with antibiotics.

Sources: Iowa State University Center for Food Security and Public Health, "Typhus Fever—*Rickettsia prowazekii*," last updated February 2017, http://www .cfsph.iastate.edu/Factsheets/pdfs/typhus_fever.pdf; European Centre for Disease Prevention and Control, "Facts about Epidemic Louse-Borne Typhus," accessed August 2, 2022, http://www.ecdc.europa.eu/en/epidemic-louse-borne -typhus/facts; Victoria A. Harden, "Typhus, Epidemic," in *Cambridge World History of Human Disease*, ed. Kenneth F. Kiple (Cambridge: Cambridge University Press, 1993), 1080–84.

arrivals, while Garrigues struggled to house, feed, and clothe them in addition to the patients already being cared for.

When a sickly vessel like the *Venture Again* arrived, pastoral tranquility gave way to the pell-mell horror of dead and dying bodies amid the effluvia of an overcrowded ship. The creak of rigging rang out along with the bargemen's shouts, echoed by sailors on the other ships already "riding quarantine" in the stream. Hungry children cried for their mothers, some of whom had not survived the voyage. From the miserable passengers transported to the hospital came soft moans and incoherent muttering—one of the hallmarks of typhus being what was called a "passive delirium"—accompanied by shallow, rapid breathing. Their bodies gave off a sour, fetid odor, and their bloodshot eyes stared uncomprehendingly from behind fever-reddened faces. A dusky purplish rash covered trunk, limbs, and neck. Their muscles twitched spasmodically, although they were nearly too weak to move.[13]

Evacuating patients from the ship and burying any dead who had not been dis-posed of at sea were critical priorities for Hall and his men, followed by unload-ing the cargo, whitewashing the ship, and the rest. Back at the hospital, Garrigues immediately requisitioned tents to be pitched on the lawn outside the main building for healthy passengers who had arrived on other vessels undergoing quarantine. The typhus patients had to be treated—most commonly with wine, and occasion-ally with opium or bloodletting—and their clothing washed. This time the ef-forts of the station's physician and steward paid off; at least 36 of the 49 desper-ately ill Welsh immigrants recovered and began their new lives in their new city.[14]

At the Lazaretto, weeks of uneventful routine were punctuated by urgent bursts of activity. Most of the manual labor fell to the six Lazaretto bargemen, who after the rowing and the unloading and the carrying and the whitewashing and the grave digging earned a ration of rum and a rest—until the next sighting downriver.

When, as expected, ships bearing people sick with yellow fever arrived from the West Indies, the scene at the Lazaretto was more chaotic, the sensations more vivid and horrifying, than with a typhus ship. Yellow fever patients emitted a putrid, fishy odor similar to that of typhus patients, but the repulsive stench was intensified by projectile vomiting and the uncontrollable evacuation of bloody, tar-like stools, all of which covered the ship, the sickroom, and the cloth-ing with a viscous soup of excreta. When the vomit kept coming and turned a dark chocolate color from the dried blood in the stomach, observers knew that the end was near.

More common than outbreaks of typhus or yellow fever were the mundane inconveniences and frustrations occasioned by a vigilant quarantine policy. Those who found themselves subjected to it were none too pleased about it, and the an-noyance was not limited to sailors and maritime travelers. When Vice President Aaron Burr's eighteen-year-old daughter, Theodosia, and her new husband, South Carolina governor Joseph Alston, traveled south from New York in October 1801, they planned to spend two or three days in Philadelphia. Widespread reports of a yellow fever outbreak in New York changed their plans. Philadelphia's Board of Health not only required all vessels from that city to be detained at the Lazaretto, but also posted guards on all roads entering Philadelphia County and ordered them to keep out people and goods from New York. "The good people [of Philadel-phia] have taken it in their heads that there was literally a plague in New York," the young bride complained in a letter to her brother. She and her husband were forced to cross the county line "by stealth" and ride around the northern and western fringe of the city on their way to Washington, where they dined with

President Jefferson in the White House.[15] (Mrs. Alston's indignation proved justi-fied, as the feared New York epidemic never materialized.)[16]

But sea captains and merchants complained most frequently and most bitterly about Philadelphia's quarantine—even when they were not detained. Any delay was intolerable, no matter the cause. In the new Lazaretto's very first month of opera-tion, an anonymous source went to the *Aurora* newspaper with the allegation that Lazaretto physician James Hall had delayed seven vessels for two full days by failing to visit and inspect them promptly upon their arrival at the station. When the board investigated the charges, it found that the ships had arrived on a Friday afternoon in conditions so windy that it was not safe for Hall to go out to them, and that all seven vessels had been inspected and permitted to proceed by seven o'clock Saturday morning. (The remainder of the two-day delay was caused by unfavorable winds.)[17]

James Hall, the first physician at the Tinicum Lazaretto, almost made it through one full quarantine season before an unknown illness killed him in mid-September 1801. Governor Thomas McKean appointed Dr. Michael Leib, a Demo-cratic firebrand and leader of the German American community, to replace Hall at Tinicum. There was only one problem: at the time, Leib was serving in the House of Representatives in Washington, 140 miles away. Federalists mocked Leib's qualifications—saying that by appointing him "physician," McKean had done "what genius or education could never do"—and protested that one man could not possibly perform the duties of the two jobs simultaneously. The governor defended his appointment, citing Leib's "patriotism, talents, and attachment to our revolu-tionary and republican principles," but the legislature passed a bill over McKean's veto prohibiting the simultaneous holding of state and federal offices. Leib chose the US Capitol over Tinicum Island.[18] McKean's next choice, distinguished Revolu-tionary War veteran Nathan Dorsey, would serve at the island in Leib's place.

In 1801, disease outbreaks were limited to ships detained at the Lazaretto. This was exactly the result that the new station was designed to accomplish. The city was spared another attack of yellow fever in the summer of 1801, despite a brisk trade with many West Indian ports. But while Hall and Garrigues had their hands full containing disease on Tinicum Island, the Board of Health continued to have trouble finding its public voice.

The quarantine season of 1802 dashed any hopes that the new regime would be trouble-free.

Chapter Four

Exodus (Again) and Compromise, 1802–1803

John Edwards died just three days after falling ill. He lived on Artillery Lane, between Front and Second Streets, just a block and a half from the wharves. A ship carpenter, he had been working on the brig *Esperanza* at Stewart's Wharf, above Vine Street. On July 4, 1802, he was seized with a "chilly fit," an intense headache, distorted vision, and severe pain in his back and limbs. The chills turned to fever, then back to chills. He vomited over and over. Jaundice came over him and, finally, the copious black vomit that sealed his fate.

The next day, biscuit baker John Crosley died with similar symptoms, and the day after that, it was the turn of a young cooper's apprentice named Henry Miller. All three lived or worked in the immediate vicinity of Vine Street Wharf. By the end of July, the disease had spread through much of the Northern Liberties (the township north of Vine Street near the river) and down Front Street into the city proper.[1]

Mid-August to mid-October had been the deadliest time in previous epidemics, but in 1802 there had already been 63 cases and 25 deaths by August 1. The Board of Health was facing its biggest crisis since the 1799 epidemic, when board president Edward Garrigues had fiddled as Rome burned around him. The only holdover from the 1799 board was William Donaldson, a lumber merchant and Democratic-Republican party activist in the riverside district of Southwark. He would not be a bystander to this epidemic.

Donaldson had occupied a front-row seat to Garrigues's inaction as a member of the Board of Health—and had been an activist board member ever since. He person-ally investigated ships, wharves, and neighborhoods, and he repeatedly advocated more thorough disinfection of vessels.[2] Now Donaldson and the board were, once again, being petitioned by the College of Physicians to forbid contact with the infected houses and to evacuate healthy residents from that part of the city to the countryside.[3]

On August 5, 1802, the board heeded the College's entreaties. After its investigative committee reported a resurgence of cases near the Vine Street Wharf, the board issued a public statement warning citizens of what they called a "CONTAGIOUS DISEASE . . . as malignant . . . as any which has hitherto afflicted this city." The board phrased the next sentence very carefully: "In consequence of an impression of this nature, the Board of Health is impelled by motives of duty and regard for their fellow citizens, to warn them of the approaching danger, and to entreat those whose health will permit, immediately to withdraw from the City and Districts; by which means we hope to be instrumental, under Providence, in preserving to the community the lives of many useful and valuable citizens."[4]

They may as well have shouted from every street corner, "Run for your lives!"

The exodus began immediately. Roads out of the city were choked with families in flight, their furniture and belongings stacked hurriedly onto carts. Benjamin Rush, lamenting "uncommon degrees of terror and precipitation," considered the board's advice overblown and hasty. Still, two-thirds of those who lived between Third Street and the Delaware River fled the city, along with many others living farther from the danger zone. Homes and shops were shuttered. Newspapers moved their operations as far from the riverside districts as possible and asked their subscribers to leave forwarding addresses when they left town. All those who had nowhere to go—no country house, no family or connections outside Philadelphia—were left behind. Needless to say, other port cities immediately declared a quarantine on all traffic from Philadelphia or banned it outright. For the rest of the summer, no Philadelphia merchant could hope to do any significant business outside the city. Travelers from Philadelphia were unwelcome everywhere.[5]

The malignant fever continued on its pitiless path. Those who remained in the city sought whatever relief and medical care they could find. Many went hungry. In August the disease extended southward along the riverfront, to Chestnut Street Wharf, then below Dock Street, and then below South Street. It continued unabated through September and on through late October, when the first hard frost extinguished it. Death estimates ranged from 307 to 835. Hundreds more sickened but survived.[6] The death toll had not reached the thousands, as it had four times in most Philadelphians' memories, but that was meager consolation to the survivors.

Early on in the new quarantine regime, it became clear that along with strict enforcement came unforeseen consequences. In late May 1802, the brig *Samuel* and the sloop *William* arrived at the Lazaretto from New Orleans with passengers who lived in western Pennsylvania. After being told they would be detained for fifteen days, the passengers appealed the Lazaretto physician's decision to the Board of Health. Their argument was that they could not be a danger to the health of Philadelphia or its adjoining districts if they never set foot in or near the city. The board played it by the book: fifteen days. The passengers continued to press their case, arguing that they were healthy but that continued confinement aboard their crowded vessels would soon make them sick. After a few days, the board relented. The rules it had recently adopted would, it said, "operate with singular inconvenience, and probably with some danger to the health of the crews and passengers of small vessels under quarantine" who lived in "the remote parts of this state." "It may be expedient," the board concluded, to discharge them "whenever such indulgence cannot be attended with any risk to the health of this city and districts."[7] In this case, the desired end could be achieved without inflicting unnecessary harm and inconvenience.

No such calculus guided the doctors, who still argued among themselves. The contagionists of the College of Physicians blamed the 1802 outbreak on the ship *St. Domingo Packet*, which regularly plied the route between the island of Hispaniola and Philadelphia and had arrived at the Lazaretto on June 9. One seaman and one passenger aboard the vessel had died of fever before it departed from Cape-François in Saint-Domingue (today Cap-Haïtien, Haiti). When the ship arrived in Philadelphia, its steward fell ill and died under mysterious circumstances. Captain John Wilbourn told those inspecting his ship at the Lazaretto that the steward's death was due to "the piles"—hemorrhoids. Unpersuaded by this claim, Lazaretto physician Nathan Dorsey detained the *St. Domingo Packet* for disinfection and observation. During this quarantine, when another sailor became "slightly indisposed" and was admitted to the Lazaretto hospital, Dorsey and the board extended the ship's detention for five days. On June 28, nineteen days after its arrival, with the sailor recovered and no further signs of illness aboard, the *St. Domingo Packet* was permitted up to the city.[8]

During the epidemic, Dr. William Currie turned detective. Reconstructing the earliest stages of the outbreak, he claimed to have traced nearly every one of the first 197 cases either directly to the *St. Domingo Packet* or to the immediate vicinity of Stewart's Wharf at Vine and Front Streets. His meticulous sleuthing turned up stories like those of Richard Essex and John Crosley, who worked in Brown's Bake House next to the wharf. The two men knew the *St. Domingo Packet* well, as the ship regularly docked at Stewart's Wharf. Curious Philadelphians occasionally stopped by to ogle the ship's figurehead, the carved likeness of Toussaint Louverture, "the Black Napoleon," who in the 1790s had led the rebellion of enslaved people in Saint-Domingue. Soon after the ship was released from quarantine and tied up at its customary wharf, Essex told Crosley that Toussaint had "come back," and the two went to investigate. Crosley noted with amusement that the Black general had turned white, as the likeness had recently been painted to avoid giving offense to the French military authorities. They paid dearly for their curiosity: Essex contracted yellow fever and recovered, while his son (who brought him his meals at the bakery) and Crosley were dead within two weeks.[9]

Currie insisted that his documentation of the path of the disease—from person to person within each household, from street to street, from neighborhood to neighborhood—proved yet again the contagious character of yellow fever. If only healthy people had been protected from contact with the first cases as well as with those patients' lodgings and belongings (and the *St. Domingo Packet*'s cabin, which Currie claimed had not been disinfected at the Lazaretto), the epidemic could have been averted. Currie singled out for praise the Board of Health, which "had no alternative" but to recommend that Philadelphians flee to the countryside. "Influenced by motives which do honor to their humanity," he reflected, "they honestly and judiciously acknowledged the truth." After some short-term economic damage, Currie believed that Philadelphia's port would benefit in the long run, as merchants near and far learned that they could trust the board's pronouncements about the city's health. And Currie had no doubt that the board's recommendation had made a difference. The epidemic had been "manifestly restricted in its progress" by the "sudden and early desertion of the inhabitants."[10]

Board of Health member Dr. Charles Caldwell, a student of Benjamin Rush's and an ardent anticontagionist, was having none of it. "Rash, precipitate, and out of all proportion to the cause" was his assessment of the board's unprecedented action. He especially resented the contention that the board's order to flee the city had saved lives, calling the move "worse than common error." The carnage of 1798 had proven definitively, in Caldwell's view, that the mass desertion of the city did nothing to mitigate yellow fever's death toll, because the disease was not contagious. Furthermore, the relatively moderate body count in 1802 convinced Caldwell that what they had just experienced was not true yellow fever, but a milder cousin, the ordinary "fall fever of the city."[11]

Did the board's early recommendation to leave town limit the death toll from yellow fever in 1802? Currie said yes, and Donaldson may have comforted himself in thinking so, but Caldwell and others scoffed at the idea. It is true that many more deaths occurred after the exodus than before, but then again, who could say how many would have died if more people had stayed? The contagion question was no closer to resolution, and the effectiveness of the quarantine regime at the new Lazaretto was thrown into doubt just a year after its seemingly successful launch.

The only apparent point of clarity was that the Board of Health had yet to win the full confidence of the people of Philadelphia.

The "radically new" quarantine system that Governor Thomas Mifflin had urged on the state legislature after the calamity of 1798 had gradually fallen into place. Nothing of significance happened at the Lazaretto without the Board of Health hearing about it, and no decision of any consequence was made there without the board's approval. Until 1879, when the mail was superseded by the telegraph, mail went back and forth between the quarantine station and the board twice a day.

But the board's broad new responsibilities went well beyond quarantine: vital statistics, water supply, vaccination, street cleaning, privy cleaning, nuisance abatement, sewerage, housing, industrial establishments, burial grounds, and the city hospital, among others, fell under its purview. While disagreements over the handling of these responsibilities sometimes busied board members, it was the Lazaretto that proved to be the board's preoccupation, especially during warm-weather months. In the off-season, when tropical diseases were not considered a threat, the port physician inspected vessels as they tied up directly in the city. The Lazaretto was open during quarantine season, which always lasted at least from June 1 to October 1, although reports of disease at West Indian ports or unseasonably warm weather often caused the board to open the Lazaretto early or keep it open late in the year. Board members met once a week in the off-season and every day during quarantine season. During epidemics they often convened twice daily. Their headquarters was at the Health Office on Walnut Street near Front Street, where the governor-appointed health officer was responsible for investigating public complaints and violations of the health law, as well as for enforcing Board of Health resolutions in the city.[12]

For most of the nineteenth century, twelve men sat on the Board of Health. Members were appointed by the governor until 1818 and were elected by the municipal councils of the city and adjoining districts after that. At least two, but never more than four, physicians were always among the members. Most board members fit the classic profile of the nineteenth-century civic leader: a politically connected merchant, manufacturer, lawyer, or other professional who was expected to take part in public affairs by virtue of his position in the community. A member was also likely to serve on other civic or charitable boards, such as the Board of Guardians of the Poor, the Board of Charities and Corrections, the Pennsylvania Abolition Society, and the Humane Society, as well as on the boards of such potentially lucrative enterprises as banks, insurance companies, and bridge and canal companies.

The board's quarantine deliberations were occasionally contentious, especially in the early years, when the specter of epidemic disease loomed on the horizon every summer. In 1805, for example, Dr. James Reynolds resigned from the board after an altercation in which he had been "cruelly beaten and mauled" by one of his colleagues, according to the press.[13] (No outlet reported who had been the alleged assailant.) The board relied on its medical members for special expertise from time to time (as when examining patients to determine whether they were ill with an ordinary fever or something more worrisome), but physicians did not exercise disproportionate influence on important decisions. The board generally conducted itself as if public health policymaking belonged as much to enlightened laypeople as to medical doctors. Minutes from the Board of Health in this period show its members spending more time on paperwork and procedures than on discussing how to protect public health—perhaps as a result of anxious caution. Members of the board were conscious of their heavy responsibility when it came to quarantine, and the high-stakes art of quarantine enforcement was rarely clear cut. In difficult cases they deemed it safest to appoint committees, conduct investigations, follow established protocols, and leave a clear procedural record behind.

The seriousness and resolve of the board's members did nothing to repair the breach between the two entrenched and stridently polemical camps: those who saw yellow fever as contagious and imported, and those who believed it to be neither of those things. How could the board make meaningful decisions when even its careful record keeping and respect for protocol couldn't protect it from recriminations both internal and external?

The first hint of an answer came from an unlikely source.

Charles Caldwell blamed the disease on Philadelphia's climate and the accumulation of decaying matter. Caldwell was incurably irascible and thin skinned, with an ego to match his imposing height and massive head. He never missed a chance to pick a fight or take offense. For example, Rush had been generous to Caldwell for years, but Caldwell broke with his mentor because he believed Rush had not sufficiently supported him for a professorship he wanted at the University of Pennsylvania. Recurring disputes and petty resentments did not prevent Caldwell from courting public support for his causes, however—occasionally with success. He was an early proponent of vaccination with cowpox to prevent smallpox, and his advocacy in the press helped bring to fruition the plan to clean up Philadelphia by tapping the Schuylkill River for municipal use. He went west in 1819 and enjoyed a long and illustrious career teaching medicine in Kentucky, never laying down arms in the war against quarantine, that "erroneous," "destructive" "false idol" "founded on . . . superstition and prejudice," not to mention "bigotry and delusion." (Caldwell's own credentials in bigotry were robust; he helped build and propagate the American brand of scientific racism that served as one of the pillars of the institution of slavery.) He was especially proud of his role as the first advocate of mesmerism—treating mental and physical illness by manipulating "animal magnetism"—in the Mississippi Valley, and he claimed to have introduced phrenology to the United States. Lecturing on this putative science, which associated mental faculties with the size and shape of the skull, he told his students: "Gentlemen, there are but three great heads in the United States: one is Henry Clay, another is Daniel Webster, and modesty forbids me from telling you who the third is."[14]

But in 1802, when Philadelphia found itself in danger of falling back into the yearly cycle of epidemic, panic, and flight, this insufferably vain young doctor stumbled on a deceptively simple idea that held within it the promise of peace—or at least a lasting truce. After laying out yet again in a pamphlet and newspaper columns the case against the contagiousness of yellow fever and in favor of a policy of civic cleanliness instead of quarantine, Caldwell baldly stated that after ten years of fruitless and paralyzing debate, doctors were not going to reach consensus on the contagion question anytime soon. Rather than keep fighting, why not ensure that both sides win?

Caldwell proposed that the Board of Health be reorganized to include at least one physician from each side of the yellow fever controversy. That way, he reasoned, each side would be motivated to cooperate with the other: the contagionists would know that they would get their strict quarantine if they agreed to clean up the city (which no one opposed), and the proponents of local origin would know that they would get a cleaner city if they would go along with some kind of quarantine at the Lazaretto. Caldwell's prescription for the board was straightforward: Simply act as if both sides are correct! The single most intemperate doctor in the contentious world of Philadelphia medicine had put forward what he called "an amicable compromise."[15]

After the 1802 outbreak ended, Caldwell went on to propose that quarantine at the Lazaretto move away from lengthy detentions and instead emphasize thorough disinfection of vessels and cargo. This suggestion struck a chord with William Donaldson, who in his years on the board had surely heard his share of grumbling about Lazaretto delays from his fellow merchants. A warrior in the rough-and-tumble of Philadelphia politics, Donaldson was preparing to run for sheriff. He understood the appeal of a policy that advertised aggressive action and promoted security without unduly hindering the port's trade.[16] Caldwell's reform might lead the way forward to a quarantine that was simultaneously more efficient and less burdensome, and if the compromise carried Donaldson's imprimatur as well as Caldwell's, so much the better for Donaldson.

A Regime of Vigilance "to Banish from among Us Even the Apprehension of Disease"

As the quarantine season of 1803 approached, the Board of Health resolved to hew to the Caldwell-Donaldson compromise in protecting the city from disease. Thanks to a new state health law, the board now seated five members, not the twelve of previous years. (It would remain at five until 1817.) The compromise did not succeed in banishing yellow fever from Philadelphia—at least not at first—but the five-man board was determined: vigilance would tame disease. And vigilance would be modulated only when there was no imminent threat of an epidemic and when the board's bedrock commitment to vigilant quarantine was not in question.

Governor Thomas McKean appointed pro-quarantine lawyer John Kessler and hardware merchant James McGlathery to the newly trimmed board. He balanced them with two physicians, both of whom were committed to the local origins of yellow fever and opposed to lengthy detentions. The first was Rush's ally Felix Pascalis, and the second none other than Charles Caldwell. McKean's final appointee was the only holdover from 1799 and from the previous year, William Donaldson, who was elected president at the board's first meeting.[1] With Caldwell at the table and the savvy politician Donaldson presiding, the stage was set for enacting Caldwell's compromise on yellow fever—something previously unimaginable.

Donaldson knew that the board needed to send a strong and clear signal to the public, who had fled the city in alarm during the outbreak of the previous summer. Thus, in a statement published in all the city's major newspapers and bearing the unmistakable imprint of Donaldson and Caldwell, the board took an unusually frank tone in renewing its commitment to keeping the city safe and healthy. The result is the closest thing to a founding compact of the Board of Health that was ever set forth. First, the board did not pretend, as Governor Thomas Mifflin had five years earlier, that a consensus had emerged on the causes of yellow fever. The statement acknowledged that a serious difference of opinion remained between those who believed that the disease was imported from abroad and those who believed it originated locally. Donaldson and his colleagues decided not to come down on one side or the other but rather to hedge their bets—to act aggressively as if *both* propositions were true: "In our daily intercourse with you we discover that different persons still entertain different opinions respecting the origins of our late malignant diseases, and that their apprehensions are directed to different quarters, as the source from where they may assail us . . . It belongs not to us to aspire to the characters of umpires, in a dispute where difficulties stand opposed to difficulties, and in the estimation of many, arguments meet with such equal force."[2]

The board's response to the doctors' decade-long stalemate was both a stroke of genius and a desperate last resort. Instead of the paralysis of *either/or*, the board chose the liberation of *both/and*:

> It is our determination to guard against [yellow fever] with our best energies whether it be the offspring of *external* or *internal* causes, or arise and spread by their joint cooperation. While we pledge an assurance that those who believe exclusively in the importation of malignant fever, shall find no ground to charge us in default in the business of quarantine and purification, we flatter ourselves that the defenders of domestic origin will have no reason to complain of our inattention to the removal of nuisances.

From this point forward, Donaldson and his colleagues on the board recognized that the only politically tenable approach was to acknowledge the public's demand for both aggressive quarantine *and* cleaner streets. "By thus taking as auxiliaries to our own judgments the opinions, fears, and wishes of the public," the 1803 compact stated, the board would "endeavor to close every suspected avenue to danger, both from within and from without."[3] The board's compact might be seen as an early version of the environmentalist "precautionary principle": until there is definitive scientific evidence one way or the other, we must act as if a *suspected* threat is *in fact* dangerous.[4]

The board wisely made "the public" a partner in the defense of the city. Indeed, the statement insisted on this tactic, inviting "fellow citizens" to share "useful information" with the board, even as it promised not to make decisions merely "to gratify the wishes or silence the clamors of censorious individuals." The board would not subject Philadelphians to the plague quarantines capriciously enforced by European autocracies for centuries. Rather, American democratic ideals gave birth to American quarantine, rooted in law and justified by the people's trust. Without it, the board would be effectively disarmed:

> We entreat you to repose in us, so much of your confidence as may be necessary to enable us to perform our duty with promptness and facility. On no other terms can our official situation be tolerable to ourselves, on no other condition can our labors be useful to you. Distrust is the bane of that respectful consideration, and of those friendly reciprocities, which ought to subsist between the people and even the lowest of their public servants.[5]

Finally, Donaldson and Caldwell's 1803 compact proclaimed the board's determination to fight on every front, and to act on the people's fears, even when they were unwarranted. "Even admitting many of these opinions [on the spread of yellow fever] to be erroneous, and the fears which accompany them visionary and unfounded," the board explained, "still, as reason is inadequate to their immediate extinction they must be treated with the tenderness and regard which are due to realities." Unchecked fear had a nasty way of *becoming* dangerous reality:

> It is important that we should be able not only to prevent the actual occurrence, but if possible to banish from among us even the apprehension of disease. For next in point of mischief to the prevalence of malignant fever in our city is the perpetual dread of it in the minds of inhabitants. Such a dread, if suffered to exist, not only paralyzes the spirit of industry and enterprise at home but is apt to break out in rumours, which soon find their way abroad, that we are actually subject to the ravages of disease.[6]

The Board of Health generally did not make grandiose public statements. But the board intended its May 1803 compact to convey that it wished to engage with, and be transparent to, the public:

> In entering on the duties of an appointment, which from its connection with your health, your interests, and everything that renders life desirable, must operate powerfully on your hopes and fears, we feel incumbent on us to disclose to you the leading features of that system which we mean to pursue, in our endeavors to discharge so important a trust. When we consider the smallness of

our own body, the extent and variety of our duties, the magnitude of their objects, and the weight of responsibility attached to our functions, we experience
sensations of the most serious nature—sensations inseparable from a consciousness that our reputations are in some measure staked on the issue of our
transactions.

In words that recall Thomas Paine's "These are the times that try men's souls," the
board invokes the "circumstances which render our situation delicate and our duties arduous." The statement's somber tone carries a faint echo (albeit in a minor
key) of the great founding texts of the nation: "A decent respect to the opinions
of mankind requires that they should declare the causes which impel them to the
separation," wrote the Founders, whose Declaration of Independence concluded
with these words: "We mutually pledge to each other our Lives, our Fortunes and
our sacred Honor."[7]

Members of the board saw themselves as public servants facing a challenging
task, yes, but also as heirs of the Enlightenment and guardians of Philadelphia's
future. In 1803, the prosperity of America's port cities—all of which had experienced severe yellow fever attacks in the past decade—and the American experiment itself were endangered.[8] In defending them, the Board of Health would be
guided by the eighteenth-century values that had guided the Founders: reason,
democracy, transparency, and a spirit of improvement.

The first order of business called for new rules and new procedures to maintain vigilance at the new Lazaretto. Micromanaging the Lazaretto's operations, the
board voted on whether to permit the Lazaretto physician's wife to leave the
grounds for church on Sunday, and on whether a business partner should be allowed to approach the Lazaretto gate to converse with a captain under quarantine.
Indeed, the entry and exit of every single person to and from the Lazaretto grounds
at any time was subject to debate and approval by the board. Board members debated whether members should be permitted to read during meetings.[9] They announced and recorded every piece of correspondence addressed to the board. They
discussed at great length the amounts of fees, fines, and penalties; how to recover
them; and when to forgo or refund them.

But what might look like the triumph of form over substance, or like a meticulous charade of governance, actually testified to a renewed seriousness of focus.
The state legislature and the Board of Health had come to a hard-earned realization: when it comes to quarantine, details matter, and one can't be too careful. The
board met every day during the quarantine season, and every day, lives were at

stake. To deviate from the rules even slightly was to court disaster. The board's acute awareness of the danger fueled its determination to follow the rules to the letter, and every instance of strict enforcement bolstered its self-image as the duty-bound, inflexible protector of Philadelphians' health.

The essence of quarantine was simple: prevent any potentially infected person, ship, or article from entering the city until a certain period had elapsed, or until the ship and cargo had been properly disinfected. In principle, this was what quarantine meant in the fifteenth century, what it meant in the nineteenth century, and what it still means today. It involves, first, attentively detecting the warning signs of danger; second, carefully limiting dangerous contact within the quarantine space; and third, conscientiously policing the boundaries separating the quarantined from the general population. Vigilance on shipboard in the river, at the Lazaretto gate, and at the board's Health Office in the city: vigilance, vigilance, vigilance.

Making a sound decision about whether to allow a ship to proceed to the city relied partly on what the physician observed, and partly on what the physician learned from the ship's captain. But what happened to vigilance when a captain was less than forthright in answering the Lazaretto physician's questions about illnesses or deaths in the port of departure or during the voyage? The board added another layer of scrutiny by insisting that the physician and the quarantine master follow up the evasive or dishonest captain's interview with at least two more interrogations of people on the vessel. And when a ship was permitted up from the Lazaretto and the board later learned of a "malignant disease" prevailing at its port of origin? Then the ship, along with its passengers, cargo, and baggage, was immediately sent back down from the city to the Lazaretto.

The board had heard rumors of a previous epidemic being caused by a patient hidden by the crew in the cargo hold, so the physician and quarantine master were reminded to be "careful and minute" in their inspection of the vessel. All passengers and crew were to be mustered on deck for visual examination. Anyone who was "indisposed" at the time of the inspection was to be visited below, and any crew member working up in the rigging was to be called down for examination.[10]

Early on, it came to the board's attention that the fence securing the perimeter of the Lazaretto property extended to the river's edge only at high tide. (The Delaware rises and falls more than five feet, on average, at the Lazaretto.) Theoretically, quarantined people could wait for low tide and simply walk past the end of the fence to freedom. The board promptly ordered the steward to hire a carpenter to extend the fence to the lowest tide line to prevent escapes or unauthorized contact with the outside. Another fence was built along the head of the US Customs wharf next door, where cargoes were unloaded for storage, to prevent "improper intercourse" between ship personnel and visitors on shore. The board issued repeated reminders that communication with anyone outside the Lazaretto was to take place only through the aperture in the main gate, and only with advance written permission of the board.[11]

Anonymous sources alleged that in 1802, Lazaretto officers had allowed contact between vessels under quarantine, access to the gate from the wharf, and entry to and exit from the Lazaretto grounds without permission. The board could not fire the physician or the quarantine master, as they served at the pleasure of the governor, but it threatened to report the alleged violations to the governor unless the officers enforced the rules more strictly. Chastened, they seem to have cleaned up their act: it was not long before the board was praising them for catching the owners of the sloop *Sally* in the act of visiting their vessel while it was moored in the river under quarantine. The officers confiscated the owners' boat and confined the two men on their sloop for the duration of its detention.

A few years later, however, the board again had reason to criticize officers at the Lazaretto. A fight broke out between two sailors aboard a schooner under quarantine; one threw the other overboard, and he drowned. The Lazaretto officers turned the murderer over to the police, much to the "apprehension and horror" of the board. In the board's reasoning, strict enforcement of the quarantine regulations (including the removal of all boats from detained vessels) would have prevented the culprit's escape from the schooner, and he could have been turned over for justice when the quarantine was lifted. Meanwhile, his imprisonment risked spreading infection to the prison population. In such cases, the board insisted, the quarantine imperative should trump the justice system, at least temporarily.[12]

Passengers under quarantine were often allowed to leave the Lazaretto by posting bond, on the condition that they stay away from the city of Philadelphia until their quarantine expired. Violators exposed themselves both to forfeiture of the bond (which could be as much as $500 per person) and to criminal prosecution. The board vigorously pursued rumors of bond violations picked up from maritime and commercial grapevines. Rewards of up to $50 were offered for the apprehension of violators. Because most port cities' health laws barred bonded passengers from any city or town, Philadelphia's board was in regular contact with New York's quarantine authorities. Each city captured and returned violators of the other city's quarantine bonds for prosecution, often at the expense of considerable time and energy.[13]

In early 1805, with funding from the state legislature, the Board of Health erected a new building at the Lazaretto after an unusually heavy influx of German immigrants on typhus-infected vessels. Informally called the Dutch House—thanks to a common confusion between the words Dutch and Deutsch (German)—the building was needed to house healthy passengers and healthy sailors under quarantine. When construction for the building came in far under budget, the board saw an opportunity to crack down more effectively on quarantine violations. They bought a guard boat and hired a captain to patrol the river during the night, preventing contact between vessels and taking away detained vessels' boats.[14]

Parallel interrogations, searching vessels for hiding places, confiscating boats—some of the board's precautions seem to verge on paranoia. But every rule, every crackdown, happened for a reason. Violations and attempted violations were real, and the consequences were potentially disastrous. Subterfuge, evasion, even conspiracy could never be ruled out. Danger always loomed. The terribly high stakes kept nerves ragged, both at the Lazaretto and in the office of the Board of Health.

Perhaps the most consequential step the board could take was the simplest one of all: with the stroke of a pen, it could extend the length of the quarantine season. Yellow fever, the disease that haunted all Philadelphians, was strictly a warm-weather disease, so maintaining the Lazaretto year-round would have been a colossal waste of money and a needless drag on the port's business. Nevertheless, every revision of the state health law gave the board the authority to begin quarantine operations early or extend them past the official closing date. And the board did not hesitate to do so. A suspicious case arriving at the port, rumors of an epidemic in a Caribbean port, or even something as innocent as unseasonably warm weather could trigger the decision to open the Lazaretto early or keep it open late. When the danger seemed to come from only a few places, the board extended the season selectively; for example, when reports reached Philadelphia in late November 1804 of a yellow fever epidemic in the southern Spanish cities of Cadiz and Malaga, the board immediately ordered all vessels from those ports to stop at the Lazaretto for inspection until further notice. It did the same in 1819 for seven ports in the southern United States, the West Indies, and North Africa.[15] Again and again, the board demonstrated a determined and united vigilance.

In the summer of 1803, late in the season, "a disease of a malignant aspect" appeared near the Chestnut Street Wharf. By September 12 it had spread enough to alarm the Board of Health, while rumors, as usual, had spread even faster and farther. The outbreak was confined to four narrow city blocks between Market and Walnut Streets, and between Front Street and the river. The small scale of the outbreak allowed Donaldson and the Board of Health to stick to their policy of full disclosure while turning down the volume on their recommendation of the previous year. The disease had shown no signs of contagiousness, Donaldson announced reassuringly in a public statement, and a "general removal" of residents from the city was "by no means advisable." Be that as it may, he urged residents of the small "diseased district" to leave immediately, and he informed residents that all vessels would be removed from the adjacent wharves. The tone of the statement was unusually frank, like that of the May compact—full of "deep regret" at having to share bad news, and acknowledging the heavy responsibility that came with discouraging Philadelphians from "placing their safety in flight."[16]

Donaldson and the board were prepared to carry that weight. They promised the public honest and timely updates if the fever spread beyond its initial boundaries, but as it turned out, there was no need.[17] New cases stopped before the weather turned cold, and by October 20 the board felt confident announcing the outbreak's end. The 1803 outbreak had petered out three weeks after the board's statement. One estimate put the number of dead at 195.[18] Again, a far cry from the terrifying numbers of the 1790s but still enough to fuel the public's fear.

Was the board's enforcement overzealous? Not only passengers, sea captains, and crew, but even the Lazaretto physician occasionally thought so. As doctor on the spot, the physician might argue, he had the needed medical training and opportunity for firsthand observation to decide when detention was called for. But the same health law that provided for the governor of Pennsylvania to appoint the Lazaretto physician also subjected the physician to the ultimate authority of the Board of Health. When Dr. Nathan Dorsey delicately broached the question in a letter to the board at the beginning of the 1803 quarantine season—may I use my discretion in enforcing the health law and the board's resolutions?—the response was an unequivocal no. On several occasions, Dorsey detained vessels only to be ordered by the board to liberate them. When he asked the board to confirm that it considered three Caribbean ports to be "infected" (and that therefore vessels from those ports ought to be detained), the board refused and then went so far as to write the governor asking for an amendment to the health law endorsing the board's exclusive authority to declare ports infected or healthy. The board's decisions were final and absolute.[19]

Philadelphia's business community, too, felt the sting of the stricter quarantine regime at the new Lazaretto. The Chamber of Commerce protested to the governor in 1804 that vessels and goods were being delayed "beyond what the law directs, or the necessity of the cases requires," and that the board was "imposing hardships" on citizens and their property not warranted by "either the letter or the spirit of the law." The chamber's Exhibit A was the ship *New Jersey*, detained for a full month at the Lazaretto after a voyage from Batavia (today Jakarta, Indonesia) laden with coffee and pepper.

When the *New Jersey* arrived, the Board of Health ordered the ship's cargo to be landed at the Lazaretto for inspection; if the cargo was in good condition, the vessel would be permitted to proceed after disinfection. Instead of submitting the necessary customs forms for the unloading of the cargo, however, the *New Jersey*'s owners spent their time lobbying the members of the board to liberate their ship. Only after the board allowed the owners to bring the ship to a wharf in Southwark for the discharge and inspection of the cargo did it learn that several of its crew had suffered at Batavia and on the voyage to Philadelphia from a suspicious fever. The information had not been disclosed to the Lazaretto physician.[20] At that point, any chance of avoiding a lengthy delay vanished.

In defending itself to the governor against the chamber's charges, the board claimed to have no illusions about what lay behind the dispute. "This is a contest of interest against principle," it wrote. "Any man must have uncommon public spirit who would sacrifice twenty thousand dollars profits on a cargo for the public good." Even if merchants generally approved of the idea of quarantine after yellow fever had devastated Philadelphia's trade in the late 1790s, "when the individual finds his own interests affected, he is apt to complain of the hardship."[21] The board understood that the contest of interest against principle was built into the very idea of quarantine, and it was prepared for the battle.

Merchants' grumbling usually went hand in hand with their private lobbying of the board (by mail or in person) for more lenient treatment. Occasionally, though, they went to court for relief. One captain, pleading poverty, demanded forty-four dollars in damages from the board for the detention of his schooner at the Lazaretto. The Board of Health flatly rejected the premise of his demand, reasserting its immunity from such claims, while at the same time acknowledging that the schooner in question was delayed an extra day by a miscommunication between the board and the Lazaretto physician. Taking into account the captain's description of his woeful financial situation, the members of the board voted to pay him twenty dollars.[22]

When the Board of Health's members disagreed among themselves or with the Lazaretto officers, its delicate and unpopular job was further complicated. In 1803, the new Lazaretto's third year of operation, a 3–2 vote determined nearly every quarantine-related decision the board made, including Lazaretto physician Dorsey's request for leeway in declaring quarantine. Board president Donaldson sided with the localist physicians Caldwell and Pascalis in advocating shorter detention of vessels, cargo, and passengers. The minority, Kessler and McGlathery, continually voted for stricter quarantine.[23] Nevertheless, the Caldwell-Donaldson compromise—in which the board took its quarantine responsibilities seriously and paid special attention to the disinfection of vessels and cargoes as well as to policing filth in the city—kept the peace.

The deep and consistent split on the board in 1803 was unusual, but internal debates were not. Quarantine was almost never strict enough for Dr. William Currie, who served on the board from 1804 to 1809, and his dissents from board decisions were legion.[24] Members rarely aired their dirty laundry in public, however, and consequently the board spoke to Philadelphians and to the outside world with a single voice. Those who found themselves on the wrong end of quarantine often complained and pressed their case, but they seldom officially challenged the board's authority.

The 1803 board remained true to its May vow even with a consistent majority skeptical of quarantine. Members often voted to detain vessels for extended periods—especially when they arrived at the Lazaretto with illness aboard. The ship *Fanny* from Cape-François (Haiti), for example, was kept out for the entire six-month quarantine season. When two men visited another detained vessel in violation of the quarantine, the board voted to confine them for the duration of the ship's detention.[25]

The new regime of vigilance carried the day throughout the fractious season of 1803.

The very next year, however, the viability of the new vigilance would be challenged by the arrival of vessels from Europe jammed full of immigrants, most hungry and many ill, who swelled the Lazaretto beyond its capacity to properly shelter and care for them. As quarantine days dragged on endlessly, and ships sat at anchor awaiting release to the city, the weary immigrants—anxious to begin their new lives in a new land—apparently rose up in protest over their confinement.

The trying ordeal of the 1804 season triggered a new phase in the board's approach to quarantine. It began to discover the virtues of "expedience": firmness tempered by flexibility.

PART II / Managing the New Normal, 1804–1847

Chapter Six

"Expedient" Measures and Rioting Redemptioners, 1804

Nobody enjoyed quarantine. It was always an unpopular policy, even among those who agreed that it was occasionally necessary. Quarantine affected not just the sailors and passengers who were detained at the Lazaretto, and not just the ship owners and the consignees of the goods that were delayed, but also the businesses and customers who depended on those goods, and those whose jobs depended on those businesses. All of them disliked quarantine. But in the endlessly repeated protests against quarantine over the years, almost nobody contested the *right* of the state to temporarily deprive people of their liberty in the interest of public health.

The Anglican moral philosopher William Paley, whose work was widely assigned in American schools and colleges in the nineteenth century, saw quarantine as the classic case study in the paradox of liberty. His example involved a passenger detained on returning to England from the Middle East, where bubonic plague outbreaks were common. The quarantined Englishman might resent his detention, Paley argued, but he "would hardly accuse government of encroaching upon his civil freedom." On the contrary, he might even "congratulat[e] himself that he had at length set his foot again in a land of liberty." In Paley's view, the resolution of the paradox of freedom-through-detention lay in the "manifest expediency" of quarantine.

The temporary suspension of liberty was "expedient" if it was *intended to achieve a specific and limited civic goal* and if it was *appropriate to that goal*. In quarantine, denial of freedom actually made freedom possible. "It is not the rigour," Paley concluded, "but the inexpediency of laws and acts of authority which makes them tyrannical."[1]

For most of the twentieth century, the right of government to restrict individual liberties in the name of the public's health was unquestioned and virtually unlimited. More recently, however, ethicists and lawmakers have tried to balance state authority with a concern for the protection of individual rights. The result has been the widespread acceptance of the "least restrictive alternative" principle: whenever public health measures threaten individual liberties, privacy, or other rights, authorities should choose the path that achieves the desired health goal with as little infringement of those rights as possible.[2] The members of Philadelphia's Board of Health in the early nineteenth century would have recognized this principle; in fact, they probably took it for granted. It was rehearsed and refined every day at the Lazaretto.

In a nation that aspired to be a paragon of liberty in the world, quarantine could be accepted, and even embraced, only to the extent that it was seen as *expedient*. The expedience doctrine proved to be perennially useful in quarantine decisions because it allowed the Board of Health some flexibility without undermining its authority or its principles. Members of the board did not have to agree on the rightness—or wrongness—of a course of action, as long as there was something *expedient* that could be done.

One early invocation of expedience by the Board of Health stands out from the others, as it stretched the board's usual protocol: instead of accommodating aggrieved passengers or ship owners, the board accommodated unwarranted public fears. It happened in 1809, amid rumors of disease in Havana. The ship *Cleopatra* and brig *Eliza* both arrived at the Lazaretto on July 14 and performed a ten-day quarantine as prescribed by the physician and approved by the board. But instead of permitting the vessels up to the port when their quarantines were over, the board made special arrangements for their coffee and sugar to be brought up to the city, and for them to be reloaded with new cargoes at the Lazaretto before heading back out to sea. The reason? The "agitated state of the public mind" over reports about Havana, the board felt, made the arrival of any ship from that port in Philadelphia "inexpedient," whether it had performed quarantine or not.[3]

The ship *Mary Ann* also sailed from Havana to Philadelphia that summer, but no special arrangements were made to accommodate it. It was detained at the Lazaretto for three long months, for no other reason (in the board's explanation) than "the state of the public mind of the citizens of Philadelphia." Public worry had to be accounted for as much as public health. When the brig *Neptune* from St. Thomas (Virgin Islands) was permitted up to the city, the captain was ordered to leave one passenger at the Lazaretto: a sick boy. His disease was not contagious, the board explained, but if he came to the city before his symptoms abated, "apprehensions" might arise "in the minds of the citizens."[4]

The board's mission was not just to prevent epidemics but to manage "the public mind." Sometimes that required sounding the alarm; other times, it meant reassurance; and quite often, it called for both at the same time. It was not an easy task.

Members of the Board of Health were coming to understand what scholars today call "social efficacy."[5] Keeping disease out was essential, but it was not enough. Anxious people, traumatic memories still fresh in their minds, needed reassurance that vigilance was constant and unwavering. Even measures that did little to protect public health could at times be effective in shoring up public confidence in the new regime of quarantine.

Even while the Board of Health was preoccupied with preventing disease outbreaks and managing the public mind when epidemics threatened or appeared, the thorny problem of managing the Lazaretto during the quarantine season remained a constant. At any moment a ship might arrive at Tinicum Island with dozens or even hundreds of sickly immigrants aboard.

As Pennsylvania and other British American colonies continued to grow throughout the eighteenth century, hundreds of thousands of immigrants arrived from the British Isles, German-speaking lands, and France. Many of them were too poor to pay for their passage and were forced to indenture themselves as servants on arrival until their passage could be paid off. These immigrants, known as *redemptioners*, were continually subject to abuse by recruiters and sea captains, who were paid by the body and who regarded food rations as a cost to be minimized. (The traffic in redemptioners thrived throughout the seventeenth and eighteenth centuries, and eventually slowed to a trickle after about 1820, when some large European ports began requiring would-be emigrants to prove that they had the resources to pay for their passage. But even then, the underlying economic incentives did not change, and even fare-paying immigrants who could not afford to bring their own food continued to be crowded into overstuffed cargo holds and denied adequate rations.)

In the mid-eighteenth century, the Pennsylvania Assembly had passed two laws intended to protect the redemptioners by regulating the number of passengers per ship and requiring a minimum square footage per passenger. But the arm of Pennsylvania's law did not reach as far as the European ports of embarkation, and the new rules proved impossible to enforce.

Seeking better lives, the immigrants kept coming. When they arrived at the Lazaretto, the sick and healthy alike had to be housed, clothed, fed, and washed, and the sick had to be treated in the Lazaretto hospital. Healthy passengers sometimes stayed aboard their ships, but when the vessels needed to be disinfected or when conditions aboard were simply too crowded or unhealthy, they had to be accommodated at the Lazaretto, either in the Dutch House or in tents pitched on the station grounds.

Days or weeks with relatively few detained ships could turn without warning into an overwhelming onslaught of desperately needy arrivals. The Board of Health could not afford to buy supplies or to pay nurses and other staff to be on duty when they were not needed—"just in case"—but it also had to respond immediately with beds, tents, food, clothing, and medical care when the need arose.

In 1804, the ship *Rebecca* arrived at the Lazaretto from Amsterdam with close to 400 passengers aboard. Most were impoverished Swiss German redemptioners. The word *redemptioners* contains a hint of spiritual uplift, but the riot of the *Rebecca's* redemptioners at the Lazaretto in 1804 shines a light on the ugly underbelly of America's immigration history. It had been a decade since American participation in the slave trade had been outlawed, and it would be another six decades before slavery itself would be consigned to history, but in its shadow, another form of human trafficking continued to thrive with little public outcry, even in the capital of the abolition movement.

Make no mistake: even if, as some historians have argued, the conditions on the redemptioners' journeys were as bad as or worse than those of the infamous Middle Passage, there are hugely significant differences between slavery and voluntary (even if coerced) immigration.[6] The redemptioners were treated like animals, were sold (sometimes at auction), and were subjected to sometimes violent corporal punishment, but they were not slaves. They were not captured by force. They were not shackled. Their bondage did not last a lifetime, and their children were not born into servitude. Enslaved Africans and their children endured an entire world of degradation that even the most ill-treated European immigrant never experienced.

Comparing shipboard conditions for enslaved people and redemptioners cannot capture the full extent of either group's suffering or dehumanization. But the plight of the passengers aboard the *Rebecca* does highlight the cruel victimization of vulnerable migrants from Europe, which has been largely lost to public memory. The patriotic mythology of the Statue of Liberty—"I lift my lamp beside the golden door"—has always been at best a very partial representation of America's immigration history. Viewed from the Lazaretto, where redemptioners fortunate enough to have survived their journeys were disgorged half-dead while ship owners collected their handsome passage fees, the myth seems almost obscene. The *Rebecca's* journey was longer than most, but in its grinding privation, it was quite ordinary.

It was more than the call of freedom or flight from want that brought Johan Christen and his shipmates to Philadelphia via the Lazaretto.[7] Immigrant indentured servitude was a sophisticated and extremely profitable industry, designed to turn the hopes of the poor into cash. Like most redemptioners, the *Rebecca's* passengers came from German-speaking lands—precisely those territories targeted by the human traffickers of the late eighteenth and early nineteenth centuries. They were recruited by Newlanders (Neuländer)—earlier German-speaking American immigrants who were paid by the shipping companies to travel back to the homeland and lure new migrants to follow them across the sea. From Aarau and Tübingen to Bad Dürkheim and Darmstadt, the Newlanders crisscrossed the most promising regions—promising in the sense that many of those living there lived in poverty and had already moved at least once, in search of safety or security, or because they were forced to by soldiers seizing their homes and land. Dressed in their finest clothes, complete with ruffles, wigs, and jewelry, recruiters touted America as a place of easy riches. They "conduct[ed] themselves as men of opulence," one victim complained,

> in order to inspire the people with the desire to live in a country of such wealth and abundance . . . They would convince one that there are in America, none but Elysian fields abounding in products which require no labor; that the mountains are full of gold and silver, and the wells and springs gush forth milk and honey; that he who goes there as a servant, becomes a lord; as a maid, a gracious lady; as a peasant, a nobleman; as a commoner or craftsman, a baron.

"Now, as everyone by nature desires to better his condition," the rueful emigrant concluded, "who would not wish to go to such a country!"[8]

The Newlanders, who had no trouble finding vulnerable marks, were paid by the head, while would-be emigrants paid at every step. A Newlander might extort his own fee or volunteer to take possession of the traveler's cash for "safekeeping." All worldly possessions were packed into trunks as the journey down the Rhine began. Each city or principality along the way—several dozen in all—charged its own customs duty as delays and expenses mounted. It could take weeks to reach Rotterdam or Amsterdam, where the waiting continued.

Even those who had left home with money in hand were by then often broke or in debt. And that was the point. When the time finally came to board an America-bound ship and set sail, both the (now-plundered) trunks of belongings and the Newlander who had promised to be on the same ship and to safeguard money and valuables were often nowhere to be found. The ship's captain or his agents often paid off the emigrants' debts, adding the amount—plus interest, of course—to the fare for the passage. Little wonder that the Newlanders came to be known as Seelenverkäufer—"soul-sellers."[9]

Each person or family agreed on a fare with the captain before departure. In this human cargo trade, bodies were money, and sea captains had every incentive to cram as many of them aboard as possible. Emigrants were "packed like herring in a box," it was said at the time—averaging 300 passengers in the smaller vessels (under 200 tons cargo capacity) and reaching up to 800 passengers in the larger ships (250 to 300 tons capacity). Some passengers were forced to sleep on deck, exposed to the elements.[10] Belowdecks, even the cleanest vessel quickly turned foul when crowded with so many sweating, itching, eating, belching, flatulating, excreting, unwashed bodies. Heavy seas or routine seasickness layered the sour stench of vomit over the palette of other unpleasant odors.

Odors were not the only thing shared among the passengers. That these human herring boxes were hothouses for ship fever was well known long before investigations of bacteria and insect vectors reshaped medical science. What today we call epidemic typhus spread wherever chronically hungry people were crowded together in filthy conditions without clean clothing or washing facilities. The redemptioner vessels offered the disease an ideal breeding ground. "The lice abound so frightfully," said one German passenger on a redemptioner's ship in 1750, "that they can be scraped off the body."[11]

Wind and weather determined the length of the passage. In unfavorable conditions, cheek-by-jowl in the fetid cargo hold, passengers felt the hours drag by like days, the weeks like lifetimes. Sickness and death were inescapable. "There is on board these ships terrible misery, stench, fumes, horror, vomiting, many kinds of sea-sickness, fever, dysentery, headache, heat, constipation, boils, scurvy, cancer, mouth-rot and the like," one passenger lamented, "all of which come from old and sharply salted food and meat, also from very bad and foul water, so that many die miserably." A rock-hard biscuit or two and a few ladles of a brownish liquid that once resembled water often made up a day's full diet. Captains strictly rationed supplies and apportioned a whipping or beating to anyone who demanded more—and even so, passengers constantly complained about the quality and quantity of food and water. If the voyage was unexpectedly long, and the food and water ran out or spoiled, then the human cargo simply went hungry and thirsty. With an eye on the bottom line, the captain could not afford to be softhearted. Illness and death were costs of doing business; besides, in many cases, if a passenger died past the halfway point of the journey, surviving relatives were required to pay the deceased's full passage anyway.[12]

Six decades after his journey, Johan Christen—or John Christian, as he became known in Berks County, Pennsylvania—wrote about it in his memoir. Time had smoothed over some of the most painful details, but he still recalled most of it vividly. He had left his village of Frenkendorf near Basel in northern Switzerland at age 18 with hundreds of other emigrants from the region, which had been impoverished by high taxes and the depredations of Napoleon's army. His fare was sixty-five dollars. To journey to Amsterdam, young Christen and his compatriots spent seventeen days packed aboard a flat-bottomed boat with no room to lie down. Then they waited for a ship to take them to America, "the land of milk and honey" that they had heard so much about.[13]

Three hundred seventy-four people crowded aboard the Rebecca, which was built to ship cargo, not passengers. Christen and his shipmates were "crowded together between decks like so many pigs." And there they festered on one meal a day, for two weeks, not sailing anywhere, as the undersupplied ship replenished its provisions. Once they finally got underway, the first storm caused dreadful seasickness among most of the passengers, and from then on, healthy bodies were hard to come by. Headwinds and constant storms delayed the Rebecca's progress through the North Sea and English Channel, but in the open ocean, twelve days of good weather brightened spirits considerably.[14]

Then came the fierce headwinds that announced a storm unlike anything any of them had ever seen. The "mountain high" waves tossed the ship about like a child's toy. After a few hours, the ocean's fury tore off all three masts and pulled the vessel over until it lay on its side, on the verge of capsizing. The ship took on a huge amount of water, and the middle hatchway was stuck open by a broken yardarm, flooding the jam-packed passenger hold. Quick work by the crew cut away all the rigging that was pulling the ship over toward its broken masts and righted the hull. The dismasted *Rebecca* was then at the mercy of the waves, as all on deck lashed themselves to the rings on board, and the passengers below were tossed about mercilessly along with their chests and trunks and other belongings. After two and a half days, the wind abated enough to allow the hatches to be opened and the terrified emigrants finally to get some air and light, but the rough seas continued. The crew and some of the able-bodied passengers were eventually able to splice together a rudder and two makeshift masts.[15]

The *Rebecca*'s bad luck went on and on. Eight days of headwinds gave way to nine days of no wind whatsoever. After finally reaching the lighthouses of Cape Henlopen and Cape May at the entrance to the Delaware Bay, and taking on a river pilot to guide it the rest of the way to Philadelphia, the ship was blown back to the ocean for five more days. No one is to blame for bad weather, of course, and the *Rebecca* had more than its share of that. The overcrowding and underprovisioning of the ship, however, were the deliberate decisions of Captain Low, under pressure to carry as much human cargo as possible and to minimize expenses. As supplies dwindled, one meal a day was reduced to a fraction of a meal. Water rations were cut to a quart per person per day. Anyone who wanted to eat was required to give half of this scant water ration to the cook.

Around the time rations were cut, a few passengers began to feel ill. It started as a slight chill, accompanied by a splitting headache and intense pains in the arms and legs. Not long after came a high fever and utter prostration; the sick were unable to move, had barely enough energy to speak above a whisper, and even lost their appetites. After four or five days, pink blotches broke out on their abdomens, then on the rest of their torsos. The spots turned red, then purple, then a dark reddish brown, and eventually spread to their limbs. Their loved ones watched in horror as the rash covered their entire bodies, leaving only their faces unmarked. Sordes (pronounced SOR-dees), a thick dark paste-like deposit, coated their tongues and crusted over their teeth. Their bodies gave off a foul stench. From time to time their arms and legs twitched uncontrollably. Delirium gave way to what looked like a drunken stupor (the word *typhus* comes from the Greek root for smoke, cloud, or stupor): eyes dull, cheeks flushed, demeanor seemingly careless or indifferent. If flies began to collect on their faces, they may not have shown any sign of noticing. A few days after the reduction in rations, the deaths began. There would be sixty-four burials at sea before the voyage was over.[16]

Christen's account of the ship's journey indicates that 17 percent of the *Rebecca*'s passengers died during its voyage. On the *Venture Again* in 1801, 52 percent had died. On the ship *Hope* from Amsterdam in 1817 (see chapter 8), it was 18 percent (or 27 percent, if you count those who arrived critically ill and died at the Laza-retto). Historians disagree about how representative the horror stories are, and these immigrant ships may be outliers in the vast sea of such vessels in the eighteenth and early nineteenth century. One small sampling of fourteen vessels carrying German immigrants between 1727 and 1805—the only ships that kept careful records—showed overall mortality during the voyages of just under 4 percent, with child mortality just over 9 percent.[17] But to the steward, quaran-tine master, physician, nurses, and bargemen at the Lazaretto in the station's early years, receiving a ship like the *Rebecca* was all too common.

It took the *Rebecca* fifty-six storm-tossed days to make it to Philadelphia—that is, *almost* to Philadelphia. (Eight weeks was not an uncommon duration for an Atlantic crossing at the time.) After all that travel—from the village to the Rhine, slowly downriver to Amsterdam, the waiting for departure, then the endless days at sea—one final obstacle stood in the redemptioners' way before they could reach their destination: the Lazaretto. When they finally arrived at the quaran-tine station on Tinicum Island on August 16, 1804, some had already been travel-ing for more than four months. The Lazaretto physician immediately informed the Board of Health that the *Rebecca* was in "very foul" condition. Christen counted sixty-four deaths during the voyage, but Captain Low told the physician that there had been only two deaths. Seventeen more passengers died not long after arrival. The sick among the surviving passengers were sent to the Lazaretto hospital, and the board immediately requisitioned a supply of tents on the station grounds to house the others so that they could be liberated from their fetid float-ing prison.[18]

And there the redemptioners stayed. Two days after their arrival, wealthy Phil-adelphia merchant Samuel Coates—who was either the *Rebecca*'s owner or the owner's agent—was granted permission to meet with the ship's captain. The pur-pose of the meeting was not to get to the bottom of the ship's foul condition or the captain's treatment of the redemptioners, but simply to collect the money owed— calculated per passenger—for the journey. The surviving passengers, so close to their destination, stewed in the summer heat and humidity. They had already been there for two and a half weeks in their makeshift tent encampment when the ther-mometer climbed to 96 degrees in the shade.

On day 25 of the passengers' quarantine, Samuel Coates advertised in the Phil-adelphia dailies "about one hundred Redemptioners, principally Swiss, arrived from Amsterdam, by the ship *Rebecca* . . . consisting of a Sugar Boiler, Masons, Joiners, Shoemakers, Tailors, Farmers, Saddlers, Gardeners, a number of Women, and Boys and Girls, to be disposed of." Four days later, the Board of Health denied Coates's request to permit the ship and its human cargo up to the city.[19]

Johan Christen shared a tent on the Lazaretto grounds with three other healthy young single men, although it is hard to imagine how four men could make do with a small amount of straw and a single blanket. One night a powerful thunderstorm soaked everything, and it continued raining steadily for days afterward. It was impossible to keep dry, and after sleeping on wet straw for several nights in a row, Christen fell ill and was admitted to the Lazaretto hospital. There he was given a strong calomel purgative—to "clear out the chimney up and down," he recalled ruefully—followed by "Peruvian bark" (quinine) powder mixed in porter, which made him feel much better. Christen had nothing but praise for the care he received—"no better attention could have been bestowed on me anywhere"—but, restless and confined in the not-quite-prison of quarantine, he had had enough.[20]

From his hospital bed Christen could see down into the basement, where every morning the bodies of those who had died during the night were laid out. The sight filled his 18-year-old mind with dread, and as the days dragged on, he began to feel that he had to get out of there. As his fever receded and his strength returned, he was allowed to walk around the grounds, where he noticed a fence board with all but one of its nails missing. Christen borrowed a gimlet from the baker and surreptitiously dug out the remaining nail. Early one morning, he gathered his few remaining belongings, shoved the fence board to one side, and slipped through to freedom, leaving the rest of his impatient and exhausted shipmates behind.[21]

On September 26 (day 41 of the *Rebecca*'s quarantine), another large immigrant ship arrived with sick passengers aboard: the *Fortune*, from the German North Sea port of Emden. Its sad story was all too familiar: the crossing had taken an excruciating ninety days, during which twenty passengers had died; forty-one were sick on arrival. The Board of Health sent the sick to the Lazaretto hospital and ordered that "the remainder shall be accommodated in the other buildings at the Lazaretto, and that if these shall prove insufficient, the most healthy and robust of the men shall be placed in tents."[22]

The troubles of the *Fortune*'s survivors did not end at the Lazaretto, however. A number of passengers happened to be on board the ship when a sudden storm struck. The violently gusting winds blew the ship completely off its moorings and capsized the huge vessel in the river just a hundred yards from the Lazaretto wharf.

Three of the *Fortune's* unfortunate passengers drowned, including two fathers who left destitute families behind with no means to support themselves.[23]

As tragedy compounded misery, the board needed an expedient way out of the dangerous crowding at the Lazaretto. Its solution was to allow the *Fortune's* owner to take one hundred of its passengers up to the city, on four conditions: the passengers had never been ill, their baggage and clothing had been "well cleansed and fumigated," they were transported "in a pure vessel," and the vessel would anchor in the river—not at a wharf—north of the city, no nearer than Vine Street.[24] Exceptional circumstances, the board often found, called for carefully crafted exceptions to the rules. The economic and human cost of quarantine could be reduced, as long as no risk was posed to the health of the city.

Even with the release valve of one hundred *Fortune* passengers, the Lazaretto boiled over. The riot happened during the week between the *Fortune's* arrival on September 26 and the long-awaited end of the *Rebecca's* forty-eight-day quarantine on October 3. Maybe the arrival of hundreds of new hungry immigrants was the spark that lit the flame. Maybe the fact that some of the newcomers were housed indoors, with proper beds, struck those who were not as unfair. Maybe the tents simply became too crowded. Maybe food rations were reduced, or the weather turned suddenly cold, or someone uttered an ethnic slur. Maybe it was not even a riot at all. What we know for sure is that sometime between September 26 and October 3, a group of quarantined passengers caused $200 worth of damage at the Lazaretto (more than $4,000 in early twenty-first-century terms).[25]

Without specifying the nature of the damage, the Board of Health initially charged the owners of the *Rebecca* and the *Fortune* $100 each to defray repair costs. When Samuel Coates, ever solicitous of the bottom line, protested that $100 was too much, Lazaretto steward George Budd shot back that the figure "would not compensate for the entire injury sustained" and insisted on full payment. When the board asked about the amount charged to the *Fortune*, Budd said that $50 would be fair, since the *Rebecca's* passengers caused most of the damage.[26]

There may be a perfectly ordinary explanation: carelessness with a fire, a drunken quarrel that got out of hand, or a single bored malcontent bent on causing trouble. But the surviving accounts of those days tell of the soul-sellers' perfidy, the redemptioners' long journeys and endless delays, the agents' rip-offs, the

herring boxes, the meager rations and filthy water, and the stench, vomit, diarrhea, and ship fever. After the waiting—endless waiting—followed finally by
landfall and arrival and then *seven weeks* of quarantine, it is easy to see conditions
for a riot falling into place on Tinicum Island. A combustible crowd of desperately
poor redemptioners who had cheated death may have gradually regained some of
their strength at the Lazaretto. Almost anything could have set them off. Anything
could have triggered a violent howl of indignation and outrage and blind fury—
an uprising that ended as soon as it began, leaving only the faintest trace in the
historical record to testify to the fragile physical and emotional state of a group
of new Americans in 1804.

Chapter Seven

A Mischievous Boy, 1805

Even when the Lazaretto was overwhelmed with yellow fever cases from the West Indies and shiploads full of German redemptioners suffering from ty-phus, the Board of Health congratulated itself on the "vigor" of its quarantine and its "strict attention" to disinfection, which had kept Philadelphia safe. It also took advantage of the opportunity to ask the governor for money to erect a new building at the station to accommodate more passengers away from the unhealthy confined shipboard air. The request was granted, and building of the Dutch House began.[1]

A two-part refrain sounded continually in the Lazaretto's early decades: we are under threat, and we are successfully keeping the threat at bay. The Board of Health needed to keep Philadelphians' fear and their confidence in balance. If citizens lost sight of the epidemic threat, their support for a strict quarantine and other burdensome health policies might dissipate; but if their fear overcame their belief that the proper authorities had the threat under control, chaos could ensue. Rumors, commercial hesitancy, and flight—even when they fell short of all-out panic—caused nearly as much harm as an epidemic. And political support for an institution that depended on state appropriations was always both vital and fragile.

The board conducted its "public mind" campaign through Philadelphia's daily newspapers. That indispensable communication channel was always open, and the audience was large. (By 1811, Philadelphia would have eight daily newspapers, with a total circulation of more than 8,000.)[2] Before the beginning of each quarantine season, the newspapers published the board's announcement with the key details of the quarantine regulations. Every time the rules were revised, the newspapers published the board's announcement. When a ban was imposed on travel or trade from a particular city because of a disease outbreak, the newspapers published the board's announcement. When officials from rival ports circulated rumors about an outbreak in Philadelphia, the newspapers published the board's denials.[3]

Maintaining this channel of communication served several purposes. It ensured that merchants, sea captains, and others involved in maritime travel and trade knew the rules. It also enlisted the services of readers as potential informants who were kindly requested to contact the Health Office if they became aware of any violations. Keepers of boardinghouses, taverns, and stagecoach offices were especially invited to help "in detecting and exposing conduct which may involve the most important interests of the city."[4] But the newspapers also allowed the Board of Health to regularly advertise its vigilance.

The board found it useful to renew the founding Caldwell-Donaldson compact from time to time through the press, usually near the beginning of a new quarantine season. It often began with self-congratulations for the "exalted state of health" the city had enjoyed since the last epidemic, and went on to explain the board's approach to quarantine. The 1804 appeal emphasized that the board had "endeavored to subject commerce to the least restraints compatible with the public safety"—the equivalent of today's "least restrictive alternative" ideal—while bragging about the strictness of ship inspections and the "inflexibly rigid" nature of quarantine when it was imposed. It also solicited public support for its policies, arguing that the "occasional . . . inconvenience" imposed on merchants was far outweighed by the economic and human costs that another epidemic would entail. "It is trusted, we shall receive the support of *all* in the practice of the legal restraints necessary to the safety of *ALL*," Dr. James Reynolds, secretary of the board at the time, concluded drily.[5]

The year-end reports of the Board of Health to the governor and of the governor to the legislature provided another opportunity for self-congratulation and cultivation of public support. (The board and the governor made sure these were reprinted in the Philadelphia dailies, of course.) An epidemic-free year could be attributed to "the vigilance of the Board of Health and the officers of the Lazaretto." The board reminded the governor that every time a sailor or passenger suffering from a "malignant fever" was hospitalized at the Lazaretto without the illness subsequently spreading to the city, another silent argument had been made in favor of Philadelphia's quarantine.[6]

Investigating and fighting rumors about possible disease outbreaks occupied an inordinate amount of the board's time. As always, the stakes were high: an epidemic in another city meant the suspension of all trade and travel from that city for weeks. And time was of the essence: if there was yellow fever in New York, Baltimore, or Charleston, even a brief delay in taking action could increase Philadelphia's vulnerability. But hasty measures based on unfounded reports not only caused economic damage all around, but also exposed Philadelphia to counter-rumors and retaliatory bans. Regular correspondence with health officials in all major American seaports allowed rumors to be investigated and at least some measure of trust to be established.[7]

If Tobias Smith, Peter Young, and Elizabeth Young had been paying attention at all to the Board of Health's persistent efforts to engage the public in keeping disease away from the city, they surely would have realized that sneaking down to the Lazaretto in midsummer to sell goods to the fleet under quarantine was asking for trouble.

Front Street, Lombard Street Wharf, Vine Street Wharf, Chestnut Street Wharf: it was always the same areas. Every outbreak of yellow fever in Philadelphia's history did the bulk of its damage inside a narrow strip of the city along the riverfront, between Vine Street in the north and Christian Street in the south, and between Second Street and the Delaware River. Eventually the Board of Health began to use the shorthand designation "the infected district."[8]

Partisans of the contagion theory seized on this spatial clustering to press their case: yellow fever was always imported in ships from the West Indies, spread from them to the wharfside houses closest to the ships, and from there to the surrounding neighborhood. Those on the other side of the debate pointed to this same evidence with just as much conviction: this was the most overcrowded part of town and the filthiest. Anyone who had walked those streets in the summertime could tell you that a disease originating in accumulations of decaying matter would find its most welcoming home there. In this way yellow fever's peculiar geography, which might seem to be valuable evidence about the disease's origins and prevention, did nothing but entrench each side more firmly in its position.

Eleven-year-old Tobias Smith did not have much to lose when he was confronted by investigators from the Board of Health in early August 1805. He was known to be "idle and mischievous." He was probably an orphan; if he wasn't, he was destitute and had been given up by his parents. At age 6 he had been placed in Philadelphia's almshouse, where he lived for a few months before the managers sent him out as an indentured servant to Samuel Crisman. Crisman and his wife kept a "grocery, dram, and huckster shop" (that is, a not entirely respectable dry-goods shop and bar) at the Catharine Street Wharf in Southwark. Tobias had been with the Crismans for five years when he was thrust into the public spotlight as a person of interest in a Board of Health investigation about violations of the quarantine law at the Lazaretto.[9]

A sailor's life would have been the likeliest career for an unruly orphan like Tobias, whom the Crismans found hard to handle. And according to those who knew him, that was indeed his plan. When Samuel Crisman did not have enough work for the boy, he hired him out to a boatman to help bring oysters up from the Delaware Bay. Later, Crisman signed Tobias on to crew aboard the brig *Ceres*, due to depart in early August 1805 for the port of Santiago in Cuba. The boy spent two weeks aboard the *Ceres* in port as it prepared for the voyage, returning to the Crismans' for meals and to sleep. The lure of the sea may have led him on the fateful journey—or journeys—that landed him in so much trouble. Several versions of the story can be pieced together from the sworn statements of fifteen witnesses, who frequently contradicted themselves and one another.

Maybe Tobias's thirst for adventure and penchant for mischief started everything. The risk of getting caught made the adventure all the more exciting. Or maybe the boy and 20-year-old Peter Young, both members of the rootless urban rabble whose chief occupation was idleness and who had no prospects and no stake in the social order, simply could not be bothered with Philadelphia's determination to protect itself from disease while remaining a busy commercial seaport. Maybe it was the bad influence on Tobias of Young, who did odd carpentry jobs for Crisman and lived with his wife above the shop. Maybe it was Crisman himself who instigated the outings and deserved the blame.

When Young was questioned about his activities, he gave several different versions of events. On Sunday, July 21, 1805, he told Crisman that he had procured a boat and was going to the Lazaretto to visit his brother, who was stuck in quarantine on his return from Port-au-Prince, Haiti. (The boat was likely a small craft, perhaps with oars and a small mast and sail.) He told one member of the Board of Health that he had "been through the fleet" at the Lazaretto on that Sunday, but he denied seeing any sick people or boarding any "sickly vessel." (The Lazaretto steward, also present at that interview, recalled Young saying that the outing happened on Sunday, July 14, and that he had later proceeded to land at Thompson's Point in New Jersey, on the shore opposite the Lazaretto on the far side of Little Tinicum Island.)

Young was interrogated by two more board members the following day, at which point he claimed that on the twenty-first, he had gone with Crisman,

Crisman's wife, and more than twenty other guests downriver. They landed at Little Tinicum Island, then at Thompson's Point. One of the board members later swore that Young had "solemnly denied" having boarded any vessels or having come "within the precincts of the Lazaretto"; another board member recalled hearing Young say that the party had landed at the Lazaretto shore. Young's wife, Elizabeth, said the outing with the Crismans and their many guests had happened on the fourteenth, though Peter had told her at the time that he had gone down only as far as Fort Mifflin, some 5 miles upriver from the Lazaretto and Thompson's Point. In her report to a board member, Elizabeth added helpfully that her husband was "fond of company and addicted to idleness, was often on board vessels along the wharves, and had been frequently out late at night."

Crisman acknowledged the large group cruise to Thompson's Point, "for refreshment," on Sunday the fourteenth. When interviewed by the board's Dr. William Currie, he declined to name any of his guests. The following Sunday, the twenty-first, Crisman said, Peter and Tobias went downriver on the pretext of visiting Peter's brother—a story Crisman said he did not believe.

Questioned on at least three separate occasions, Tobias Smith never changed his story. Whether he felt defiant, terrified, or simply baffled by all the fuss, he repeatedly told the Board of Health investigators the same thing: He had gone downriver in a boat on Sunday, July 21, with Peter and Elizabeth Young. "A great way down the river"—Tobias didn't know if it was at the Lazaretto or not, but it was opposite a large white house—the Youngs boarded a vessel and stayed there for nearly an hour, leaving Tobias waiting on the boat. Then the three returned home, arriving around sunset. (The Lazaretto would have been the likeliest place for a vessel to be at anchor downriver. There was no large white house at the Lazaretto, but there may have been one at Thompson's Point on the opposite shore.)

Investigators' accounts of Tobias's testimony diverged on only two points. In Dr. James Reynolds's version, Tobias said that they had actually "been on shore" at the white house—a detail missing from other versions. And Dr. William Currie reported that Tobias "was certain" that the vessel was opposite the Lazaretto. But neither of the two physicians put much stock in the boy's account anyway. According to Reynolds, his testimony was "so confused, either from the effect of disease or natural imbecility of his intellectual faculties, that nothing satisfactory could be ascertained." Currie claimed that after Tobias returned to the Crismans', the boy denied to his master "every syllable" of what he had told the doctor. The doctor seemed to see the creature before him as some kind of feral child whose utter ignorance of manners and morality was exasperating, whether or not his conduct had been criminal. He did not consider the possibility that the boy was afraid he would be punished by Crisman if Crisman learned that he had cooperated with the board's investigation.

Why all the fuss over a mischievous 11-year-old orphan? Why did the Board of Health undertake such an extensive investigation in the first place, and publish its lengthy report in the newspapers six months after the events? The details mattered because less than a week after their possibly illicit expedition, Tobias Smith and Peter Young were bedridden with debilitating headaches and back pain, extreme fatigue, nausea, alternating chills and fever—the classic symptoms of yellow fever. (Elizabeth Young apparently escaped illness.) The Crismans called a doctor, who notified the Board of Health. The board immediately ordered the two patients sent down to the Lazaretto hospital. Four days later, Peter Young was dead. The board knew what the rest of the city did not yet know: a crisis loomed. What happened in the next few days and weeks would determine if the two youngsters remained isolated cases—merely another unfortunate urban anecdote—or if the sadly familiar scenario of mistrust, panic, exodus, hospital overflow, and emergency relief operations would once again play out in Philadelphia.

When the Crismans' doctor reported the two cases on July 30, the Board of Health moved quickly. Drs. Reynolds and Currie were dispatched to Catharine Street to see Tobias and Peter for themselves. What they saw led the board to order the two patients down to the Lazaretto as a precaution. That same day, Reynolds and the board's president, Ebenezer Ferguson, issued a press release on their colleagues' behalf. If they had learned anything from earlier calamities, it was this: whether or not swift action and full disclosure actually helped limit the spread of yellow fever, the *appearance* of swift action and full disclosure was imperative to maintain public trust. The board's press release assured residents that the patients had been isolated—Tobias and Peter at the Lazaretto, and another Crisman apprentice (who showed milder symptoms) at his father's house away from the city. The Crisman family had been evacuated to the country, and their house was to be "immediately and carefully purified." Reynolds and Ferguson punctuated their statement with an earnest promise: "Our fellow citizens it is trusted will regard this communication as a pledge of the ingenuousness which shall in all cases govern the conduct of the Board, and whilst we offer them our congratulations on the perfect exemption which (with this exception) they enjoy from every malignant disease, they may be assured of the earliest information of danger."[10]

The board's credibility rested on vigilance, transparency, and trust, but the spread of yellow fever depended on proximity. And so the same sad, exhausting story began to unfold yet again in the wharfside districts of Philadelphia and Southwark. Chilly fits, sudden headache, fever, delirium, jaundice, black vomit. House by house, block by block. Rumor. Fear. Flight.

The contagionist majority on the Board of Health, led by Dr. Currie, urged the "immediate removal" of all residents in the vicinity of Catharine Street Wharf and called for accommodations to be set up for the sick and their families in the country. They warned those in other parts of the city against "visiting or transacting any business in the infected streets." But most Philadelphians ignored the board's injunctions. By September 20 the fever had spread throughout much of Southwark, along the southern fringe of the city proper, and up Water Street as far as Walnut. Cooler weather in October seemed to dampen its intensity, and it was extinguished entirely by All Saints' Day.[11]

Over the months the epidemic struck about 1,200 Philadelphians, killing more than 300 of them. It was up to the Board of Health, after the fact, to reconstruct the chain of events that sparked the outbreak. Dr. Reynolds, for one, suspected that Tobias and Peter were part of an illicit "contraband commerce" with ships under quarantine at the Lazaretto, which flouted the law and continually threatened the health of the city. One newspaper reported that the two had been smuggling coffee from quarantined vessels, and that the authorities had seized a portion of the coffee.[12] With hundreds dying, rumors flying, and memories of the 1790s still fresh, it was imperative that the board lay out for public consumption a thorough and plausible account of the epidemic's origin. Whether or not anyone was ultimately prosecuted, Philadelphians needed to see their leaders in control.

After several rounds of interrogation of many witnesses to the outbreak's earliest stages, Currie and the board fingered Tobias Smith and Peter Young as the culprits who had brought the yellow fever from the Lazaretto to the city. (The official version had them boarding or having contact with the schooner Nancy, recently arrived from the port of Santo Domingo [today the capital of the Dominican Republic] with several yellow fever casualties aboard.) The board's annual report lamented the public's widespread disregard of its warnings, which it attributed to a growing but mistaken belief that the disease was not contagious. Nevertheless, the board congratulated itself for its aggressive response, which it credited with saving many lives and averting a wholesale calamity.[13]

Benjamin Rush, Charles Caldwell, and other anticontagionists just as confidently identified the source of the outbreak as a large pile of putrefying oysters left on the Catharine Street Wharf for the entire month of July. Neighbors complained of being sickened by the "putrid effluvia," but the Board of Health refused to have them removed. Caldwell insisted that Tobias Smith and Peter Young had never been at the Lazaretto, and that no cases of yellow fever existed there anyway at the time they were supposed to have visited. In his view, residents were more reluctant to leave their homes and more eager to return than in previous years, and he believed that the board's heavy-handed approach was seen as "odious" and "despicable" by the public, which therefore ignored the fervent warnings and pleas.[14]

Poor Tobias Smith was in the wrong place at the wrong time.

Currie said that the boy "did not know what sin meant, or that there was any harm in telling a lie." Maybe. But it is also possible that Tobias saw some advantage in feigning ignorance to Currie or was just terrified by the ordeal of illness and interrogation. Perhaps the boy wanted only to punctuate his monotonous life at Crisman's store with the momentary stimulation of a downriver adventure. He probably did not know anything about the niceties of the Pennsylvania health law or quarantine regulations. But Peter Young's yellow fever was fatal while his was not, and the Board of Health in the fall of 1805 desperately needed a clear narrative of importation and contagion, along with an identifiable guilty party if at all possible. (Beyond the very public accusation in the newspapers and the attendant public opprobrium, there is no evidence that Tobias Smith or Elizabeth Young were prosecuted or punished for their role in the 1805 epidemic.)

Yellow fever retreated from US mid-Atlantic ports after 1805 and all but disappeared after 1820. Most northeastern US seaports, which had tightened their regulations after the flurry of epidemics in the 1790s, still enforced some kind of quarantine, although with variable stringency. The kind of milder outbreaks that spared most Philadelphia neighborhoods were becoming familiar to residents soon after the new Lazaretto opened in 1801. Still, in 1805 memories of the 1790s remained fresh, and two young men who brought fever to the city after successfully slipping through the safety net around the Lazaretto easily revived fears over the potential for mass casualties and chaos, which continued to lurk beneath the surface.

Chapter Eight

"This Inhuman Traffic," 1817

G ermans continued to flock to Philadelphia at a rate of more than 1,000 per year during the early years of the nineteenth century, and Philadelphia's Board of Health continued to struggle with the extraordinary demands of caring for them. During the peak years, fully one-third of German migrants were re-demptioners or other servants arriving mostly destitute, many near death.[1]

In response to the persistently dreadful plight of immigrants who arrived as redemptioners, a group of German immigrants had joined in 1764 to form the German Society of Pennsylvania. With only marginal success, the society fought to help new arrivals and protect immigrants from the worst effects of the entrenched system of redemption and servitude. They helped many indigent newcomers begin their new lives, but they could not stop the profitable fleet of deadly herring boxes.[2]

Thomas Jefferson's Embargo Act of 1807 and the Napoleonic Wars all but turned off the immigration faucet, but pent-up demand for emigration and an agricultural catastrophe that began in 1816 opened it back up. Well over 4,000 Germans came to Philadelphia in the year 1817 alone—more than 40 percent of them redemptioners.[3]

On their ill-fated journey aboard a ship bound from Amsterdam to Philadel-phia in that 1817 wave of migration, hundreds of passengers came close to revolt-ing against the captain and the crew. This ship was called *Hope*, and hope was nearly lost—many times over. Much of the *Hope*'s misfortune can be traced to factors beyond human control, but the decisions made by the vessel's owner, cap-tain, and crew before and during the voyage show just how expendable they con-sidered its cargo to be.

In 1816 Europe suffered what has come to be called "the year without a summer," a very cool year after a massive volcanic eruption in Indonesia spewed ash into the atmosphere over much of the world. Dire food shortages followed, and many Europeans, faced with a choice between starving and emigrating, were forced to leave their homes.

In the early spring of 1817, this is what 26-year-old Rosina Gös and her family did. Rosina and her husband, Matthias, also 26, and their 4-year-old son, George, left their village of Sasbach on the edge of the Black Forest, just across the Rhine from the French city of Strasbourg. It is possible that she did not know it yet, but as she undertook this long and perilous journey, Rosina was pregnant. Along with other emigrants from their region, the Gös family headed down the Rhine toward Amsterdam. The Black Forest group met another group of emigrants along the way, from the Aargau district in northern Switzerland. Among the second group were 34-year-old Jacob Hilfiker, his wife, Maria, and their 18-month-old son, Rudolph. Three hundred and fifty strong, the emigrants set sail for Philadelphia from the island of Texel just north of Amsterdam on May 8, 1817.[4] The wind was favorable, and Captain Geelt Klein of the Dutch ship *Hope* was looking forward to a smooth, quick, and profitable passage.

The good luck lasted just a few minutes. As soon as the *Hope* made it out into the North Sea, the wind disappeared, and for the next eight days, the jam-packed ship floated aimlessly, either absolutely still or fighting a headwind. When the wind finally picked up on May 16, the ship made quick progress into the English Channel. Noticing that the delay had made a severe dent in their food provisions, the passengers asked the captain to land somewhere in England to replenish the supplies. He refused, telling them they had plenty of food for the rest of the journey.

They soon found themselves in the open ocean in strong winds. On June 4, a ship from Morocco sailed near and greeted the *Hope* with a barrage of gunfire, setting out a boat with a boarding party. Captain Klein mustered the crew and as many passengers as possible on deck, arming them with the ship's entire supply of guns and swords. This show of strength deterred the pirates, who promptly made a half moon around the *Hope* before sailing away.

Not long after the *Hope*'s confrontation with the pirates, a violent storm appeared with little warning. Battered mercilessly for two full days and nights, the ship nearly had its masts snapped off, and almost all the sails and ropes were torn down. The costly damage and the delay for emergency repairs was bad enough; even worse was the effect on Captain Klein, who became so terrified of further damage—which would cost him money—that for the rest of the journey, as soon as the wind grew strong, he ordered the sails lowered. He gave up entirely on the topmost and side sails. The ship slowed to a plodding pace.

After seven weeks at sea, the passengers expected to see the North American mainland any day. They were confused when they saw mountains, until word spread that they were looking at the Azores, the Portuguese island chain barely a third of the way across the Atlantic. The migrants' spirits were crushed. They looked at their meager food supplies in despair. Ever since the North Sea delay, Klein had reduced all food and water rations by a third. Realizing that they faced the real prospect of starvation, the passengers pulled together enough energy to turn hopelessness to anger. They demanded that the captain land in the Azores and buy food. "We were close to a revolution," survivor Adrian Märk later recorded in his account of the journey. When a gang of passengers threatened the captain, Klein linked arms with all his crew and faced down the mutineers. There would be no stopping for supplies.

As June turned to July, and the *Hope* crept slowly westward, the immigrants' hunger-weakened bodies were powerless to fight off illness. Ship fever spread throughout the cargo hold, which was serving as the "passenger cabin." A man from the Aargau group had been hired as the ship's doctor, but he had been given almost no medications and was all but powerless in these conditions.

The deaths began with a family from the Black Forest group, whose youngest son, the family's sole survivor, could only watch as his loved ones' bodies were weighted down with shot, sewed into sailcloth shrouds, and dropped overboard to sink into eternity. A few days after the first deaths, a ship from Liverpool sailed near. Hearing of the widespread hunger and illness aboard the *Hope*, the English captain offered food and medicine. Klein refused the offer. The *Hope*'s passengers, so weak they could not stand upright, watched the other ship sail away, its passengers dancing gaily on deck.

It had been eight weeks since Amsterdam. There was no more meat, no more butter, no more cheese or even vinegar or liquor. Captain Klein was now allowing half a daily ration of water every three or four days. The bread was "moldy and inedible," Adrian Märk recalled. The captain had stopped distributing wood for cooking, so the remaining rations of peas, barley, and rice were useless. Adults received only a drinking glass of soup per day. Illness was everywhere, and the pace of death accelerated. Not a day went by without at least one sailcloth casket being dumped into the sea. To make matters worse, it was discovered that thirty of the thirty-two water barrels allocated to the passengers had sprung leaks. Those well enough to do so were reduced to collecting rainwater that had accumulated on deck; it smelled like asphalt and garbage, and no matter how thirsty they were, many could not keep it down.

Märk recalled simply, "Our misery was great."

Four times in the last two weeks of July, the ship got tangled in huge patches of seagrass. Another storm tossed the *Hope* around for four days, forcing the starving Germans to stay belowdecks surrounded by ship fever, and pushing them back eastward as if taunting them. By now all but three of the crew were also sick, and there were not enough able-bodied hands on deck to guide the ship safely through the storm. Finally—the weary passengers thanked God for at last hearing their desperate prayers—the weather calmed, and five days of favorable winds carried the *Hope* swiftly toward the American mainland. One night a light was spied in the distance, and Captain Klein had a big lantern hung at the top of the storm mast. Within the hour a boat arrived carrying the pilot who would guide the ship through Cape Henlopen and Cape May, up the Delaware Bay and River toward Philadelphia.

As he boarded the ship, the pilot blanched with horror: the crew and passengers looked more dead than alive. Sensing the urgency of the situation, he overrode Klein's timidity and ordered all sails hoisted. Only a few passengers were able to stand on deck and take in the scenery. Märk's heart surged with relief and awe at the sight of the New World, with the "dark green oak woods" and "beautiful meadows and plantations" on the banks of the Delaware. The *Hope* sped upriver, making up for lost time, and reached the Lazaretto on August 7. It had been ninety-two days since the departure from Texel. In Märk's words, "the healthiest of us looked like dead."

The unprecedented influx of Germans to Philadelphia in 1817 was well underway when the *Hope* finally arrived. Even before the redemptioners' riot of 1804, Lazaretto officials had found it impossible to accommodate so many people in quarantine at one time. They had the Dutch House now, to house healthy passengers, but nothing could have prepared them for the 1817 season, when Germans came to Philadelphia at more than double the rate of 1804.[5]

The first ship that Lazaretto physician George Lehman and quarantine master Christopher O'Conner inspected on August 7 was the *Johanna & Elizabeth* from Amsterdam, carrying 421 redemptioners and other migrants. Because of the overcrowding Lehman found aboard, he detained the vessel, admitted the sick to the Lazaretto hospital, and sent the remaining passengers to the Dutch House. Next he inspected the *Hope*.[6]

During the official questioning, Captain Klein reported just a few cases of illness aboard. Dr. Lehman had been on the job for all of two months. Just 24 years old, he was barely four years out of the University of Pennsylvania medical school, but his political connections to Democratic governor Simon Snyder had gotten him appointed to the Board of Health in 1816 and to the Lazaretto position the following year. He would go on to serve for nineteen years on Tinicum Island, more than three times longer than any other doctor in the Lazaretto's history. When he finally retired, he had seen it all. But on that August morning in 1817, he did not need years of experience. He had only to open his eyes to dismiss Klein's protestations out of hand. He had never seen anything like the groaning mass of gaunt, pale creatures he found aboard the *Hope*. The ship had left Amsterdam with 346 passengers aboard. Of those, 48 had been buried at sea; and 10 or 12 more arrived showing just the faintest signs of life and did not survive long enough to be admitted into the Lazaretto hospital, which immediately filled up with the most desperate cases. About 120 were so sick that they were unable to eat or drink. "Most of those remaining," Lehman reported, "were so feeble and exhausted that they could with difficulty walk to the house provided for their reception."[7]

What the young doctor saw and felt aboard the *Hope* might have resembled the experience of the young quarantine doctor Lauchlin Grant in the historical novella *Ship Fever* (1996):

> Into the hold: again, again. Already Lauchlin felt as though he knew that place by heart. The darkness, of course; and the rotting food, and the filth sloshing underfoot. The fetid bedding alive with vermin and everywhere the sick. But a last surprise awaited him here. He inched up to a berth in which two people lay mashed side by side. He leaned over to separate them, for comfort, and found that both were dead.
>
> He vomited into a corner, a place already so filthy he couldn't make it worse. Then he scrambled up the ladder and hung breathing heavily over the rail. It was too much, it was impossible. He would go home at once, on the next steamer out, and when Susannah chided him he would tell her that this was not what he had bargained for: this was madness, he could be of no help. All the instruments he'd learned to use, all his theories and knowledge were worth nothing here. These people needed orderlies and gravediggers and maids and cooks, not physicians, not science. They needed food, sleep, baths, housing, priests.[8]

Lehman had a job to do, and it was getting more overwhelming by the minute. He immediately sent word to turn the passengers from the *Johanna & Elizabeth* around and send them back aboard their ship for the time being. It was crowded and dirty, but it was palatial compared to what Lehman saw on the *Hope*. Those passengers from the *Hope* who were least acutely ill were sent to the Dutch House. Amid the chaos and sickness, stepping over corpses and soon-to-be corpses, Lehman could barely stifle his anger. Reflecting on that moment a day or two later, he wrote: "Justice and humanity demanded that the *Hope*, in her wretched situation . . . should be first attended. She is a living sepulcher. The slave trade has been abolished, as contrary to the laws of God; so should this in-human traffic. Three, four, and five hundred poor and ignorant creatures, are stowed in one vessel, conveyed to a far distant country, living on provisions that we would sometimes hesitate to give our beasts." The quality of the *Hope*'s bread became notorious. Coarse and sour even when not moldy, it was roughly ground from the chaff and the hard outer layers of whatever grain it came from, with little actual flour. Lehman said even hogs would not eat it. A newspaper said a piece of it "would cause the blood of every human person to chill." Another ob-server called it "the worst I ever saw."[9] But what chilled Lehman's blood was a system that generated profits from misery through what amounted to the pur-chase and sale of human beings. The ship owner or captain or consignee might be perfectly villainous or perfectly virtuous. It was not the individual but the structure of human trafficking itself that caused such suffering, ship after ship, year after year.

Lehman, O'Conner, and Lazaretto steward James McGlathery had little time for philosophizing. A couple of days after the *Johanna & Elizabeth* and the *Hope*, the ship *Vrow Elizabeth* arrived from Amsterdam, also full of German redemp-tioners (477 total passengers). Then came the *Xenophon*, likewise jammed full of redemptioners: 484 passengers had left Amsterdam, and 49 (mostly children) had died en route. With the approval of the Board of Health, Lehman ordered the *Johanna & Elizabeth* disinfected as quickly as possible and then sent up to the city with all her healthy passengers. But that still left well over 1,000 passengers at the Lazaretto. (The hospital was designed to accommodate up to 48 patients. The Dutch House could probably hold another 100, perhaps 200 in very close quar-ters.) Most were destitute, and many were starving and sick. After an emergency meeting with Lehman, O'Conner, and McGlathery, the Board of Health reported that "a more distressing scene has not been witnessed at the Lazaretto since its establishment."[10]

For two weeks the Lazaretto's employees were in constant motion—there was so much to do. Of course, the board immediately ordered the vessels under quar-antine to be cleaned, whitewashed, and fumigated as extensively as possible, with special procedures prescribed for the *Hope*.[11] But what about all those people?

Meeting their immediate material needs not only was a humane imperative; it could also prevent discontent from boiling over into violence. Steward McGlathery had been a member of the Board of Health in the early years of the Tinicum Lazaretto, and he remembered how much trouble provisioning could cause. So did George Budd, a current member of the board in 1817. He had been the Lazaretto steward in 1804, when the *Rebecca*'s redemptioners had rioted. The board and the quarantine officers were determined not to allow that to happen again.

The high fences surrounding the station were occasionally breached, so it was concerning but not unusual when a passenger from the *Hope* named Swigelar escaped from the Lazaretto with his children during their quarantine. Whenever there was an "elopement," the Board of Health put out word in the city through either informal channels or newspaper notices, sometimes offering a reward, and often the escapee was caught and returned to quarantine. What Swigelar did, however, was unheard of. After making his way to Philadelphia, he left his children there and went *back* to the Lazaretto (likely sneaking in through the same hole in the fence). There he was accused of "using such conversation as tended to excite mutiny and dissatisfaction among the passengers." After the harrowing journey of the *Hope*, it should not have been hard to stir up discontent. As soon as McGlathery got wind of this agitation, he put Swigelar under detention at a nearby tavern, where he could not be a disruptive influence on the quarantined masses. (The board sent out a messenger to find his children and place them under proper care.) The troublemaker was later moved to an isolated room in the Lazaretto that was used as a prison when needed. This confinement changed Swigelar's attitude, and within two days he was released "after making proper concessions for his misconduct."[12]

McGlathery and the Board of Health had their hands full housing, feeding, clothing, and caring for all those Germans. The Dutch House was not big enough to accommodate more than a fraction of them, and even all the tents in Philadelphia might not suffice for the others. A board delegation met with the US customs collector for the Port of Philadelphia, who agreed to allow the board to temporarily house passengers in the huge customs warehouse next to the Lazaretto, normally used for storing and ventilating potentially contaminated cargo. The Health Officer (charged with enforcing the board's policies in the city) hired an emergency assistant physician and two nurses in the city and sent them down to the station right away. All tents in the city hospital's possession were requisitioned and sent down. A committee was appointed to make plans for setting aside a wing of the city hospital for the Germans if necessary. A delegation from the board met with the German Society of Pennsylvania to solicit their help in providing relief for the miserable newcomers.

After McGlathery reported that he could not possibly feed so many starving mouths, the board hired a baker to help him. When he needed more food and supplies, the board told him to purchase them and keep a separate account, to be charged to the Philadelphia consignees of the *Hope*. Lehman reported an urgent shortage of medicines, and the board's secretary procured them and sent them down. More nurses were needed—German-speaking ones—and the board hired them. Extra nurses and provisions continued to be requested, and supplied, through the expiration of the quarantine season in October.[13]

Shortly after the *Hope*'s arrival, the board ordered "twenty rough coffins" to be "sent down forthwith." Five days later, they ordered twenty-five more. A month later, twenty-five more. Forty-eight of the *Hope*'s passengers who were alive (if only barely) on arrival at the Lazaretto died there, bringing the ship's full death toll to ninety-four. Given what we know about the voyage from eyewitness descriptions, it is surprising not that so many died but that 252 passengers somehow *survived* and were restored to a semblance of health at the Lazaretto. Some were hospitalized for as long as two months.[14]

The Gös family from the Black Forest—pregnant Rosina, Matthias, and young George—survived. Baby Maria Anna, whose name would soon be Americanized to Mary Ann, was somehow born safely, either at the Lazaretto or not long after the family's quarantine ended. They became the Gase family of Pennsylvania; a second daughter, Elizabeth, followed four years later. Rosina lived to age 66, and Matthias and the children all survived into their late seventies. Sometime in the 1820s, they moved to Perry County in south central Ohio, then in the 1830s to Seneca County in northwestern Ohio, where many of their descendants live today.[15]

The Hilfikers from Aargau—Jacob, Maria, and little Rudolph—also survived, and settled in Montgomery County north of Philadelphia, where four more children were born over the next ten years. That generation eventually scattered throughout Pennsylvania, Indiana, Illinois, and Nebraska. (Their descendants include the clothing designer Tommy Hilfiger.)[16]

Adrian Märk was detained for four weeks with his wife and three children. After recovering from her serious illness, his wife shared a room with a woman who was despondent after the grueling ordeal she had been through. Her threat to commit suicide so traumatized Märk's wife that she fell ill again, and their nursing baby subsequently died. Märk nevertheless credited the medical care and "very good food" they received at the Lazaretto for saving many lives. The family stayed in Philadelphia only three weeks, then bought a carriage and horses and headed west across the mountains, settling in Pittsburgh, where Märk found work as a hatmaker.[17] Their surviving shipmates, like the survivors of the *Venture Again*, the *Rebecca*, the *Fortune*, and the thousands of other vessels inspected at the Lazaretto, left no record of their experience there before they continued their American journey and started new lives in Philadelphia, on the western frontier, or wherever else the tides of fortune and circumstance took them.

Members of the Board of Health, now back up to twelve in number, set out to recover the exorbitant costs incurred at the Lazaretto because of the *Hope* disaster. As the *Hope*'s consignee, the Philadelphia merchant firm of Glazier & Smith was responsible for costs associated with its passengers' board and medical care while in quarantine. After the firm did not respond to a request to send down clothing for the *Hope* survivors, the Board of Health sent a delegation to investigate.

On August 20, two weeks after the ship's arrival, Glazier & Smith informed the board that after a "disagreement with the captain," the firm no longer considered itself the consignee of the *Hope*. This complicated matters considerably. Another delegation visited the Dutch consul, who insisted that because none of the passengers was a Dutch citizen, he had no stake whatsoever in their welfare, but because the ship was Dutch owned, he would defend the owners' interests vigorously. A three-month legal wrangle ensued in which the board's solicitor reaffirmed the collective responsibility of the *Hope*'s owners, captain, and consignee for quarantine-related costs, and the board tried to apportion those costs to the appropriate parties.

Two board members spoke with Captain Klein at the Lazaretto in early September, as the *Hope* was being prepared to come up to the city. They told him he would be billed not only for the supplies needed to outfit the ship, but also for all supplies furnished to passengers and sailors while at the Lazaretto. Klein acknowledged the former but pretended not to understand the latter. The board finally calculated the total amount due: $2,980.13. It billed Glazier & Smith $404.56 for the expenses incurred while that firm was the consignee of record, and the balance to the "captain or owner." Glazier & Smith paid their bill and promptly began negotiating on behalf of the Dutch owner. A payment plan was eventually arranged whereby the board received full payment, plus interest.[18]

The German Society of Pennsylvania took little comfort in this financial resolution. As bad as the *Hope* disaster was, it was also a symptom of a larger problem that needed to be addressed. As part of their effort to "assist and relieve" the German immigrants, the society sent its member John Keemle to the wharves as an interpreter. He was able to get candid firsthand reports from the new arrivals, just out of quarantine, about how they had been treated, and he was angry enough to challenge the captains of various ships face to face. Keemle bemoaned the cruel treatment that had reduced his fellow Germans to "the lowest state of poverty and wretchedness" and that forced the society to come to their aid lest they "perish in our streets for want, which as a Christian and enlightened people," he said, "we cannot tolerate."[19]

The passengers on the ship *Vrow Elizabeth* complained bitterly of harsh treatment at the hands of Captain Blackman. He withheld bread for days on end. He kept them on salt rations as if they were still at sea, and the salt-preserved meat was too salty and tough to chew or swallow. He regularly demanded more money from the passengers for nonexistent expenses or for services that were included in their fare, like medicine and cooking. When Keemle confronted him, Blackman admitted matter-of-factly, "Yes sir, they are all against me," then waved him off, saying that as a foreign subject, he was answerable only to his own country's laws. Keemle shot back that he was mistaken, and that he would abide by Pennsylvania's laws or be banned from the Port of Philadelphia. Blackman's response was to complain to Keemle that he had been forced to refund $1,000 in unjustified fees. In the captains' eyes, Keemle reported back to his colleagues at the German Society, they were the only law aboard their vessels.[20]

After visiting several other immigrant vessels and interviewing their passengers and captains, Keemle finally saw the *Hope* after it had come up from the Lazaretto. He asked Captain Klein about Dr. Lehman's report that hundreds of "famished and emaciated beings" had been taken from his ship. Klein "blustered out, 'Poh, poh, who cares for the doctor there? I am a subject of a foreign power.'" Keemle bristled ("I grew warm," he confessed to his colleagues). At last, his indignation boiled over. "You are mistaken," he spat out at Klein. "We will let you know that you shall conform to our laws and regulations, and if you do not like them, away with you from our shore! Who the devil sent for you?" Later, Klein demanded a ten-dollar fee "for expenses incurred at the Lazaretto" from each of the redemptioners he had brought. The German Society promptly filed suit and forced him to refund the money.[21]

Keemle's indictment of the captains and their employers was harsh. No doctor on board. Medicine chests barely stocked enough for ten or twelve patients. (One captain told passengers who asked for medicine, "*Geht und kauftein schnaps!*"—"Go buy some liquor!"—which he then sold to them.) Keemle went on: the captains and employers were "lost to every sense of feeling for the sufferings of their fellow creatures"; "If they can only get their money, enjoy themselves, and gratify their infernal passions, it is all they care and look for." As for the immigrants, many told Keemle they had lost everything during the Napoleonic Wars ("Bony's ambitious bloody war") and sought only to improve their lot in "a peaceable and happy country." Instead, they "fell into the hands of avaricious merchants and cruel-tempered captains, who treated them as bad as Bony's soldiers did." Keemle calculated that if ship owners provided adequate food and supplies, and boarded fewer passengers per vessel, they could still make a healthy profit from the immigrant trade. But he concluded that only a new law with tough penalties, strictly enforced, could remedy the evils that he had described.[22]

When the *Hope* finally left Philadelphia to return to Amsterdam in late December 1817, Geelt Klein was at the helm. When the ship next crossed the Atlantic in the spring of 1818 en route to Baltimore, however, it was captained by a man named Hancock. Adrian Märk reported in his account that Klein had been fired and fined one hundred dollars for his misconduct.[23]

By the first week of October 1817, the last of the Amsterdam ships had finished their quarantines, all but twelve of the patients in the Lazaretto hospital had either died or recovered, and operations were winding down for the year. Because of the unprecedented volume of patients and healthy passengers, the quarantine season had been extended to October 15. McGlathery, the 44-year-old steward who had somehow managed to feed, clothe, and supply many hundreds of sick and hungry Germans week after week, and keep order at the overwhelmed station, could finally breathe a sigh of relief that the chaos was over. But his labors had taken their toll, and the exhausted steward was stricken with a sudden fever. By October 7, just over a week before the season was to end, James McGlathery was dead—the last casualty of the ill-fated journey of the ship *Hope*.[24]

The scandalous shipboard conditions and tragic death toll of German redemptioners in the quarantine year 1817 would prompt Pennsylvania's legislature to pass a new law the following year regulating the importation of immigrants, and the US Congress followed suit soon afterward with the Steerage Act of 1819. Both laws aimed to remedy the worst abuses of the redemptioner trade—for example, by strictly limiting the charges captains could levy on immigrants beyond the fare for their passage and by providing a minimum allotment of space and supplies per passenger on immigrant ships.

The Steerage Act improved shipboard conditions only marginally, as traders in emigrants exploited loopholes in the law to continue piling passengers on top of one another in herring boxes that lacked both light and ventilation. Most immigrant vessels were built for cargo, not passengers. Captains of ships carrying American timber or cotton to Britain, rather than make the return trip under ballast, could simply lay down some boards as temporary flooring between the ships' beams and add rows of shelves (described as barely larger than dog kennels) with some straw on top for bedding. A money-losing trip was instantly transformed into a profitable opportunity, as one kind of cargo was exchanged for another.[25]

No, it was not US legislators who managed, finally, to bring the traffic in redemptioners virtually to an end after 1820—it was the Dutch. Spurred to action by the continuous flood of destitute migrants into port cities like Amsterdam and Rotterdam, Dutch authorities began requiring all who wished to enter those cities to prove that they had enough money to pay for their sea passage. Going forward, would-be immigrants were able either to pay for their passage themselves or to borrow their fare from family and friends already in America.

Chapter Nine

Fencing in Yellow Fever, 1820

A fter staying away for fifteen summers, yellow fever finally came back. This time the fervent anticontagionists, including George Lehman, who had begun his service as Lazaretto physician in 1817, and Board of Health president Samuel Jackson, were in charge of quarantine.[1] If the justification for quarantine was contagion, then it would be reasonable to expect the likes of Lehman and Jackson to relax quarantine operations at the Lazaretto and to oppose limitations on commerce and on people's movements in the name of public health. Instead, they maintained quarantine as usual at the Lazaretto, and fenced off entire neighborhoods in the city to limit yellow fever's spread. Clearly, the question of contagion was more complicated than it appeared.

In the summer of 1820, Hodge's Wharf, just below Race Street, was festering in a stew of soap suds, plaster of paris, kitchen refuse, and human waste. A pile of plaster had been left on the wharf several years earlier, and thanks to the wharf's poor drainage, all the garbage disposed of by nearby residents became trapped in the plaster and fermented there. This local filth trap would later fall under suspicion as a contributing factor in the epidemic's origin and spread.

On July 2, when the brig *Susan* arrived at the Lazaretto from Santiago on Cuba's southeast coast, it was carrying that island's two most profitable exports, both harvested by enslaved Africans, and both destined to stimulate the palates and minds of Philadelphians: sugar and coffee. During the twenty-five-day voyage, passenger Christopher Geisse of Philadelphia had sickened and died with symptoms strongly suggestive of yellow fever. Dr. Lehman ordered the ship detained and thoroughly cleaned, and all sailors' clothing and personal effects unloaded, landed, and disinfected. The Board of Health ratified the physician's decision when it received his report the next day. On July 10, eight days after its arrival at the Lazaretto, the *Susan* was permitted up, and the next day it sailed to the Port of Philadelphia, docking at Pratt's Wharf, immediately adjacent to Hodge's Wharf.[2]

About a week later, a chilly fit along with debilitating head and back pain struck James Jackson. Jackson, a young man who lived in a boardinghouse on Water Street near Hodge's Wharf, had recently found work making and repairing sails at Keen and Drais's sail loft. A day or two after Jackson fell ill, the same symptoms came over John Hays, a sailor who lived nearby on Water Street and had been looking for work on the wharves. Port physician Alexander Knight reported Jackson's death to the Board of Health on July 26, adding that there were two women "ill with fever of a suspicious aspect" in the same neighborhood, next to Race Street Wharf.

There had been sporadic yellow fever cases in the city since the last epidemic in 1805, but four suspicious cases at the same time in a two- or three-block radius were cause for alarm. The board named a committee to visit the area and inspect Keen and Drais's sail loft; it also told Dr. Knight to send the two women to the Lazaretto immediately. The familiar machinery of the public response to an epidemic—illness, rumor, investigation, patient isolation, public statements, newspaper polemics—had been set in motion. Board president Samuel Jackson, a physician and professor at the University of Pennsylvania, soon became the public face of the city's response. Jackson was convinced that yellow fever always originated locally, and he consistently denied the possibility of both importation and contagion.[3]

The sailmaker Daniel Drais told the board's committee that his shop had recently taken in sails from both the *Susan* and the schooner *Catharine & Jane*, recently arrived from Port-au-Prince, Haiti. He confirmed that all his hands, including James Jackson, had worked on the sails of the *Catharine & Jane*. The *Susan*'s foresail, he said, had been stored in the cargo hold during the voyage, then aired out when the hold was opened at the Lazaretto, but it had not yet been unfurled at his loft. Drais added the telling detail that James Jackson had slept on the *Susan*'s foresail in the loft. (Later, when Samuel Jackson wrote up his lengthy report on the episode, Daniel Drais changed his story, claiming that James Jackson "never had anything to do with" the *Susan* or its sails. Dr. Jackson personally inspected the foresail in question in Keen and Drais's loft and found it "perfectly sweet and clean.") As a precaution, the board ordered all the *Susan*'s sails sent down to the Lazaretto for disinfection.[4]

Chills, shooting pain behind the eyes, fever, extreme lassitude—the cases mounted, slowly but surely. Eight more definite, and two possible, in the area around Hodge's Wharf in the last week of July. Nine of the first twelve cases were fatal. On the last day of the month, the board took the unprecedented step of forcibly evacuating the vicinity of the wharf and putting up fences around the area to prevent entry. All residents were asked to leave, and access to the areas was prohibited. Fever refugees were accommodated in the west wing of the city hospital and in an unoccupied building near the Schuylkill River. Guards were posted at the fences, and Health Office workers got rid of as much of the "offensive matter" on the wharf as they could manage.[5] Merchants anxious to continue their trade besieged the board with requests to remove goods in storage from their riverside warehouses—initially to no avail.

And suddenly, it stopped. No new cases.[6] The board asked doctors to report any suspicious illnesses, and it investigated the inevitable rumors, but there was nothing. Quick, aggressive action—some might have considered it overreaction—had put a stop to the epidemic before it even got started. Dr. Jackson and his colleagues may have heaved a sigh of relief, but they knew better than to let down their guard. It was, after all, only the beginning of August.

Thirty-year-old Christopher Beatty had arrived on the *Georgia Packet* from Charleston, South Carolina, on July 18, "laboring under fever of a suspicious character," as Lazaretto physician Lehman put it. Dr. Lehman soon rendered the verdict: bilious remitting fever—in common parlance, yellow fever. Lehman updated the board dutifully on Beatty's condition: "considerably worse" on July 21, still "seriously ill" the next day, but "considerably better" on July 24, and "convalescent" the day after that. Two and a half weeks after his arrival and ten days after his illness began to subside, Beatty had had enough of the Lazaretto. He made his getaway under cover of night on August 4, leaving an unpaid bill for board and medical care of $13.75. The board ordered health officer William Mandry to hunt for Beatty in the city and took out an advertisement in the newspapers, offering a twenty-dollar reward for his apprehension. Beatty was described as five feet, eight inches tall, with blue eyes, sandy whiskers, and a "genteel appearance," wearing a dark blue coat, black waistcoat, and white pantaloons. The reward went unclaimed. There is no record of his capture.[7]

On August 9, with the manhunt for Beatty in full swing, Samuel Jackson was asked by two fellow physicians to consult on a worrisome case: that of Jesse Smith, an accountant who worked in an office on the Walnut Street Wharf. Smith had been ill for three days, and Jackson found his symptoms strongly suggestive of malignant fever. The doctor learned that Smith's clerk was also ill but recovering, and that the two men had recently picked up a shipment of sugar from Hodge's Wharf. Jackson may have reasoned (or fervently hoped) that these two men would be the last to take ill from the initial outbreak near Race Street. But then came Mr. Forsyth and Mr. Edwards and Mr. McLeod and the young son of a Mr. King: all were taken sick within a few days of Smith, all resided and worked in the neighborhood of Walnut Street Wharf, and none was known to have visited the vicinity of Hodge's Wharf. Jesse Smith died the day after Dr. Jackson's visit, as did Forsyth, and Edwards the following day. Jackson now faced a possibility that filled him with foreboding—"that there was some mischief lurking about Walnut Street Wharf."[8]

On Sunday, August 13, Dr. Jackson went back to Walnut Street to see a Mrs. Duffy, who complained of a violent headache and severe pain in her back and limbs. Her abdomen was excruciatingly sensitive to the touch, and Jackson found her skin hot, her face flushed, her eyes red and swollen, and her tongue "furred"—that is, crusted with a whitish layer of mucus, food particles, and dead epithelial cells. Mrs. Duffy had "eaten heartily of lobsters" on Saturday evening, then was seized with vomiting and high fever in the night. She may have blamed the lobsters, but Jackson knew better, especially when he learned of Abraham Barker's illness in the same neighborhood. The truth he dreaded was "no longer to be doubted": the malignant yellow fever was back.[9]

The next day Jackson rushed to convene an impromptu summit of the city's leading physicians before the Board of Health. They counted a total of seventeen cases so far in the Walnut Street Wharf neighborhood. The doctors and the board resolved unanimously to evacuate the infected district and prevent access to it with barricades, just as the board had done half a mile north, at Race Street, two weeks earlier. Quick, decisive action and aggressive enforcement: Samuel Jackson was determined not to repeat the hesitancy and prevarication that had bedeviled past Boards of Health. By Tuesday evening the fences were up, and most of the residents had already left.[10]

But the cases did not stop. Reports of new illnesses reached the board in an ominous drumbeat: nine more between Monday morning and Tuesday evening, and then a steady trickle of two or three per day over the next week and a half. Jackson and other members of the board found reassurance only in the fact that as of Saturday, August 26, all the new cases were located in the four blocks immediately south of Walnut Street Wharf, between Water Street and the river.[11]

But that was about to change.

Two weeks after Dr. Jackson had visited Mrs. Duffy, a colleague asked him to visit three of his patients in the Wharton household on Front Street—a full block west of Water Street—between Walnut and Chestnut. Jackson examined the two boys and the family's servant and found in their symptoms "unequivocal" evidence of yellow fever. On Monday, August 28, the boys' sister fell ill. (All three siblings died within three days; the servant recovered.) That same day another case was found in the Drinkwater family next door, and then another in the same house on Tuesday—this one so violent that William Drinkwater became comatose immediately after feeling unwell and died the same evening in convulsions. A young apprentice boy next door to the Drinkwaters on Front Street took sick with a milder case at the same time. His was the seventh case on Front Street in three days. As soon as the Wharton cases were reported, the board had Front Street evacuated and barricaded between Chestnut and Dock Streets.[12]

The parts of the city declared off-limits were expanding in tandem with new cases. On August 29, a young boy fell ill on Duke Street in Northern Liberties, a mile north of the Walnut Street Wharf. Rumors alleged that the boy and his father had been "pilfering the stores" on the fenced-off wharves. There were twelve more cases over the next week, all of which could be traced with some confidence to the vicinity of Walnut and Water Streets. Then, in the space of three days, four new cases appeared in Laetitia Court, off Market Street between Front and Second, and three people fell ill in the area of Second and Shippen Streets in Southwark.

Seven more cases, two previously untouched neighborhoods—the board's sense of control was crumbling. And now the press had gotten wind of the brig *Susan*'s voyage from Cuba with a yellow fever patient aboard, its eight-day quarantine at the Lazaretto, and its subsequent arrival at Pratt's Wharf, near where the first cases in the outbreak appeared. The *Franklin Gazette* demanded a full accounting from the Board of Health, including details of disinfection procedures at the Lazaretto and a list of members who had voted in favor of permitting the *Susan* up after such a short detention.[13]

The heat had been turned up.

For the first time in fifteen years, public alarm was building toward panic, amid whispers that doctors distrusted the Board of Health and were refusing to report the cases in their practice. As the board's president, Dr. Jackson published a reassuring statement in the newspapers. He did not deny the existence of an outbreak, but he denounced the rumors that he called "wholly destitute of foundation" and "a gross perversion of the truth" for spreading "the most groundless apprehensions to the manifest detriment of the community." To prove the board's commitment to full disclosure, Jackson reviewed the current status of each confirmed or suspected case of malignant fever in the city, one by one. "There is a strong probability," he concluded, "that the present week will present a declension of the disease." If it did not, he pledged that the board would warn the public promptly of any worrisome developments.[14]

Not everyone—even within the Board of Health—found Jackson's statement convincing. Three members were moved to file an official dissent for the record, although they refrained from publishing it. The fever was slowly spreading through the city, they warned, and the board was frantically chasing after it, expanding the fenced-off districts and evacuating neighborhoods piecemeal as new cases were reported. "The eastwardly winds that have prevailed," the dissenters claimed, "have extended the course of the disease beyond its former limits, and . . . the citizens in the immediate vicinity are not out of danger." They refused to be party to a dishonest reassurance: "Should the people of the neighborhood remain, and fall the victims of this . . . disease, let it be remembered, there was a voice raised against this delusive address."[15]

In an attempt to put rumors to rest, the board issued a public statement at their September 4 meeting, denying any animosity or mistrust between Philadelphia doctors and members of the board. An honest difference of professional opinion about a few fever cases had been turned by "newspaper clamor and popular rumor" into an incipient public scandal, the statement explained. As if the board did not already have enough to worry about, another troubling item was on the agenda that busy Monday. Philadelphians had been looking forward with great excitement to the launch of the US Navy's newest warship, the 74-gun *North Carolina*. Steamboat entrepreneurs were offering tickets at fifty cents each (twenty-five cents for children) and promising the best viewing locations opposite the Navy Yard in Southwark, where the 200-foot-long behemoth would make its public debut. An artillery salute would greet the ship's entry into the water, followed by a public celebration.[16]

Huge crowds were expected along the nearby wharves—precisely what the Board of Health wanted to avoid amid a burgeoning epidemic. To make matters worse, a partial solar eclipse was expected shortly before the hour of the launch: two o'clock on the afternoon of Thursday, September 7. Curiosity about this rare celestial event would surely swell the crowds. The board begged Commodore Alexander Murray, longtime naval veteran and commandant of the Philadelphia

Navy Yard, to delay the launch until the fever receded and a full-throated celebration could be had. Murray would have none of it. A delay, he said, would
cause "great detriment to the public service," and the launch would go ahead as
scheduled on Thursday afternoon. Still, the board would not give up. It took to the
newspapers yet again on Wednesday to "earnestly recommend" that Philadelphians "refrain from assembling to view the launch."[17] Even when events seemed
to be conspiring against them, Jackson and his colleagues were determined to be
aggressively proactive. No one would be able to say that they had not done everything in their power to block the fever's advance.

On the afternoon of the seventh, the launch went forward as planned, "amid
the cheers of an immense concourse of citizens." The *Franklin Gazette*, which had
criticized the Board of Health continually since the beginning of the outbreak,
groused that the board's warning had kept the crowds smaller than they would
otherwise have been, and insisted that another fifty such launches would be less
harmful to the city's health than the entry of a single vessel from an infected
port—a not so subtle allusion to the brig *Susan*.[18]

Even as the Board of Health focused on detecting new cases and extending the
fenced-off districts, it had not neglected quarantine. Shortly after the first case
was observed near Hodge's Wharf, the board ordered the detention of every vessel on which a death "not from an accidental cause" had occurred during its
voyage—regardless of the nature of the illness. In early August, the board sent a
delegation to the Lazaretto to investigate the thoroughness of its disinfection
procedures. (It came away quite impressed and simply urged quarantine master
Henry Kenyon to keep up the good work and to ignore the complaints of the detained captains.) Another delegation was sent down on September 3 to investigate allegations of unspecified "improper conduct" on Kenyon's part. Again the
board members found nothing amiss, although their trust in the quarantine
master may have been shaken after the visit, as they did ask Kenyon to report
back to them with the details of his disinfection of certain vessels. During the
outbreak, requests from those detained at the Lazaretto to be permitted to post
bond and self-quarantine in the countryside outside Philadelphia—which had
been routinely granted in other years—were denied.[19] In the board's view, the
Lazaretto remained a crucial bulwark in the city's defense, even after an epidemic had broken out.

The outbreak in the city demanded the board's attention every single day.
On the day of the *North Carolina's* launch, Laetitia Court near Market Street was

evacuated and fenced off. The board ordered all houses and cellars in the court thoroughly cleaned and disinfected. Reports of new cases continued to trickle in—two to four per day—from Duke Street in Northern Liberties, from Shippen Street in Southwark, and now from Second Street in the couple of blocks just south of Market. If all these reports were true, the total area involved in the outbreak now encompassed more than forty large city blocks in the economic heart of the city. The board debated a resolution encouraging residents of the affected parts of Second Street to "remove immediately with their families" but, unable to reach an agreement, tabled the measure for the time being.[20]

Guards strictly policed the fenced-off "infected districts." One unlucky guard fell ill with the fever, but he recovered, and the board paid him wages for the duration of his illness.[21] Merchants needing access to their sequestered warehouses flooded the board with petitions pleading economic hardship and requesting permission to remove their goods. At first denying nearly all the requests, the board began to grant some of them as the volume mounted and the outbreak waned, but under strict conditions: only certain goods could be removed from certain locations, no more than two people could be involved, the goods had to be transported by water, and the like. In one of the infected districts, the guards arrested a small boy who admitted he belonged to a group of young thieves who were pilfering from the evacuated homes and stores. A few days later a storekeeper named John Smith was caught in the act of removing goods from his store without the board's permission. Both scofflaws were turned over to magistrates for prosecution.

After September 15, reports of new cases slowed to a trickle, and the board began routinely approving requests from those who wanted access to the infected districts. Still, on the sixteenth, the board was not yet willing to go so far as to grant a petition from the residents of Laetitia Court to have the fences keeping them from their homes removed. Some days now saw just one new case, and more and more days saw none. Strictness remained the watchword at the Lazaretto. To investigate possible local causes of illness, two board members visited the neighborhood of Second Street near Shippen Street, where they found the family of one fever patient airing bedding and laundry from their windows and in their yard. (That practice would have to stop.) On the twenty-first, the board ordered the houses on Laetitia Court recleaned and ventilated in preparation for the fences coming down.[22]

When the firm of Maris & Evans asked permission to remove twelve hogsheads of molasses, nine pipes of wine, and one hundred dry horsehides that month, the board granted their request—excepting the firm's stored hides, which, along with coffee and rags, were considered particularly dangerous. That same day, the board allowed the cargoes of all four vessels arriving at the Lazaretto to be brought up to the city—again excluding the hides.[23]

Friday, September 22, found the Board of Health finally prepared to declare the epidemic over. "The malignant fever having disappeared from the City," its public address began, "the Board cannot refrain from congratulating their fellow Citizens, that all cause of alarm has ceased to exist, and that . . . the danger of a desolating epidemic has been averted." "A measure of prudence" led the board to keep the fences up for the time being, but it promised to remove all barriers to free movement "as soon as it appears compatible with safety." The previous day had seen one new case reported, and the next day saw two more. The board voted 7–3 to remove the fences enclosing the district near Race Street and Hodge's Wharf on September 27, two months after they were put up. That week, a handful of new cases were reported around the city.[24]

Had the board declared victory too soon?

Two weeks after the board's triumphant address, the other fences were still standing, and the guards were still on duty. Residents and merchants of the infected district near Walnut Street Wharf had been kept from their homes for seven and a half weeks. They were tired of waiting, and on October 5 they sent a delegation to plead their case to the board. Always sticklers for protocol, the board refused to meet with the citizens, but it agreed to consider a written communication from them. The delegation complied, asking politely "at what time the board intended to remove the fences" from their neighborhood. Mindful of the drip, drip, drip of new fever cases since their declaration of victory, the board refused to commit to any date for reopening access to the area. Two days later not only were the fences not removed, but they were expanded to enclose a *larger* area. Finally, on October 10, another citizens' committee petitioned to have the fences removed, and the board agreed. New cases still continued to appear sporadically, especially near Duke Street in Northern Liberties, but fewer and fewer people took ill until, by the end of the month, when cold weather set in, the chilly fits, sudden head and back pains, fever, vomiting, and all the misery that came with them were no more.[25]

Board of Health president Samuel Jackson, having already prematurely declared the outbreak over, now boasted half-heartedly that the board's aggressive action had averted a real epidemic. One hundred twenty-five residents of Philadelphia and the adjacent districts had fallen ill with the malignant fever, and eighty-three of them had died.[26] The death toll was much lower than in previous epidemics. No one was in the mood to celebrate, although the members of the Board of Health surely were relieved it was over.

Philadelphians had gone fifteen years without seeing their loved ones or neighbors die amid spasms of black vomit. While everyone shared the sense of relief that far fewer had died than in the bad old days, the sight of fenced-off streets and shuttered warehouses, as well as the familiar feeling of dread in the pit of the stomach, brought back chillingly awful memories.

Chapter Ten

"Detained on Account of Her Hides"

C aptain Thomas Harrison did not take kindly to waiting. When he arrived at the Lazaretto on the morning of July 23, 1821, from Puerto Plata and Monte Cristi in Santo Domingo (today the Dominican Republic), he wanted to be released swiftly so that he could be on his way to the city. Harrison was a man who valued speed; he bragged about outracing other vessels between Philadelphia and Cape Henlopen and Cape May, where the Delaware Bay opens into the Atlantic.[1] In contrast, Lazaretto physician George Lehman was a man who valued caution; he detained Harrison's schooner because he had heard reports of disease in Santo Domingo.

In a letter sent from quarantine, the impatient captain described his arrival and detention to his employer, Philadelphia merchant William Boone. Harrison reported that all aboard the vessel were in good health. Why, then, wouldn't Lehman allow him to go ashore at the Lazaretto?[2] Later that day Harrison wrote Boone again, to update him on the business he had transacted on the voyage. After just a few hours at the Lazaretto, Harrison, clearly irked, begged Boone to intercede with the authorities on his behalf. In his frustration Harrison portrayed the Board of Health as a mysterious and sinister governing body composed of "Black Judges": "If there is any possibility of so doing, I wish you would try the Black Judges and see if they will not let me on shore." "State the case as feelingly as possible," he urged. "Tell them I am just spliced [married] and it is absolutely necessary for my health to go on shore."[3] If Harrison thought he could arrange a conjugal visit during his quarantine, he was sorely mistaken. And if he was that impatient after less than a day at the Lazaretto, he had not seen anything yet. Business and pleasure would both have to wait.

Five days later the board remained deaf to Boone's plea, insisting that the reports from Santo Domingo justified caution even if the captain and his crew remained healthy. Their position struck Harrison as absurd, and he shared his frustration with Boone:

> I am very sorry to hear of your unsuccess and am very sorry to hear that the Board are so stubborn and that such learned men as Doctors pretend to be should suppose that so vast an Island as St. Domingo contained but one climate. You may tell them from me that I can prove that there is as many Different climates in the Island of St. Domingo as there is on the Continent of America . . . and that Puerto Plata is and has been . . . a more healthy place than any part of the City of Philadelphia containing the same number of inhabitants in its most healthy time.

Harrison went on to enumerate for Boone the goods and gold he had lost on the voyage to a pirate attack. He couldn't very well make that money back as long as he was stuck in the limbo of the Lazaretto. On July 30, Captain Harrison reported to Boone that he had found a customer for his limes—if, that is, Boone could get the Board of Health to release them—and that now, a week after arrival, he was "completely out of patience."[4]

Plenty of seamen endured far longer detentions at the Lazaretto without complaint—quarantine was a fact of life, after all, and no one was exempt—but Harrison's letters surely expressed the impotent exasperation of generations of seagoing men doing their time under the yellow flag of quarantine. The fatigue of the journey, the baselessness of the decision, the ignorance of the authorities ("such learned men as Doctors"), the uncertainty about how long it would last, the sheer boredom, and the thought of loved ones, so close and yet so far—it was all too much to bear.

As he fumed through yet another endless day anchored off Tinicum Island just 13 miles from home, Thomas Harrison would not have been amused if someone had pointed out to him the irony of his schooner's name: *Hamlet*.

The prince of uncertainty and delay.

A French doctor had arrived in Philadelphia a few months before the *Hamlet*. Thirty-eight-year-old Nicolas Chervin was on a mission to expose quarantine as damaging to commerce, yes, but also as absurd and ineffective. He would have fiercely championed Captain Harrison's cause.

Chervin was nearing the end of a New World odyssey, having spent the better part of eight years investigating yellow fever in its native habitats, from the Caribbean Basin to the Gulf of Mexico and the seaport cities of the United States.

The evidence he gathered was intended to answer one question, and one question only: Is yellow fever contagious? Chervin had long before answered that question in his own mind: no, yellow fever was *not* contagious, it had *never been* contagious, and it could not under any circumstances *become* contagious. Therefore, any policy based on the idea that yellow fever was or could be contagious was misguided and ought to be done away with. Contagion meant quarantine, quarantine meant contagion, and if there was no contagion, there was no need for quarantine.

But he was battling entrenched notions. Nearly every major seaport in Europe and North America enforced some kind of quarantine in the early decades of the nineteenth century. Chervin was aghast at the pointless waste of it all, and at the medical ignorance ("such learned men as Doctors"?) that spawned it. If he could somehow prove by undeniable empirical facts that yellow fever was not contagious, then surely governments would see the error of their ways.

Chervin surveyed physicians in every US city he visited: Had they observed yellow fever in person? Did they believe it to be contagious? Working his way northward through New Orleans, Charleston, Norfolk, Washington, Baltimore, and Wilmington, he compiled lists of local doctors and sent each one a letter explaining his request. He asked them to write their responses on paper of uniform size with extra-wide margins so that all the doctors' responses could be bound together. He even asked them to provide duplicates so that he could ship a full set of responses back to France separately from his personal affairs, in case one set fell victim to the hazards of sea travel. City by city, the replies piled up.

His years of chasing the horrid disease throughout the Western Hemisphere had thrown Chervin into the midst of several epidemics, but his journey finally brought him to the most crucial of his New World destinations: Philadelphia. Yellow fever had visited the birthplace of American medicine more frequently and more devastatingly than any other city. The fate of the contagion doctrine and of the quarantine system that depended on it would be sealed here. He arrived in April 1821 and lost no time sending out his inquiries across the city.[5] If Philadelphia's long-divided medical community could somehow speak with a single voice on the contagion question, Chervin's holy grail might be within reach.

The timing of Chervin's arrival was propitious. Had he arrived in Philadelphia a year earlier, the city's physicians would have had to cast their minds way back—fifteen years ago—to their previous firsthand experience of yellow fever. But the summer of 1820 had given them a reminder, so the scourge was fresh in their minds when Chervin surveyed them.

Throughout May and early June, Philadelphia's physicians responded to Chervin's letter. Former Lazaretto physician Thomas Mitchell: "It is not contagious." Current Lazaretto physician George Lehman: not contagious. Board of Health president Samuel Jackson: not contagious. Philip Syng Physick, John Redman Coxe, Nathaniel Chapman—all professors at the University of Pennsylvania and the leading lights of Philadelphia medicine: no, no, no. Even the old warrior William Currie hedged his bets, emerging from his semiretirement to make his voice heard: yellow fever, he wrote Chervin, "is only contagious . . . in situations where the air is confined and rendered impure by exhalations from . . . putrifiable substances." Only one Philadelphia doctor declared without qualification that yellow fever was contagious: Samuel Powel Griffitts, a College of Physicians member and veteran of the 1793 battles. Four others equivocated, joining Currie in suggesting that the disease could become contagious under certain circumstances. The fifty-one other respondents rejected contagion outright. Many denounced quarantine in their replies. A "farce of inconsistency," said one. "Utterly useless and unnecessary" and a cause of "great inconvenience and ill will," said another.[6]

Chervin's survey found only seven physicians in the entire country who considered yellow fever contagious. Ten more believed that it was contagious under certain circumstances. One hundred ninety-two said it was not contagious.[7] Benjamin Rush, dead nine years, would have felt vindicated.

But quarantine, which those same doctors said was based on contagion, was alive and well. The evidence didn't add up. David Hosack, the New York–based leader of the few remaining contagionists, recommended evacuating patients' homes and preventing residents from entering the neighborhood when yellow fever was suspected. That is precisely what the strongly anticontagionist Board of Health had done during Philadelphia's 1820 outbreak, while also keeping a close eye on quarantine operations at the Lazaretto. How could the Board of Health have fenced off the infected districts, and how could quarantine have survived, when medical opinion so overwhelmingly rejected contagion? The answer lies belowdecks, in the dark, dank recesses of the arriving ships' cargo holds.

While in Philadelphia in 1821, Dr. Chervin almost certainly visited the Merchants' Coffee House at the old City Tavern on Second Street below Chestnut. Here in the bustling heart of the city, he would be well situated to collect information about business transactions and other goings on. He would drink his coffee—which was imported, likely from the West Indies—and plot the end of quarantine with his yellow fever contagion survey, all while failing to recognize that his mission would ultimately prove irrelevant because of what was taking place all around him: commercial goods of all kinds were bought and sold here via auction and other means. Around the corner on Chestnut Street, curriers Robert and Thomas Barnes were just the closest of dozens of firms in the leather-goods trade, which demanded a regular flow of animal hides into the Port of Philadelphia. Across the street, Hurley's Paper-Hanging Warehouse competed with a throng of businesses who depended on the importation of rags for paper manufacturing.

Instead of corresponding with prominent physicians about the contagiousness of yellow fever, if Chervin had visited the Lazaretto on Tinicum Island and observed its daily operations, he would soon have realized that his crusade was aimed at the wrong target. While ships like the *Hamlet* were detained because of reports of disease in foreign lands, and other ships because they arrived with sick passengers and crew, what sustained the practice of quarantine for most of the nineteenth century was not belief in contagion. It was belief in the danger posed by potentially infected *cargo*. Three kinds of cargo in particular could always be counted on to sound the alarm at the Lazaretto: coffee, hides, and rags.[8]

At Tinicum, Dr. Chervin might have learned about the brig *Fortitude*, which had arrived at the Lazaretto from Santiago, Cuba, during the yellow fever epidemic of 1820. It carried sugar, tobacco, tortoise shell, and candied fruit and nuts, all of which were allowed up to the city within a few days of arrival. The vessel itself and its eighty-one bags of raw coffee beans, however, were detained for two weeks, taking its place in a long parade of ships quarantined primarily for what lay in their cargo holds.[9]

Chervin had good reason for opposing quarantine, and many shared his feelings about it. A decision to impose quarantine affected lives and fortunes; it caused inconvenience and boredom on one end of the scale and severe financial loss on the other. But did it prevent illness and death? Making a detention decision required wisdom, experience, and scrupulous attention to various permutations of danger or safety. Maybe the vessel and cargo were sound, but a passenger was sick—might the illness be harmless? Or perhaps the passengers and crew were healthy and the vessel sound, but with rotting cargo; or filthy vessel and cargo, healthy passengers and crew. Or everyone and everything healthy and sound, but reports of widespread illness at the port of departure.

Often the decision rendered was that the cargo had to be unloaded so both it and the vessel could be ventilated and disinfected—"cleansed and purified," in the formulaic language of the Lazaretto physician and the Board of Health. The vessel, cargo, and passengers could be detained for periods ranging from a day to two weeks, but in some cases quarantine lasted a month or more, or until the end of quarantine season. After receiving the Lazaretto physician's report, the board might declare that cargo could be sent on to the city while the vessel and passengers were detained, or that passengers could proceed to the city in lighters or by road while the cargo and vessel were detained. Or a number of other combinations. Not surprisingly, merchants and others continually implored the board to release cargo, to permit vessels to return to sea without approaching the city, and to release passengers or allow communication with them.

Amid this thicket of potential health hazards and heavily freighted decisions, through contentious epidemic years and calm years with relatively little illness, cargo was the most discussed and most anxiety-inducing topic in the Lazaretto physician's reports and the board's deliberations.[10] And while rags frequently drew the attention of city health authorities, public enemies numbers one and two among goods shipped to Philadelphia in the first half of the nineteenth century were coffee and hides. The preoccupation with these common articles of trade helps explain why anticontagionists enforced the quarantine laws: contagion was not the only, or even the primary, justification for quarantine in the nineteenth century.

Coffee and hides. What two commodities could be more different? The aroma of roasted coffee is as rich and alluring as the stench of decomposing animal flesh is repulsive. The nineteenth-century tannery was nasty and rough, the coffee house urbane and cultivated. Yet quarantine officials spoke of the two items in similar terms and often treated them alike. Their common link lay in the one thing raw coffee beans and incompletely treated animal hides were both liable to do: rot.

In 1793 Benjamin Rush and others had indicted coffee in that year's epidemic. Rush located the epidemic's origins in a shipment of "damaged" coffee that had been dumped on the Arch Street Wharf, and "had putrefied there to the great annoyance of the whole neighborhood." Other eminent medical men blamed the outbreak on the arrival of a ship bearing refugees from the revolution in the French colony of Saint Domingue (now Haiti), but Rush insisted on a local origin. The first apparent cases of what Rush called "the bilious remitting yellow fever" occurred in the vicinity of the Arch Street Wharf, in persons who "had been exposed to the exhalations of the coffee for several days."[11] One of the earliest victims, Mrs. Bradford, had spent an afternoon in a house directly opposite the wharf and had been "much incommoded" by the "noxious effluvia" a few days before her illness began. Mrs. Bradford's sister fell sick after visiting her and subsequently "perfectly recollected perceiving a peculiar smell unlike to any thing she had been accustomed to in a sick room." Other victims also reported being sickened by the smell of the rotting coffee. Rush's investigation of the neighborhood's sanitary condition immediately before people fell ill revealed an additional curious detail: exposed on the wharves near Arch Street along with the "extremely offensive" coffee were "some putrid hides."[12] As early as 1793, then, coffee and hides were perceived at least by one prominent observer as uniquely disgusting or uniquely pathogenic, or both.

During the yellow fever epidemic of 1798, two Philadelphians complained to the Board of Health about coffee unloaded from the brig *Mary*, recently arrived from the port of Jérémie in Saint Domingue. Stored in a dockside warehouse, the coffee "appear[ed] to be in a very putrid state, and extremely offensive." An adjacent store contained "a quantity of hides in a putrid and offensive state"; its occupant had very recently died of a fever "which has excited great alarm in that neighborhood," and his daughter was said to be ill with similar symptoms. The board immediately ordered the disinfection of the premises, the return of the coffee and hides to the *Mary*, and the return of the vessel to the quarantine station.[13]

The focus on coffee and hides continued into the new era of quarantine vigilance when the Lazaretto opened on Tinicum Island in 1801. "Landed," "cleansed and purified," "permitted up"—the words and phrases almost take on the quality of a ritual incantation, so often do they recur in the Lazaretto physician's reports and in the board's deliberations. Routine practice for vessels arriving with coffee or hides required those goods to be "landed," or taken from the vessel to the US Customs warehouse adjacent to the Lazaretto; and the vessel to be "cleansed and purified"—that is, washed down, thoroughly ventilated, disinfected with whitewash or fumigation, and its bilgewater flushed. Only then was the vessel "permitted up," or allowed to proceed to the city.

"Detained on account of her hides," read the laconic newspaper report after the ship *Louisa* arrived at the Lazaretto in 1801 from Rio de la Plata in South America.[14] This explanation became as close to a blanket quarantine policy as Philadelphia had. The board periodically codified its anathema against hides, as it did in 1803, when it declared that all hides arriving from outside the United States were to be landed at the Lazaretto, and "the damaged separated from the sound"; after being thoroughly ventilated, undamaged hides could be allowed into the city only if they were immediately put into tan vats and not stored; otherwise they were to be "transported into the country."[15] By 1804 it was standard practice to land all hides and coffee at the Lazaretto until they were deemed safe, but the lowest grade of coffee—the "bad broken berries" called "triage"—was too dangerous even for this tough standard, "it being the determination of the Board not to suffer on any occasion the introduction of that article" into the city. Over the ensuing decades, the board repeatedly reiterated its refusal to allow vessels up with coffee or hides until those goods were "carefully inspected."[16]

Such restrictions did nothing to diminish demand for coffee and animal hides in Philadelphia, and the board had to refine its general policy to accommodate commercial demand without sacrificing safety. As tanneries proliferated on the outskirts of the original city limits (Vine Street to the north, Cedar or South Street to the south), and as Philadelphia's population expanded into those adjoining districts, the board allowed hides to be landed only north of Cohockshink Creek in Kensington or south of the North Yards in Southwark.

In a time of epidemic, hides already inside the city became freighted with danger. In 1820, when the Board of Health fenced off "infected districts" near Race Street Wharf and near Walnut Street Wharf, it refused to allow merchants in the area to remove hides from storage or vessels carrying hides to bring them up to the city. Only when the outbreak began petering out did the board begin to grant some of these requests.

Why such alarm over hides and coffee? One is an animal skin, the other the seed of a plant. They were among the most commonly imported items from the Caribbean Basin—the yellow fever zone—but that alone cannot explain the quarantine authorities' fixation. Sugar, molasses, and other goods from the West Indies were routinely permitted up without a second glance. The key to understanding the anxiety about cargo, and by extension the practice of quarantine in the nineteenth century, is to recognize the specific traits of the goods in question, and to *infer knowledge from practice*. The Lazaretto physician, the quarantine master, and the members of the Board of Health described the coffee and hides and the specific measures they took to neutralize the threat in words that reveal the nature of the perceived danger.

Damaged. Sound. Sweet. These words, most often used a century ago to denote dangerous or safe cargo, ring strange in that context today. Their nineteenth-century usage (per the *Oxford English Dictionary*) points to wetness, decay, and foul odor as the foundational elements of the quarantine concern. The word *damaged* was used, among other things, to denote "merchandise that has deteriorated in quality through . . . exposure to the elements." *Sound* meant, among other things, "free from . . . decay," while *sweet* indicated something that was "free from offensive or disagreeable taste or smell" or "not corrupt, putrid, sour, or stale." Hence, a Mr. Lynch's request to bring up a cargo of hides from the Lazaretto in 1803 was granted "in consideration of the sound and sweet state" of the hides. Presumably, having been thoroughly ventilated, they were dry and smelled, if not pleasant, inoffensive. Similarly, in 1804, the brig *Eliza* and the schooner *Betsy* were permitted up "after having their bilge water pumped out and being otherwise sweetened."[17]

Often the wetness or dryness of coffee and hides determined their fate. The board ordered the schooner *Olive Branch* unloaded and "thoroughly purified" in 1803 because it had sunk with coffee on board at Cape François (today Cap-Haïtien, Haiti). Wet coffee and hides aboard other vessels were ordered stored and dried—sometimes for months—before being released to their owners.[18] *Damaged* seems often to have meant *wet*; *sound* meant *dry*.

Wetness, of course, led to rot. The battle against rot is the essence of tanning, the process by which animal skins are turned into leather. Tanning requires fresh hides and tannin, a substance extracted from specific barks, woods, and nuts. American demand for hides in the nineteenth century far exceeded the supply of domestic animals, and most hides were imported untreated—or, at most, salted—from the Caribbean Basin and South America. Moisture and warmth promoted putrefaction, as with any organic matter, and sailing ships plying the Caribbean trade in the nineteenth century were nothing if not wet and warm. "Stagnant air, dampness, darkness, and warmth are frequently the inseparable conditions of the holds of vessels in warm climates," wrote one American physician, who warned that in these conditions, hides and other cargo "peculiarly liable to infection" could spread yellow fever.[19]

Coffee too suffered from putrefaction and was highly susceptible to shipboard decay. Furthermore, it was more commonly imported to Philadelphia from abroad than most other agricultural products—and it grew only in the tropics. Any moisture could begin the process of decaying the beans, which were shipped raw. Importers dreaded receiving coffee "damaged on the voyage of importation by dampness," for such coffee became musty, "its delicate flavor . . . much injured." A portion of nearly every shipment suffered such damage, and even after drying and polishing, it fetched a lower market price than "sound coffee."[20] The *contagion* polemic in medical circles—could diseases like yellow fever be transmitted from person to person?—has obscured the tacit consensus about *infection*, which undergirded most public health activity before the bacteriological revolution. Even the anticontagionists made a distinction between *contagion* and *infection*. That coffee merchants and health authorities used the same adjectives, *damaged* and *sound*, in these contexts hints at the thinking behind their anxiety: susceptible cargo articles + dampness + warmth = decay → infection.

Nineteenth-century coffee connoisseurs linked coffee, hides, and the conditions in the holds of sailing vessels in another respect as well: "Vessels from Central and South America often arrive with mixed cargoes of coffee and hides, in which the former has been almost ruined by absorbing the smell of the latter," one wrote. "The same effect is produced by the foul bilge-water of vessels."[21] A cycle of mutual pollution and decay repeatedly played out in a dangerously closed environment, where dampness damaged hides, hides damaged coffee, bilgewater damaged coffee, hides fouled the air, and foul air damaged hides.

From the viewpoint of the Lazaretto physician or the Board of Health, a nexus of wetness, heat, coffee, hides, and foul bilgewater threatened much more than the "delicate flavor" of concern to coffee importers. The board was charged with protecting the soundness of human bodies, and in hot and damp conditions, human bodies were just as susceptible to damage as were coffee and hides. Coffee and hides and humans simmered and stewed in and above the ship's hold—that cauldron of potential disease.

But *rags*?

Rags neither originated in the zone where yellow fever was prevalent nor bore the taint of animal origin. But rags, coffee, and hides were all permeable, or porous. Cotton, wool, and linen, also all permeable, often appeared on the official lists of cargo that authorities in various ports considered "susceptible of infection" and therefore were subject to special inspection or detention.[22] A permeable article might absorb not only odors but also infection, and might retain and convey infection across long distances.

The third most frequently detained article at the Lazaretto also represented the threat of indirect contact with the bodies of strangers, foreigners, and perhaps sick or even dead people. Scraps of used and discarded cloth of various sorts and from various sources were collected and bundled into bales, then shipped and sold to paper mills, where they were soaked until they began to break down, pounded to a pulp, and molded into thin sheets before being dried. Mill owners, consumers, local health officials—no one had any way of knowing the origin or means of collection of any given shipment of rags. Leghorn (Livorno) in Tuscany, for example, was an international center of the trade in rags, a Mediterranean commercial crossroads for centuries. Leghorn rags might once have covered the tables of those dining in Italian palaces, or they might have blanketed sickly bedridden peasants as far away as Constantinople or Cairo.[23]

Moreover, people who collected rags for sale stood on the lowest rung of the social ladder. Filthy scavengers of society's soiled debris, ragpickers were despised and feared by the respectable classes in many countries. The very nature of their work also linked them in the public mind with the transmission of disease.[24] The fear of indirect bodily contact with strangers, combined with the debased figure of the ragpicker, turned rags into a quintessentially contaminated and contaminating cargo.

Like coffee and hides, rags became especially dangerous when wet or "damaged." Even rags shipped in good condition could get wet in the hold of a sailing vessel in the open sea. Shipments showing signs of mold or found to be "saturated with water" were deemed "damaged" and were subjected to more careful inspection or even sent back to the Lazaretto if they had initially escaped detection.[25]

Shipments of rags were detained in quarantine as early as the first years of the new Lazaretto in Tinicum. Joshua and Thomas Gilpin, who in 1787 established the first paper mill in the United States on the Brandywine River near Wilmington, Delaware, waited more than two weeks after the brig *Boston's* rags were ordered landed in 1804 before the Philadelphia Board of Health voted to allow them to take possession. Even then, the Gilpins took the rags only on the condition that they be transported directly to the mill and not enter Philadelphia or "any populous town of the United States."[26]

Cargo was not usually excluded for the reason that it might have been handled by filthy or sick people. While the quarantine authorities *were* concerned about vessels arriving with sick passengers or crew members, and while they paid close attention to news of disease outbreaks in Philadelphia's trading ports, they feared rags, coffee, hides, and other cargo regardless of the health of those aboard, and even when disease had not been reported at the port of departure. In many cases, as with the brig *Expectation* from the Venezuelan port of Laguaira in 1809, the Board of Health allowed the crew to come up to the city "when they desire[d]," even as their coffee and hides were landed and their vessel disinfected at the Lazaretto. On the delicate quarantine question, contagion per se—the direct transmission of disease from person to person—was not the main issue; the possibility of *importing disease in filthy cargo holds* was.[27]

After William Currie withdrew from public life around 1815, the only respected medical practitioner who promoted explicitly contagionist views was David

Hosack of New York, "the American champion of contagion."[28] But even Hosack took care to distinguish between diseases like smallpox, invariably transmitted by direct contact, and diseases like yellow fever and typhus, which he believed could only become contagious when the air was fouled by environmental conditions or local contaminants. Hosack gradually fell silent after 1820, the last holdout among the contagionists.[29]

Even the most outspoken critics of quarantine advocated the careful screening of arriving goods. Of course, quarantine had been Board of Health member Charles Caldwell's perennial bête noire. He had urged that it be "entirely abolished," a sentiment that was widely shared if not always expressed so fervently.[30] Caldwell based his critique on a denial of contagion, which he presumed to be the only justification for quarantine and which he believed to have been thoroughly discredited (again, except—as everyone acknowledged—in the cases of smallpox and syphilis). Epidemics, he insisted, originated in air fouled by filth, under certain meteorological conditions.[31]

But even Caldwell did not propose to allow ships unimpeded access to American ports, stating that "in warm weather, especially, no vessel should be permitted to enter, whose foul condition or damaged cargo may aid in vitiating the atmosphere of the place, until the whole shall have undergone a thorough cleansing."[32] In other words, this diehard anticontagionist and leading quarantine abolitionist advocated a system not very different from quarantine as practiced at the Lazaretto. Other opponents of quarantine made similar recommendations: treat sick people, let healthy people go, and disinfect damaged or suspect cargo.[33]

The word *infection* derives from the Latin *inficere*, meaning "to put in [a dye bath, for example]," "to stain," or "to taint."[34] Quarantine-related usage shows traces of this ancestry, as the phrase "retaining infection" suggests. Once absorbed into permeable goods or the enclosed air of a cargo hold, a contaminating influence could be harmful for days, weeks, or months. Infection could be a process or a quality; in either case, the mechanism at work was as invisible and ineffable as it was deadly. All agreed that it arose or was generated in certain local conditions. Most authorities believed that it could also be transported outside of its zone of origin, especially in hot, damp, enclosed spaces. Hence the concern about vessels and cargo, and hence the unwillingness even of many committed anticontagionists to abandon quarantine. In fact, the actions of local health officials suggest that when push came to shove, getting rid of infection mattered more than determining exactly what it was or where it came from.

Because the experts rarely defined *infection* with any degree of specificity, the surest way to discern what they meant by it is to examine what they did to counteract or neutralize it. We are left to infer knowledge from practice. Disinfection—the undoing of infection—also has a history that long predates bacteriology. Epidemics called for fires in the streets, protective perfumes, and sulfur as a fumigant since the time of Hippocrates.[35] At Philadelphia's Lazaretto, "cleansing and purifying" vessels or cargo meant a combination of the following: ventilation, fumigation, whitewashing, spraying with a lime or carbolic acid solution, heating in a steam chamber, and bilge flushing with fresh water. By the 1890s, each of these practices could be justified on bacteriological grounds. But for most of the nineteenth century, they were used not to kill specific microorganisms but rather to fight an indefinable enemy that was known only by its effects. Foul odors and other signs of decay often signaled its presence, but the absence of signs of decay was no guarantee of safety. Diffuse and invisible but deadly, *infection* in the prebacteriological era can ultimately be defined only as a potentially disease-causing quality that could be neutralized or removed by cleansing and purifying.

Nicolas Chervin visited New York after leaving Philadelphia in the spring of 1821, as he was putting the finishing touches on his study proving definitively that yellow fever was not contagious—and therefore, by implication, that quarantine was a misbegotten policy. In September, just three months after Chervin left New York to visit the port cities of New England, a handful of yellow fever cases appeared in New York's seaport neighborhood. The city's mayor, Stephen Allen, confidently blamed the outbreak on "a large quantity of merchandise, brought immediately from the holds of infected vessels, and landed in the vicinity of Rector Street."[36]

All major US seaports except New Orleans (which became yellow fever's preferred US destination after 1820) enforced quarantine regulations to varying degrees. Even ports like Boston, where yellow fever rarely ventured and which became known for its lenient, commerce-friendly quarantine enforcement, excluded "damaged" cargo from the city. Some ports singled out specific categories of merchandise, such as hides or rags, for special scrutiny, while others merely prohibited "offensive" articles or goods deemed "liable to infection." New York surpassed Philadelphia as the nation's busiest seaport in the early nineteenth century, and like Philadelphia, it became the target of vehement complaints about its rigorous enforcement of quarantine, especially where cargo was concerned. Coffee, cotton, rags, and hides nearly always earned special attention at New York's quarantine ground.[37]

The situation was much the same in Europe and the Mediterranean Basin: quarantine was deeply unpopular with many segments of the population and highly controversial politically; the mainstream of the medical profession in most countries rejected contagion; and yet most health authorities nevertheless continued to advocate inspection and disinfection of cargo. Physicians and bureaucrats debated whether certain categories of merchandise were more "susceptible to infection" than others, but most ports seem to have paid close attention to cargo, and to have regularly subjected certain commercial commodities (including hides and rags) to detention and disinfection.[38]

Both critics and defenders of quarantine located the origins of disease outbreaks in damp, dark, crowded, filthy, and unventilated places. Those who believed in strictly local generation saw such conditions in densely populated urban neighborhoods, while importationists found them in shipboard cargo holds, but there was an underlying common denominator: a pathogenic quality that originated or thrived in certain places under certain conditions.[39]

The impatient Captain Harrison of the schooner *Hamlet* had no time for arcane medical debates. In his mind, the matter was simple: the region he had sailed from was healthy, and his sailors were healthy, so there was no reason whatsoever to detain them and their cargo. But the Board of Health had a far more complex calculus to perform. The carnage of the 1790s continued to weigh on their minds, and just as importantly, on "the public mind." The better health of recent decades eased fears but also lowered the threshold of public tolerance for any yellow fever whatsoever. Outbreaks like that of 1820 ratcheted vigilance back up to levels that brought nothing but frustration to merchants and sailors like Thomas Harrison.

Chapter Eleven

"Brought to Our Shores by the Cupidity of Others," 1847

T hree decades after the hopelessness of the *Hope*, the great Irish famine drove another human tsunami westward across the Atlantic toward the Delaware River. Earlier waves of sick and hungry immigrants had stretched the Lazaretto's capacity and resources beyond their limits. The station's staff and Board of Health members were all tested as they struggled to fulfill their responsibilities. One crisis after another prepared those who surmounted them to confront the next one, but no preparation could make up for staffing and supplies that were inadequate to meet the basic needs of so many desperate immigrants all at once.

Old hands—anyone who had been around the station since the days of the redemptioners' riot—might have had reason to think that the Irish famine exodus would finally cause the Lazaretto to collapse under this new burden. They would have been wrong.

Instead, when the waves broke on its shore, the station somehow managed to keep functioning instead of falling apart in chaos. In 1804, Johan Christen, who had arrived aboard the redemptioners' vessel *Rebecca*, believed he got sick from sleeping in a tent at the Lazaretto during a rainstorm. He was so eager to leave that he escaped through the Lazaretto's fence, but even he was grateful for the care he received: "No better attention could have been bestowed on me anywhere." Adrian Märk of the *Hope* praised the "very good food" and "useful help" that "sustained" him and his fellow survivors at the Lazaretto.[1]

If there is one surprise in the litany of nineteenth-century immigration, it is the role of the Lazaretto. What many a beleaguered immigrant found there was not a barrier to entry, but a temporary safe haven.

All through the century, poor German, Irish, and other emigrants continued to seek better fortunes in the New World, while ship owners continued to profit from their poverty by overfilling their vessels and undersupplying the passengers. The appearance of cholera in 1831 and 1832 dominated headlines on both sides of the Atlantic, spreading in its wake a fear that could itself be deadly. The Irish were singled out as a focus for virulent and deep-seated nativist hatred, which periodically erupted into violence—with or without the threat of cholera to fuel it. But still they kept coming, and ship fever continued its ravages wherever malnourished people were crowded in filthy conditions.

Thirty-two-year-old James Coulter of County Fermanagh was one of the lucky ones. He got out of Ireland alive, along with his children (14-year-old Mary and 5-year-old Alexander), his 19-year-old brother, Andrew, and his 60-year-old mother, Isabella. They left in January or February of the worst year of the Great Irish Famine—the year that would later be remembered as Black '47. Two consecutive potato crop failures had set in motion a snowballing cycle of destitution, eviction, and unemployment throughout Ireland. Hunger and disease spread through the country as a punitive and overwhelmed system for providing public relief failed to do so.

The Coulter family, like so many others, were being pushed *and* pulled. Fleeing conditions in Ireland and hoping for a better life in the United States, they made their way in any manner they could. The Coulters traveled across the Irish Sea to Liverpool, where they boarded the *Swatara*, bound for Philadelphia. James's wife is nowhere to be found on the list of passengers arriving in Philadelphia. The most likely explanation is that she died either in the famine itself—a trauma that might have precipitated the family's decision to emigrate—or on the long, sad voyage to America.[2]

The *Swatara*, named after a tributary of the Susquehanna River in central Pennsylvania, was owned by the prominent Philadelphia merchant and former sea captain, Stephen Baldwin, who had commanded one of the packet ships that plied the Liverpool to Philadelphia route throughout the 1820s. Baldwin owned at least four ships, including one named after himself, and served as a director of the Philadelphia Merchants' Exchange. He was said to have been "widely known for his numerous and extensive charities, for his honorable dealings and probity of character."[3]

Bad weather during a transatlantic voyage, although unpredictable in its timing, is entirely foreseeable. But like so many other savvy, prosperous, and putatively charitable ship owners engaged in the immigrant trade, Baldwin seems neither to have planned for adverse conditions nor to have considered it his responsibility to see to his passengers' needs. The *Swatara* famine refugees paid the price. In addition to a cargo of unspecified merchandise, the *Swatara* carried 296 refugees when the ship left Liverpool in early March 1847, most of them from the northwestern Irish counties of Galway, Mayo, and Roscommon. But before the *Swatara* could even make it out into the open ocean, a violent storm damaged the ship and forced it to take refuge in the port of Belfast, on March 17. Repairs took four weeks. Meanwhile, the pounding headache, pain in the extremities, high fever, and extreme weakness of ship fever had already made their appearance among the hunger-weakened immigrants in the overcrowded steerage.

Belfast residents' alarm grew alongside rumors of a shipboard epidemic, and the city's doctors moved to investigate. In the first week of April, thirty-five patients from the *Swatara* were admitted into the city's general hospital. It quickly became apparent that the hospital could not afford to care for them within its existing budget, but the local Board of Guardians of the Poor—authorized to support only workhouse inmates—offered no help. Local doctors inspecting the *Swatara* found the entire ship "exceedingly ill-ventilated" and the passenger quarters so dark that they had to borrow a lantern to see anything. Privies on the immigrant vessels were makeshift, rudimentary, and often neglected. Huddled amid a stagnant stew of urine, feces, and vomit, the immigrants had been subsisting exclusively on the government allowance of a pound of bread a day. The doctors recommended that passengers be removed immediately from the unsanitary steerage; once that was accomplished, the compartments were to be fumigated. Local authorities found the passengers accommodations in town and gave them £30 to buy food. Henry Brown, captain of the *Swatara*, told hospital officials that Baldwin had ordered him to fill the fever victims' berths with new paying passengers and set sail again immediately. When the ship reboarded and left Belfast on April 20, two of its original passengers were dead, and typhus was progressing rapidly through the town.[4]

Conditions aboard the "floating coffins" carrying the famine refugees out of Ireland were notorious even at the time, as witnesses and survivors recounted scenes of unimaginable squalor to incredulous audiences on both sides of the Atlantic. As they described what they saw, Stephen De Vere and John Griscom might just as well have been describing the *Swatara*. De Vere, an Irish landlord and philan-thropist, wrote:

> Hundreds of poor people, men, women, and children of all ages, from the driv-elling idiot of ninety to the babe just born, huddled together without light, without air, wallowing in filth and breathing a fetid atmosphere, sick in body, dispirited in heart, the fever patients lying between the sound, in sleeping places so narrow as almost to deny them the power of indulging, by a change of posi-tion, the natural restlessness of the disease; by their ravings disturbing those around [them] . . . [T]he filthy beds, teeming with all abominations, are never required to be brought on deck and aired; the narrow space between the sleep-ing berths and the piles of boxes is never washed or scraped, but breathes up a damp and fetid stench . . . [D]runkenness, with its consequent train of ruffianly debasement, is not discouraged, because it is profitable to the captain, who traf-fics in the grog.[5]

Upon inspecting the hold of the immigrant vessel *Ceylon*, New York City health of-ficer John H. Griscom lost heart at the sight of "emaciated half-nude figures, many with the petechial eruption still disfiguring their faces, crouching in their berths . . . [S]ome were just rising from their berths for the first time since leaving Liverpool, having been suffered to lie there all the voyage wallowing in their own filth . . . The Black Hole of Calcutta was a mercy compared with the holds of such vessels."[6]

Even as the *Swatara* passengers suffered under such conditions, their journey barely underway, they were twice more forced by storms back into the nearest port for repairs. In the first week of May, dismasted for the third time, the ship limped into Derry (Londonderry to the English). "Fever is still prevalent" aboard, the newspapers reported. This time, the repairs took two and a half months, and the ship was not able to resume its journey to Philadelphia until July 21.[7]

It was during this final stretch of the long journey that Andrew Coulter, already weakened from hunger, began to have difficulty breathing if he made even the slightest exertion. His pale face took on a yellowish tint; his gums softened, swelled, and bled; and his breath turned foul. He felt extreme pain in his arms and legs, as his legs started to swell with fluid. He could scarcely form a coherent thought; it was as if his brain had turned off. Scurvy had been observed and de-scribed for centuries, especially among long-distance sailors. It had been nearly a century since British naval physician James Lind had proved that adding citrus fruit or juice to sailors' diets both cured and prevented scurvy. But that proof did no good for Andrew Coulter, suffering with scurvy *and* ship fever on the *Swatara*.[8]

Andrew's symptoms escalated in a spiral of pain and prostration: the chill, the pounding headache, the intense pain in the extremities, and then the searing fever that had already overcome so many of his shipmates grabbed hold of him, too. The petechial rash soon followed on his abdomen, then his chest, then his arms and legs—first pink, then gradually darker shades of red and brown. He grew less and less coherent and finally fell into a stupor. His brother, James, was stricken with the same progression of symptoms a few days later.[9]

What did the Coulter brothers feel during that severe stage of the illness? Was it painful? Did they fear death, or welcome any possibility of a release from their suffering? One possible version of their experience can be found in Andrea Barrett's fictional account of a typhus patient's experience during the Irish famine migration:

> She stayed on deck when the weather allowed, even though she was very ill; anything was better than the crowding and smells below. One of her brothers brought her water, the other what food he could . . . She worried about them, distantly, and prayed they'd stay healthy. But a deadly calm had come over her, a calm she knew came from her illness. Shivering that swept her body in waves, scarlet spots on her shoulders—she had fiabhras dubh, the black fever, like all the people dying below . . . [N]ow her tongue had gone quiet in her mouth, she could no longer groan, she could not resist. She was filled with a gentle resignation that, during her brief lucid moments, she recognized as fatal.
>
> Where was it she'd finally collapsed? Near the galley, she thought. Somewhere in that crowded space around the range of cooking fires, hemmed in by the cowhouse and the poultry pens and the pigsty and the heap of spare spars. Down she'd gone, with the sky overhead rushing down to greet her. Afterwards came a long stretch of darkness and a tormenting thirst. A weight arrived, pressing and crushing as the ship heaved in what must have been a storm. Feebly, during brief waking moments, she had tried to push the weight aside. The weight was first warm and then cool and then cold and very heavy. She woke when the hatches were open, letting in a pale streak of light, and found herself staring into the open eyes of Julia McCullough. They were filmy, like the eyes of a fish.[10]

The famine and the fever—whether you called it typhus or ship fever or any of the other names that tied it to crowding and privation—marched hand in hand. The worst year for both was 1847. Malnourished families crowded together in their small hovels or in workhouses were easy prey for the disease. But the famine and its mounting death toll also spurred a panicked rush of emigrants, which peaked in

Black '47 and funneled the most vulnerable by the tens of thousands into outbound vessels like the *Swatara*—floating breeding grounds for typhus. They had no choice but to wait for departure in the seedy boardinghouses of port cities like Liverpool, where many of them contracted the disease shortly before descending into the seagoing hell of steerage. If the decimated immune systems and the overcrowding were not enough, emigrants in the herring boxes beneath the hatches suffered from an absence of ventilation and sunlight, wore a few ragged pieces clothing that could not be properly washed, were not able to bathe, and were left perpetually hungry and thirsty by the meager rations of barely edible food and impure water. Misled by unscrupulous emigration agents in the ports who drummed up business by promising a quick voyage of twenty days, families packed optimistically small supplies of food. And even at that, they often had no way to cook it.[11]

Few ships encountered such long delays or such a high death toll as the *Swatara*: 28 percent of its passengers died on the way to the United States. Fees imposed by US ports meant higher fares for emigrant passage to the United States than to Canada, which is why the poorest of the poor famine refugees mostly headed for Quebec City and Montreal, even if their final destination was the United States. Historians have estimated the average shipboard mortality in 1847 at 9 percent for United States–bound vessels and 30 percent for those sailing to Canada (presumably because the latter were even hungrier and more destitute than the former).[12] The *Swatara*'s luck was unusually bad.

Generations of immigrants who preceded Andrew Coulter would have recognized the key elements of his story: poverty and bleak prospects; enticing promises of prosperity and ease; the difficult decision to leave home and family; the long, squalid, and (for many) deadly journey; and exhaustion, hope, and uncertainty on arrival at the Lazaretto. Although ethnic prejudices might have led them to mistrust or even despise one another, these immigrants shared a common and formative experience across the decades.

Owners' and captains' greedy inhumanity, as outrageous as it could be, did not cause illness, death, or even shipboard misery. All of these outcomes were built into the structure of the business, which was nothing more or less than shipping human cargo. As long as there was demand on the part of desperate would-be emigrants and little or no government regulation, the pressure to load more bodies and to cut expenses by reducing provisions was constant and irresistible. It was probably made easier when the cargo in question—German or Irish peasants, say, with "barbaric" customs and "filthy" habits—was perceived as not fully human. Well-meaning attempts at reform and regulation, such as the Steerage Act of 1819, foundered on the multiplicity of jurisdictions involved and weak enforcement that never measured up to the volume of the trafficking and the profits to be made from it.[13]

Herman Melville's 1849 novel *Redburn* delivered an angry verdict on the whole business and on its invisibility to the larger public:

> The only account you obtain of such events, is generally contained in a newspaper paragraph, under the shipping [news]. *There* is the obituary of the destitute dead, who die on the sea. They die, like the billows that break on the shore, and no more are heard or seen . . . [W]hat a world of life and death, what a world of humanity and its woes, lies shrunk into [the shipping news]!
>
> You see no plague-ship driving through a stormy sea; you hear no groans of despair; you see no corpses thrown over the bulwarks; you mark not the wringing hands and torn hair of widows and orphans:—all is a blank.

Melville lamented that legislation failed to touch the fundamental inhumanity of the system. "What ordinance," he asked, "makes it obligatory upon the captain of a ship to supply the steerage passengers with decent lodgings, and give them light and air in that foul den, where they are immured during a long voyage across the Atlantic?" He concluded with his own groan of rueful despair: "We talk of the Turks, and abhor the cannibals; but may not some of *them* go to heaven before some of *us*? We may have civilized bodies and yet barbarous souls. We are blind to the real sights of this world; deaf to its voice; and dead to its death."[14] In his indignation, Melville echoed George Lehman, the Lazaretto physician who, seeing the ship *Hope* on its arrival in 1817, compared the shipping of migrants to the slave trade and called for "this inhuman traffic" to be abolished.[15]

A gathering chorus of like-minded voices would, eight years after the *Swatara's* voyage, force Congress to pass yet another law intended to rein in these greedy practices. The Passenger Act of 1855 mandated minimum standards for space, ventilation, and food on immigrant vessels. It may have salved consciences, but as with previous efforts, virtually nonexistent enforcement and narrow judicial interpretations of the law nullified its effects. (The Passenger Act of 1882, designed to remedy its predecessor's flaws, suffered a similar fate.)[16]

The immigrants were fleeing poverty and starvation, but what awaited when their squalid and dangerous transatlantic journeys came to an end? Acceptance into American society was far from assured. In 1844, three years before the Coulter family arrived, Philadelphia was engulfed in a wave of what would today be called ethnic and religious terrorism. It began with a dispute over which English translation would be used for the public schools' daily Bible reading: the King James version (favored by Protestants) or the Douai version (favored by most of the recent Irish Catholic immigrants). When a school director asked whether forcing Catholic students to leave class in order to read the Douai version was so disruptive that Bible reading might have to be temporarily suspended, rumors flew among Protestant nativists that Rome was plotting to take over America by replacing the King James with the Douai Bible.

Already simmering antagonism toward the increasingly numerous and recently enfranchised Irish immigrants quickly boiled over. Nativists attempted to intimidate the Irish by holding rallies in immigrant neighborhoods. When the Irish made clear that they were prepared to defend themselves at all costs, rioting broke out. Organized nativist gangs rampaged through the Kensington district of Philadelphia (home of many recent arrivals), torching churches, schools, and homes. The campaign of terror later spread to Southwark, on the other side of the city, when rumors spread of the Irish stockpiling weapons for use against native-born Protestants. More than thirty people were killed in the violence, and more than one hundred were injured. Hundreds more lost their homes in the Philadelphia Nativist Riots of 1844.[17]

This was the atmosphere that awaited the Coulter family and their shipmates when, on September 13, 1847, the *Swatara* dropped anchor in front of the yellow flag at the Lazaretto a full six months after its departure from Liverpool. Two hundred twenty-seven passengers survived the journey, including twenty babies born aboard. At least eighty-nine died at sea or in the various ports of call. If, back in Belfast, Captain Brown followed Baldwin's orders and restocked the steerage with fresh bodies after ship fever created vacancies, then the number of dead may have been much higher.[18]

Lazaretto physician Joshua Jones took one look at the *Swatara* and immediately knew it was in bad shape. Before he did anything else, he ordered thirty-five prostrate passengers—two cases of scurvy, one case (Andrew Coulter) of "scurvy and fever," and thirty-two cases (including James Coulter) of "typhus fever"—admitted into the already full hospital. The next day, another typhus-stricken *Swatara* passenger, and two days later three more, were added to the hospital's rolls. There was no cure for typhus. The lives of the Coulter brothers and the other patients—the hopes that they brought with them when fleeing the famine, their current and future families, the possible generations of American descendants yet to come—all depended on the overwhelmed Dr. Jones and his nurses, already in the midst of an onslaught of patients in the suddenly very busy hospital on Tinicum Island. It was in fact the busiest year for the hospital since 1817, when so many German emigrants had fled "the year without a summer" on the *Hope* and other vessels. This time it was Irish refugees who were chased away from home by hunger. Dr. Jones admitted more than 300 patients into his hospital during the 1847 quarantine season. (The next busiest year thereafter saw 130 patients admitted.)

It cost money to care for patients, of course, and in 1847 the Board of Health billed ship owners for Lazaretto care and provisions at the rate of seventy-five cents per patient per day. The owners were not always eager to pay, and the board occasionally had to pursue collection in court. The first major "coffin ship" to arrive in that fateful season was the *North Star* on June 14, from Liverpool and Londonderry. Sixty-two patients were admitted to the hospital from the *North Star*, and several had to stay for more than three weeks. When the time came to pay the bill, the ship's owners, Isaac Lloyd Sr. and Jr. of the merchant firm Isaac Lloyd & Son, protested that the amount was too high. Like Stephen Baldwin, owner of the *Swatara*, the Lloyds made money shipping and selling cotton and sugar from the slave South.[19] Of course, everyone in the North was implicated in the slave economy—cotton, sugar, coffee, and tobacco from plantations in the South and in the West Indies were favorite consumer goods. But it seems fitting that the merchants profiting most directly from the northern market for those goods were the same ones profiting from the human trafficking of this northerly echo of the Middle Passage, with its collateral misery, disease, and death.

The Lloyds' complaint did not sit right with the Board of Health, whose Lazaretto Committee oversaw the operations of the station and was responsible for collecting its bills. The committee's chairman, Joseph Thomas, a bookseller by trade, reported its findings in dramatically expressive language that was highly unusual in the bone-dry formalism of the Board of Health minutes:

> Your committee also beg leave to express their opinion (although at variance with that of the Messrs. Lloyd expressed in their communication) that seventy-five cents per day for board of, and medical attendance upon, the class of patients usually in the hospital is not an excessive charge, as your committee are of the opinion that the poor and friendless who are brought to our shores by the cupidity of others are as much entitled, by every feeling of humanity, to proper nourishment, careful nursing and skillful medical attendance as those who by accident or otherwise are in possession of the means of having the same at their own cost.[20]

Strong words. A cynical reading might be: "I am resorting to moralistic grandstanding to defend our antiquated quarantine system (with its associated fees and charges), which may or may not protect public health but reliably generates patronage jobs and fills public coffers." Here is a more generous reading: "Just as you have chosen to profit from slave labor with your cotton and your sugar, you have chosen to profit from the trade in human cargo. You have treated your cargo like animals—or worse—because you see them as less than human. The resulting carnage is there for everyone with open eyes to see. The least you can do is pay a paltry seventy-five cents to clean up the mess you've made, without complaining that the sum is excessive." Indeed, what the board's Joseph Thomas called "proper nourishment" and "careful nursing" may have made the difference between life and death (see chapter 12).

Historians have viewed quarantine as a barrier set up in part to check unrestrained immigration to the United States. In this view, defense against epidemics was a pretext for depicting immigrants as inherently diseased, for incarcerating harmless passengers, and for preventing entry into the country.[21] But this grim portrait of quarantine is more accurate for the third wave of immigration to North America—from the 1880s to the 1920s, the Ellis Island era—than it is for most of the Philadelphia Lazaretto's existence. Although nativist prejudice awaited most arriving immigrants when they left Tinicum Island, it did not shape the institution of quarantine itself.

Nobody was ever happy to be detained at the Lazaretto, unable to leave even if in perfect health. Especially after a long and harrowing journey, to be so close to one's destination and unable to get there, sometimes for weeks, was supremely frustrating. But the survivors of the *Swatara* and the other coffin ships did not find rejection or discrimination or a forced return to Europe at the Lazaretto. Starving and prostrate in their stupor, these patients at least had the good fortune to land in a hospital whose physician was well prepared for their illness. They found food and drink and clean clothing. They found a bed with clean sheets, blankets, and a pillow—unless the station was already overcrowded, and they were healthy enough to be placed in tents outdoors. They found medical and nursing care if they were sick. They found fresh air and so much else that they had been deprived of for so many weeks.

It has long been known that it takes more than a potato blight (*Phytophthora infestans*) to kill a million people and drive a million more out of their country. It takes a particular form of land tenure based on absentee landlords intent on squeezing as much money as possible out of disenfranchised tenant farmers. It takes a government (like the British government that ruled Ireland during the famine) that attaches greater importance to tax collection and noninterference in agricultural markets than to the urgent needs of its subjects, and that accepts extreme hunger, illness, and death on a massive scale as the necessary price of progress. And it takes a ruling-class culture that sees an entire population as belonging to a different race—uncivilized, improvident, and superstitious.[22]

In its path of desolation, the Great Famine exported misery all over the world. One week during the exodus that began in 1846 might see a hundred starving and desperately ill migrants arrive at Tinicum Island (figure 4)—where the hospital was already nearly full of patients from earlier ships—along with hundreds more hungry but not yet sick. The station officers and the Board of Health faced the challenge of housing, clothing, feeding, and caring for all of them while maintaining vigilance and not allowing any sickness or contamination up to the city.

All thirty-seven typhus patients—and the two scurvy patients—who made it from the *Swatara* into the Lazaretto hospital in 1847 walked out of there on their own two feet. After so many Irish famine migrants had recovered at the Lazaretto, after

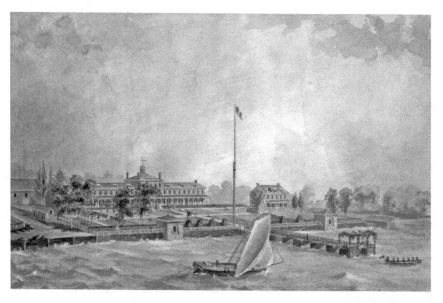

Figure 4. Bird's-eye view of the Lazaretto, ca. 1860. Watercolor by Thomas L. Cernea. Courtesy of the Philadelphia History Museum at the Atwater Kent / Bridgeman Images.

Chapter Twelve

The Care Cure

Most patients treated at the Lazaretto hospital had either yellow fever or typhus. Both of those diseases were incurable in the nineteenth century. (Yellow fever is still incurable in the early twenty-first century.) Yet somehow, *the vast majority of Lazaretto patients were cured.* Evidence from nineteenth-century outbreaks of yellow fever and typhus would lead us to expect much lower survival rates. What was the secret of the Lazaretto's surprisingly successful medical treatment?

Long before the advent of antibiotics, doctors understood that in the absence of a specific remedy against typhus, medicine's role (as one textbook described it) was "to aid the organism in its defense against infection, to moderate the symptoms which . . . may jeopardize life, to sustain by means of food and proper medication the strength of the individual, and . . . to place the patient under such hygienic conditions as will help him emerge [the] victor from the contest."[1]

Today, we call such treatment palliative care, or supportive care. These terms are often used to refer to treatments given to keep terminally ill patients comfortable. But supportive care can mean the difference between life and death.

For most of the nineteenth century, a disease was not understood to be a single stable entity with a single cause, uniform symptoms and progression, and one appropriate treatment. Each case of illness was thought to be unique, with multiple idiosyncratic causes and a shifting and often unpredictable set of symptoms. There were familiar patterns, of course—in yellow fever, in typhus, and in other diseases—but any individual patient was as likely to deviate from the pattern as to follow it.

A disease, if such a thing could be said to exist as an entity, consisted of symptoms and how they progressed, and treatment had to be calibrated accordingly.

Fever and inflammation demanded depletion by bloodletting, emetics (which in-duced vomiting), and purgatives (which evacuated the bowels). But the skillful physician also needed to know the patient's constitution and habits, and to care-fully observe the symptoms and their changes over time.[2] He needed to pay atten-tion to the patient's response to, for example, bloodletting by different means and in different amounts, to observe closely the blood itself and other bodily se-cretions, and to adjust the treatment according to these observations.[3]

Depletion by doctor mimicked depletion by nature. In illness, the body natu-rally attempted to rid itself of disease by throwing off vomit and diarrhea (and occasionally blood). Sometimes nature needed the physician's helping hand to provoke those same evacuations. The *effectiveness* of the treatment could be seen in its *effects*: for example, a good purgative succeeded in emptying the bowels. Bloodletting succeeded in reducing fever and inflammation (at least in the short term). And to the trained senses, the excretions produced could provide impor-tant clues about the progress of the illness. Keeping the four humors in balance (blood, phlegm, yellow bile, and black bile—believed in the classical tradition to be the fundamental fluids that governed human health) was nothing but a dis-tant page from the history books for the early nineteenth-century physician, but some of the remedies from that bygone age endured, along with the principle of counteracting bodily weakness and repletion. As long as patients and doctors shared a general understanding of the body and its vulnerabilities, including the basic need to correct bodily insufficiencies through stimulation and excesses through depletion, the extreme remedies that today seem shockingly reckless and dangerous were understood to be necessary and effective.[4]

The humoral system gradually disappeared from medical literature in the eigh-teenth century, but the appeal of treatment by depletion—bleeding, purging, and puking—remained as strong as ever.

Anyone who has ever donated blood knows how it must have felt to have been bled by a doctor in the early nineteenth century. After the puncture of the skin, it would be painless. A little light-headedness after a while was entirely normal. Instead of sterilized needles and plastic storage pouches, doctors used lancets—small sharp knives, some of them spring-loaded to produce quick, uniform incisions—and ba-sins to collect the blood. Basins were often marked on the inside like measuring cups so the physician could see how much blood had been let.[5]

Some doctors believed in gentle, local bleeding. Others argued that severe fe-vers and inflammation demanded a severe response. Fifteen ounces—about what we lose when we donate blood today—was usually considered a vigorous bloodletting. During the 1793 yellow fever epidemic, Benjamin Rush initially found that 10 to 12 ounces was "sufficient to subdue the pulse" and deplete the accumulated excess. As the epidemic advanced, however, he found he had to bleed more and more to achieve the necessary effect, eventually draining 60, 70, even 80 ounces from a single patient (almost half the entire blood volume of a 150-pound adult) "and in most cases with the happiest effects." Rush bled more than most, certainly, but among American physicians, tales of two-quart bleedings were not unheard of.[6]

But the cautious and the enthusiastic all agreed that the amount bled was less important than the effect achieved. Some practitioners followed Galen's advice: bleed a small amount at first, then observe the effects—pulse, fever, inflammation— and bleed more as necessary until the body responds appropriately. Others had no use for such hesitancy. Anyone who has ever fainted knows how it felt to have been bled aggressively. "Bleed until syncope" (temporary loss of consciousness) was the watchword of the true believers. Experienced doctors took pride in being able to stop bleeding just before the patient fainted.[7] Because each patient and each constellation of symptoms were different, the physician could not rely on a single formula for all cases. Careful observation and management of each patient's response to each intervention were critical.

Venesection, or opening a vein with a lancet, was not the only bloodletting technique available. Some practitioners preferred localized bleeding by the equally ancient means of wet cupping or leeches. In wet cupping, a wick or other flammable object was set afire in a cup, which was then placed upside down on the patient's skin when the flame burned out. As the air in the cup cooled, the resulting suction caused the skin to redden and swell as blood was drawn to the area. The practitioner then quickly used a *scarificator*—a set of small sharp blades—to make small incisions in the skin, and relit and reapplied the cup to draw the blood out from the capillaries. A clumsy cupper could easily cause painful burns to the patient, but experienced teachers insisted that the procedure need cause no more than mild discomfort.[8]

Another way doctors could bleed with precision was using the blood-sucking aquatic worms known as leeches, usually at the site of particular symptoms or lesions. After the patient's skin was washed and shaved, the leech was dried and then placed on the skin and induced to feed by a bit of milk or blood on the desired spot. The powerful sucker on the tail end of the leech then affixed itself, while the smaller end, the mouth end, applied its own suction, made a small triangular puncture in the skin, and began feeding. After about an hour and an ounce of blood, the sated leech simply let go and dropped off, although it could be pulled off earlier if needed. Doctors routinely used twenty or more leeches at a time on adult patients. For physicians intent on localized bleeding, leeches offered a singular advantage over wet cupping: they could be applied to internal mucus membranes such as the nostril, the ear canal, the trachea, the rectum, or the vagina.[9] (Patients' accounts of what it felt like to be nasally, rectally, or vaginally leeched are lacking, so the curiosity of present-day readers must remain unsatisfied.)

There was more to depletion than bloodletting. Certain fevers demanded that the digestive tract be regularly emptied with emetics and purgatives. Vomiting and defecation—abundant and repeated, if necessary—were the goals. Doctors relied most often on either ipecacuanha or tartar emetic to induce copious vomiting. Ipecacuanha is the root of a Brazilian shrub. Whole, it is odorless, but when ground into a powder, it has a nauseating odor so strong that it has been known to cause sneezing in some people and shortness of breath in others. Doctors administered a small dose of a chemically purified form of the powder suspended in water. In the unlikely event that vomiting did not follow immediately, the dosage was repeated every twenty minutes until the desired effect was achieved. Tartar emetic, or potassio-antimonious tartrate, is a preparation of the metallic element antimony that was sold in crystal form and administered as a powder mixed with water. Its sweetish metallic taste concealed its emetic power. Many physicians preferred it to ipecacuanha because tartar emetic "remains longer in the stomach . . . produces more frequent and longer continued efforts to vomit, and exerts a more powerful impression on the system generally." It also caused "copious discharges of bile"—all in all not a pleasant experience for the patient, but reassuring for the doctor who was looking for a thorough depletion.[10]

Purging could be just as uncomfortable. Laxatives are meant to be gentle; purgatives are not. The most widely used purgative was calomel, a mercury derivative prescribed for a range of ailments in various doses and in combination with other remedies. In treating fevers, doctors prized calomel for its fast and reliable effect on the bowels. Although its original name was "sweet mercury," calomel was actually tasteless—at first. The overpowering metallic taste came on only if it stayed in the patient's mouth. The term *calomel stools* referred to what one doctor called the "green, spinach-like evacuations" caused by its use. American doctors often paired calomel with jalap, another South American root, and painful, copious, watery diarrhea would ensue. Physicians were well aware of what mercury could do in large or repeated doses:

The first observable effects . . . are a coppery taste in the mouth, a slight sore-
ness of the gums, and an unpleasant sensation in the sockets of the teeth when
the jaws are firmly closed. Shortly afterwards the gums begin to swell, a line of
whitish matter is seen along their edges, and the breath is infected with a peculiar and very disagreeable smell, called the mercurial fetor. The saliva at the
same time begins to flow; and . . . the gums, tongue, throat, and face are much
swollen; ulcerations attack the lining membrane of the mouth . . . ; the jaws become excessively painful; the tongue is coated with a thick whitish fur; and
the saliva flows in streams from the mouth.[11]

Depletion was not a pretty business, and yet for centuries these remedies were
mainstays of every well-trained doctor's practice, especially when treating severe
fevers.

Surveying the treatment of patients during Philadelphia's yellow fever epidemic
of 1820, Board of Health president Samuel Jackson found that all were depleted
somehow; most were purged; and many were both bled and purged. Some of them
recovered, and some died; the only correlation Jackson could find between treatments and outcomes was that most of the patients who recovered had sores in their
mouths or other oral symptoms of what we would today call mercury poisoning.[12]

Because few records survive of the specific treatments administered at the Lazaretto, we are left to infer what remedies were used there from physicians' writings,
medical school curricula, published medical texts about similar patients and
illnesses from the same time, and occasional requests for supplies in the Board of
Health minutes.[13] Just before the opening of the 1847 quarantine season, for example, the Lazaretto steward wrote the board to ask for "cattail for the hospital."
Cattail roots were used in cold-water infusions or boiled in milk to soothe cough
and fever and to treat dysentery.[14]

Dr. Joshua Jones, the Lazaretto's physician in 1847, laid out his views on the
treatment of typhus in his 1829 medical thesis at the University of Pennsylvania.
Having no way of knowing, of course, that his future career path would place him
in the middle of an unprecedented onslaught of typhus-stricken famine refugees,
Jones wrote that his research convinced him that, contrary to widespread opinion,
typhus was characterized primarily not by debility but by congestion. He even
suggested it be renamed "congestive fever." The common practice in the 1820s of
treating typhus patients with remedies aimed to fortify and stimulate the body's
systems, Jones argued, was deeply misguided. In other words, this highly detailed

document gave every reason to expect that a classic depletion regimen awaited Irish famine refugees while Jones was in charge of their care: they would be bled with the lancet, bled with leeches, and bled with wet cupping; they would be given tartar emetic to empty the stomach; and they would be given strong laxatives like calomel and jalap, which would be discontinued if they produced "great distress, with copious, fetid, watery stools."[15]

And yet, according to another doctor's firsthand account, the ship-fever patients at the Lazaretto in 1847 were not depleted at all; they were stimulated.[16] There was none of the aggressive bleeding and puking advocated in Jones's thesis. A few patients were bled locally and sparingly with wet cups. Some got ipecacuanha and calomel "in very small doses"—not enough to cause vomiting or defecation, but sufficient to induce perspiration, salivation, and expectoration. The primary remedies—tonics and stimulants—used for typhus at the Lazaretto were quite the opposite of depletives. To restore the strength of the weakened body, there was sulphate of quinia, or quinine—a preparation of the bark of the Andean cinchona bush, administered in pill form or as a powder mixed with various liquids. Its intensely bitter taste could not be masked by even large quantities of sugar but was neutralized when used in combination with aromatics such as orange peel or anise. To excite the body to increased activity, or to quicken the vital functions, patients were given a punch made of spirits, wine, sugar, lemon juice, water, carbonate of ammonia (a pungent powder often mixed with lemon juice to make an effervescent liquid), and brandy. We can assume that drinking, tasting, swallowing, and then gradually feeling the effects of the tonic and stimulant treatment were incomparably more pleasant and soothing than bleeding, puking, and purging. And, in case the typhus patients were not soothed, Jones gave some of them opium to relieve pain and help them sleep.[17]

Considering the long-established and approved practice of depletion, why did Dr. Jones execute such a sharp about-face between 1829 and 1847? The change makes sense only when viewed from multiple angles. First, the original medical thesis has to be taken with a grain of salt. A thesis in 1829 was meant to be not a report of original research findings, but rather an exercise in synthesis. Its audience was not fellow physicians, but the few professors who had mentored and examined the author. The purpose was to demonstrate that he had mastered the medical orthodoxy on one particular topic from the ancients to the present day, with a special emphasis on what was taught at his own school.[18]

Meanwhile, in the middle third of the nineteenth century, a new wave of what were considered unorthodox, or *sectarian*, practitioners—botanical healers, homeopaths, water-cure practitioners, diet reformers, and others—mounted a noisy attack on the classically trained physicians, singling out for special scorn the aggressive depletive therapies, the physicians' so-called heroic treatments. Many doctors facing fierce competition in the marketplace from the new sects began to treat more gently and less heroically.[19]

But beginning in the middle decades of the nineteenth century, even established physicians in North America and Europe who had nothing to fear from the upstart sectarians resorted less often to bloodletting and other vigorous means of depletion. None of them disavowed the heroic remedies, and no significant studies claimed to prove that they were ineffective or harmful. But doctors believed, as always, that treatment had to be adapted to circumstances, and they saw circumstances changing. Urbanization and changes in occupation, doctors reported, confronted them with different illnesses—even different qualities of fever—as well as different kinds of patients, with different constitutions and habits. Treatments naturally changed accordingly, with tonics and stimulants increasingly replacing bloodletting, emetics, and purgatives.[20]

One more thing happened right under Joshua Jones's nose in Philadelphia that may have changed his thinking about typhus. While doctors had long noted that most people with typhus had fever and some kind of skin rash, they observed, too, that some patients also had severe intestinal symptoms, and that certain internal lesions were visible on autopsy in some but not all patients who died with typhus. In his thesis Jones had considered these variations to be manifestation of typhus fever, but some doctors began speaking of a typhus-like illness they called "typhoid fever."

William Wood Gerhard, who had earned his medical degree at the University of Pennsylvania just a year after Jones and had then gone off to study under the world-famous clinical researcher Pierre Louis in Paris, was on duty at Philadelphia's municipal hospital in 1836 when typhus broke out in the slums and cellars of the city's southwestern quarter, which was largely inhabited by desperately poor and malnourished free Black people.[21] In Paris, Gerhard had had plenty of opportunities to see the so-called typhoid fever, both in living patients and inside cadavers. From Louis he had learned to carefully correlate the symptoms experienced by the patient during the illness with the internal lesions visible on autopsy. The 1836 epidemic gave him the chance to do the same with the classic typhus fever. Gerhard found overwhelming evidence that typhus and typhoid fever were two distinct diseases, with different symptoms in life and different lesions apparent after death. His exhaustive study in the *American Journal of the*

Medical Sciences laid the case out clearly and convincingly.[22] Joshua Jones, it seems, had unwittingly been studying two different diseases as if they were one and the same. What is more, in fitting homage to his mentor Louis's renowned meticulous record keeping, Gerhard's own documentation of most of the epidemic's 214 patients allowed him to draw conclusions about which treatments were most effective against typhus.

Gerhard and his colleagues resorted to depletives extensively in the early part of the epidemic but pulled back from their use as evidence mounted that they did patients no good and sometimes did harm. Given the extreme prostration brought on by a severe case of typhus, bleeding was only feasible in the mildest cases, and it "never arrested the disease, nor did it apparently abridge its course." Likewise, emetics and purgatives showed no beneficial effects, and Gerhard declined to recommend their general use in typhus. Stimulants and "useful palliatives," on the other hand, proved most effective—indeed, Gerhard enthused, "wine, combined with quinine and a nutritious diet, produced an effect which was almost magical." The combination quickly revived the spirits of patients who were extremely weak and mired in delirium, while gradually increasing their overall strength. Cool sponge baths helped bring down high fevers.[23]

Camphor was also "among the most useful and powerful of our remedies," the report added. A volatile and intensely aromatic compound found in the roots, seeds, and essential oils of various plants, camphor was most often administered as a powder suspended in milk. Gerhard and his colleagues found that it immediately calmed the uncontrollable muscular tremors and twitching in typhus, and sometimes helped with the delirium as well. It did not cure the disease, but it was nevertheless useful. In fact, Gerhard took pains to call attention to the value of palliatives—"such remedies as diminish the severity of particular symptoms, and thereby materially increase the comfort of the patient." They could even be life saving, he argued. Some diseases might not be fatal in themselves, but patients could die of dehydration, "the prostration produced by excessive secretions," or of organ failure brought on by certain symptoms allowed to continue unchecked.[24]

Joshua Jones's treatment of typhus among the Irish famine refugees in 1847 bore a much stronger resemblance to Gerhard's regimen than it did to the one recommended in his own medical thesis. Medicine was becoming more gentle.

But did it work? Did *any* of it work? There is good reason to be skeptical, and yet there is one simple word that appears more often than any other in the Lazaretto hospital register for 1847–93: *cured.* It is hard not to be astonished by the carpet of "cured" appearing down the "Result" column on page after page. Eighty-eight percent of patients treated at the Lazaretto between 1847 and 1893 were listed as "cured." Yellow fever—cured. Typhus—cured. Smallpox—cured. Cholera—cured. These doctors, I thought, were lucky not to *kill* most of their patients with their bizarre treatments, and here they were, arrogant enough to assume (like the rooster whose crowing makes the sun rise) that they had *cured* them? It took an immersion in nineteenth-century medical treatises like Joshua Jones's thesis, Samuel Jackson's fever report, and William Wood Gerhard's study, as well as textbooks and dictionaries, before I was able to understand what treatment was about, and what *cure* meant at the Lazaretto.

It also took a shocking twenty-first-century outbreak of another incurable disease to remind me that the lessons of the Lazaretto are still timely today.

The nineteenth-century meaning of *cure* often did not imply that doctors or medicine were directly responsible. It was widely understood that nature healed; at best, the doctor helped.[25] Over the past century and a half, both therapeutic medicine and patients' expectations have undergone a radical transformation. As we have come to expect medicine to be able to *cure* (or at least treat effectively) nearly every health condition—even the most deadly—we have come to look back at older medical treatments as ignorant quackery: "placebos that did nothing and poisons that made you sicker."[26]

Only 10 of the 210 typhus patients admitted to the Lazaretto hospital in the 1847 quarantine season died—a case-fatality rate of 5 percent. And 1847—that overwhelming Irish famine year—was no fluke. Over the entire period covered by the Lazaretto hospital register, only 5 percent of patients admitted with typhus died. It is impossible to control for all variables in the chaos of an epidemic, and it would be a mistake to look for precise, reliable numbers in many historical accounts, but the best estimates today put the fatality rate for cases of epidemic typhus not treated with antibiotics at 10 to 40 percent. For yellow fever, the case-fatality rate at the Lazaretto between 1847 and 1893 was 22 percent. One study of six well-documented American yellow fever epidemics in the nineteenth century calculated an overall fatality rate of 59 percent, with the mildest epidemic at 25 percent and the most lethal at over 72 percent. Most epidemiologists today put the case-fatality rate for *severe* yellow fever (cases that have progressed beyond the initial mild stage to jaundice—the kind of cases most likely to have been diagnosed as yellow fever at the Lazaretto) at 20 to 50 percent.[27]

For yellow fever and for typhus, the cure rate at the Lazaretto was surprisingly high. *What was in that wine?*

There are many possible ways to explain away the Lazaretto hospital's typhus and yellow fever numbers—and its overall 88 percent cure rate for all diseases. Maybe the staff discharged some patients as "cured" who had not fully recovered and who later relapsed. Maybe the most severe shipboard cases had already died by the time many vessels reached the Lazaretto, at which point only the milder cases (with the best chances of survival) were admitted. A sample size bigger than this one at the Lazaretto (832 patients over forty-seven years) would make drawing conclusions more comfortable.

The Lazaretto numbers are not definitive, but they are at least suggestive. There was no incentive for doctors, nurses, or anyone else to inflate the hospital's cure rate, as it was not mentioned in any documents nor factored into any budgets or deliberations. And the chaotic experience of 1847 casts doubt on the idea that the Lazaretto's patients were mostly suffering from mild cases of illness. The hospital was overrun that year with famine migrants suffering from typhus. From the beginning of the quarantine season, Dr. Jones and the Lazaretto steward continually pestered the Board of Health for more nurses, more food, more supplies—more everything. They were living through a horrible reenactment of the catastrophic year of 1817. (The two years cannot be compared directly because there are no Lazaretto hospital statistics for 1817.) A hospital designed to accommodate forty-eight patients, but which most often had only a handful at a time—with one nurse on duty—suddenly had to cope with wave after wave of sick immigrants.

On fifty-three days that season, more than forty patients were under treatment, and on twenty-four days, more than seventy. Amid the chaos, short on supplies, Jones was unlikely to admit anyone who was not acutely ill. And milder cases would be discharged sooner, especially when the hospital was so crowded; no patient would be kept any longer than absolutely necessary. The more than 200 typhus patients admitted in 1847 stayed in the hospital for an average of seventeen days.[28] These were not mild cases.

Typhus patients in the Lazaretto hospital got quinine, wine punch, and the occasional dose of opium, and they also got food and drink, clean clothing and bedding, rest, and nursing care. In 1853, Lazaretto physician T. J. P. Stokes credited "very free ventilation, night and day, frequent and thorough washing, [and] generous diet in the convalescence" with curing 32 of 33 Irish ship fever patients from one vessel.[29]

We do not tend to think of these things—what today's doctors call supportive care—as medical treatment. They're ancillary, incidental aspects of health care, undeniably important but not "cures." Jones, Gerhard, Stokes, and their fellow physicians might have seen things differently. Gerhard wrote about the importance of "a useful balance wheel in preserving the harmony of the system until the disease [passes] through its natural course."[30]

The harmony of the system could also be maintained through a "farinaceous" diet—porridges and breads and other mild, starchy foods—along with beef broth, followed by a moderate mixture of vegetables and meats during convalescence. (That was the diet prescribed for Gerhard's typhus patients in 1836 and for typhus patients at the Lazaretto in 1847.) So too could actual beds preserve the harmony of the patient's system—the extra bunks, the straw for mattresses, and the pillowcases that the Board of Health bought to accommodate the influx of patients at the Lazaretto in the summer of 1847. So could the towels the board provided. So could the washing and ironing done at the station, for which the steward was continually billing the ship owners that summer. So could the muslin, the shirts, and the chemises that the board purchased in response to the Lazaretto's requisitions. And so could the care provided by the temporary nurses hired by the board and sent down every time a new immigrant vessel arrived with dozens of new typhus patients. In fact, if care was in many cases tantamount to cure, then the nurses (paid $5 dollars a week, compared to Jones's $100-a-month salary) may deserve more credit for the 95 percent cure rate than the doctor.[31]

Is supportive care still important in the twenty-first century? Comparing the survival rates of a couple of hundred typhus patients in 1847 and a couple of dozen Ebola patients in 2014 does not qualify as scientific proof of anything. But it illustrates the value of supportive care in a modern setting, suggesting that supportive care was an essential factor in the recovery of the Lazaretto's patients, and that it has tended to be scientifically undervalued.

In the winter of 2013–14, fifty people in remote Guéckédou prefecture in the West African nation of Guinea died of a terrifying disease that had never been seen before in that part of the world. Profuse bleeding both internally and through various orifices combined with violent diarrhea and vomiting to emaciate then kill the victims. On March 23, 2014, the World Health Organization confirmed the existence of an outbreak of Ebola hemorrhagic fever, part of a family of viral diseases that includes yellow fever, and one that had until then been confined to a region more than 3,000 miles away in central Africa.[32] From Guéckédou, Ebola spread unchecked into neighboring Sierra Leone and Liberia—not because the disease is "extremely contagious," as the news outlets persisted in reporting (in fact, it can be contracted only by direct physical contact with a patient's bodily secretions), but because the health care systems of the poorest countries in the world are chronically understaffed and underfunded.[33] Cases were not detected and treated early, so family members and caregivers fell like dominoes. Within weeks, it became the deadliest Ebola epidemic in history.

Reactions in wealthy countries oscillated between complacency—after all, Ebola had been defined as the quintessentially African disease—and alarm. When infected Western health workers were evacuated for treatment or when a traveler from the affected area arrived in Europe or North America and fell ill, alarm turned to media-fueled hysteria, especially in the United States. The reaction itself was nothing new; since the yellow fever epidemics of the 1790s, outbreaks of incurable and often fatal diseases of exotic origin with dramatic symptoms could be counted on to provoke some degree of panic on occasion. But a patterned public response to exotic outbreaks had become entrenched and even routinized beginning with the "emerging diseases" scare of the mid-1990s (in which Ebola, West Nile encephalitis, hantavirus, and "mad cow disease" played the early starring roles). A new cadre of virologists and disease detectives warned that globalization had shrunk the world and that the expansion of human activity into previously untouched ecosystems had placed people in contact with new and deadly pathogens that were only a plane ride away from any city in the world. "Uncivilized" people who hunt bushmeat and practice strange funerary rituals endanger "civilized" people, whose survival depends on the expertise and technology of the disease detectives.[34] This patterned response provided the context for the public reaction to a handful of Ebola cases in the United States in the fall of 2014.

But what if Ebola was incurable in the same way that typhus was incurable in 1847? Until recently, we defined Ebola as *incurable* because no specific drug had been proved effective at killing or neutralizing the Ebola virus.* But what happened to the Ebola patients who were treated in functioning, well-staffed, and well-equipped hospitals instead of in the underfunded and half-abandoned clinics of Guinea, Sierra Leone, and Liberia?

They lived.

Eleven people received treatment in the United States, including one traveler from Liberia who fell ill after arrival, two nurses who treated him, one doctor who

---

* In 2019, monoclonal antibody treatments were shown to be effective in treating Ebola. Kai Kupferschmidt, "Finally, Some Good News about Ebola: Two New Treatments Dramatically Lower the Death Rate in a Trial," *Science*, August 12, 2019.

became sick after returning from Guinea, and six health care workers and one journalist who were evacuated after first experiencing symptoms in West Africa. Of these eleven, the two patients who did not receive care immediately (because their symptoms were initially misdiagnosed) died. The nine others, who were diagnosed as soon as the first symptoms appeared, all survived. Twelve of fifteen people treated in European hospitals survived. Meanwhile, the survival rate of patients with the same "incurable" disease in West Africa was between 30 and 50 percent, far lower than the 80 to 100 percent rate in the United States and Europe.[35]

In the language of the Lazaretto hospital register, the American and European patients were "cured." They did not get a miracle drug, and they did not have any special immunity to the Ebola virus. They were diagnosed early, admitted immediately into appropriate facilities, and given supportive care. That is all.

It is conceivable (though unlikely) that those who lived would have lived anyway, even without the basic amenities that we call supportive care. But examples like these are, at the very least, suggestive. They ought to cause us to question what we mean when we say that a disease is "incurable." And they remind us to be careful about assuming a clear distinction between care and cure. There are times when it is hard to see any difference at all—when it all just looks like a "care cure."

PART III / Crisis, Statesmanship, and Decline, 1853–1895

Chapter Thirteen

"Gross and Criminal Negligence" at the Lazaretto, 1853

I t was just after sunrise on a quiet mid-July day at the Lazaretto station.[1] No vessels under quarantine, no patients in the hospital. When the three tall masts
of the bark *Mandarin* loomed into sight downriver from Tinicum Island, the quarantine station's watchman rang the bell summoning bargemen, physician, and
quarantine master to the pier. Spying the station's yellow quarantine flag, the
bark's captain dropped anchor in the channel. The six bargemen rowed Thomas
Jefferson Perkins Stokes and Matthew Van Dusen out to the ship. As Lazaretto
physician, 37-year-old Stokes was the officer in charge. After more than a year
in office, he had boarded and inspected hundreds of vessels and knew the procedure inside and out.

On board the *Mandarin*, Stokes first questioned the captain, as required by law.[2]

"Your name?"

"Robert Campbell."

"Where did you sail from?"

"Cienfuegos, southern coast of Cuba."

"When did you leave that port?"

"Seventeen days ago. Twenty-fifth of June."

"What was the state of health of that port at the time you left?"

"There were a few cases of smallpox and fever—nothing unusual."

"Is there any illness aboard at the moment?"

"No."

"Any illnesses during the voyage?"

"We lost two of our crew to fever."

"What is your cargo?"

"Sugar, molasses, and cigars."

Inspection of the crew came next. They mustered on deck, where Stokes looked them over. No obvious signs of illness or debility. All ten sailors affirmed their good health when he asked.

Meanwhile, Van Dusen inspected the ship. In an effort to make the ship appear clean and thereby to avoid detention, the crew apparently had recently washed down the deck—as was often the practice on vessels approaching a quarantine station. Nothing amiss in the cabin or galley. The sailors' quarters in the forecastle were pungent, but no more so than on any other vessel after two weeks at sea. As the quarantine master had come to expect, the cargo hold was saturated with a very unpleasant odor. The cargo itself seemed sound, but then again, sugar, molasses, and cigars were almost never subject to quarantine, because they were considered incapable of conveying infection. The water in the bottom of the hold, like the bilgewater of every other vessel plying the West Indian trade in the summertime that Van Dusen had ever inspected, was a noisome soup of foulness. His inspection finished, the quarantine master reported his findings to Dr. Stokes (figure 5).

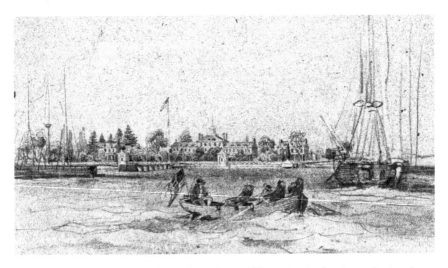

Figure 5. The Lazaretto seen from the Delaware River; in the foreground, a rowboat slightly smaller than the one in which the bargemen rowed the Lazaretto physician and quarantine master to and from vessels for inspection. Drawing by James F. Queen, 1856. Courtesy of the Library of Congress.

It was time for a decision: detain the *Mandarin* or allow it to proceed to the city? All aboard were healthy. There had been no news of any unusual incidence of fever in Cienfuegos. Vessel and cargo were sound, apart from the putrid bilgewater. On the other hand, hadn't Philadelphia learned the hard way over many decades that yellow fever often broke out in the vicinity of ships that had arrived from the West Indies in July, August, and September? And two sailors had died on the voyage. Ephraim Williams had taken sick eight days out of Cienfuegos, followed the next day by John Tuckerman. Williams died after four days of illness, Tuckerman after five—on the lower part of the Delaware River, less than 100 miles from the Lazaretto. Tuckerman died just three days before the *Mandarin* dropped anchor at Tinicum Island. Their illnesses sounded suspiciously like yellow fever.[3]

Stokes considered his options. The prudent action would be to wait and see: detain the bark for cleansing and purification, to purge it of the remnants of the two sailors' disease, and wait a few days. See if the rest of the crew remained healthy. Surely the Board of Health would approve, although Stokes knew perfectly well—and he knew the board knew—that every delay caused by quarantine was an annoyance to the commercial interests that kept Philadelphia alive. He could not detain vessels with healthy crews coming from healthy ports based on a passing doubt. For the city as well as for Stokes, the economic and political consequences of excessive caution could be severe. On the other hand, he preferred not to contemplate the consequences of allowing an infected ship to proceed directly from the Lazaretto to the port. He could simply delay the *Mandarin* temporarily and write to the board for advice; the return mail would arrive before the day's end. But he was an experienced doctor, a graduate of the University of Pennsylvania, and the governor had appointed him Lazaretto physician for a reason. The decision was his, and he played it safe—or so he thought.

He ordered the *Mandarin* detained for whitewashing, ventilation, and fumigation. The two dead sailors' clothing and bedding were burned. He saw no need to unload the cargo, and as all surviving hands were healthy, no need to admit anyone from the ship to the hospital. He reported his decision to the board in the morning mail, just as he had reported every arrival, every inspection, every illness, every quarantine decision, every death, and every patient discharge every day since he had arrived at the Lazaretto. The afternoon mail brought the board's response: Dr. Stokes was authorized to allow the *Mandarin* to proceed to the city "when in his opinion it can be done with safety to our citizens."[4] It was an exchange like any of thousands in the Lazaretto's history.

By the next morning, July 13, the disinfection was finished. The bark's crew remained in good health, as far as Stokes could tell. Captain Campbell was anxious to deliver his goods, collect what he was owed, perhaps enjoy a few days of liberty in Philadelphia, and take on new cargo. However the captain greeted Stokes's authority—whether he argued his case to the doctor, begged him for permission to proceed, or silently awaited his fate—Stokes knew from experience how deeply sailors and ship owners detested quarantine.

When Dr. Stokes allowed the bark *Mandarin* to proceed from the Lazaretto up to the Port of Philadelphia on July 13, 1853, the threat of yellow fever in the city had faded into a distant memory. A third of a century had passed since the city's last bout with the illness, and another scourge had taken its place as the most terrifying epidemic disease. Cholera had already struck Philadelphia twice in that time, and it was threatening again, sweeping westward across Europe just as it had done prior to crossing the Atlantic in 1832 and 1849. Yellow fever was a previous generation's problem. What harm could there be in sending up the *Mandarin*? Captain Campbell had reported that two of his sailors had died of "fever" en route from Cuba, but surely any lingering contamination had been neutralized by disinfection and a day's ventilation.[5]

As Captain Campbell sailed upriver from the Lazaretto on that lazy July afternoon, he had no idea that the daily and even hourly movements of the *Mandarin* would later be minutely scrutinized in an effort to understand what happened next. Dr. Stokes, little suspecting the trouble that awaited him, turned his thoughts to the next vessel headed for the Lazaretto, or perhaps to the latest news in Philadelphia Democratic politics. Ten miles northeast of Tinicum Island as the crow flies, at the Champion House hotel along the wharves near South Street, innkeeper Charles Koehler may have noticed a sour smell in the streets, but otherwise he saw no hint of the calamity that was headed his way.

The weather gave Philadelphians no quarter that summer. Relentless heat blanketed the city from the beginning of June through the end of August—several degrees above the normal averages for those months, the experts said. In the neighborhood around the South Street Wharf, the breezeless air turned more and more fetid as the weeks dragged by. At the ferry dock, one visitor reported, a sewer outlet "belch[ed] forth continually putrid masses of animal and vegetable filth accumulating around its mouth." At low tide, the sun baked this detritus into an unsavory casserole that "exhal[ed] streams of unwholesome and poisonous gases into the surrounding air." All manner of filth carpeted the wharf just north of South Street,

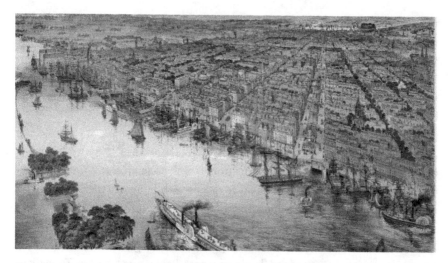

Figure 6. Bird's-eye view of Philadelphia. Lithograph by John Bachmann, 1850. Courtesy of the Free Library of Philadelphia, Rare Book Department / Bridgeman Images.

and Delaware Avenue between Lombard and South (lacking any surface drainage at all) consisted of a steaming block-long porridge of mud and waste. In the claustrophobic alleyways, even more refuse accumulated than in the streets, and accumulated river water stagnated in many a damp, confined cellar (figure 6).[6]

None of this was the best advertisement for a hotel with aspirations to "superior" quality, but then again, most visitors familiar with Philadelphia in the summertime would have been used to such sensations. Forty-eight-year-old Charles Koehler had bought the old Champion House hotel just three years earlier, boasting to prospective guests at the time that he had "fitted up" the place "in a superior manner." He promised them "the best liquors" at the bar and every manner of refreshment that would "deserve public patronage."[7] Charles's family helped him with the business. The Koehlers were a family of culture, education, and ambition. Their future looked bright.

Then came the *Mandarin*. On the evening of Wednesday, July 13, the bark arrived at the wharf immediately above the ferry dock and sewer outlet at South Street, just across the street from the Champion House. Captain Campbell discharged the crew, but he and the first mate stayed with the vessel, sleeping on board and taking their meals at Koehler's hotel. On Saturday the sixteenth, the bark moved up to the next pier, just below Lombard Street, where a crew of longshoremen unloaded its cargo. As soon as the *Mandarin*'s hold was empty, witnesses reported, it gave off "a very offensive smell." On July 19, 18-year-old Joseph Sharp, who drove a furniture-delivery cart from his stand at South Street Wharf, felt a sudden shooting pain behind his eyes and was overcome with chills, then fever. The next day, the same chilly fit and shooting pain struck Captain George Robinson of the brig *Effort*, docked one pier north of the *Mandarin*; Robinson had also been taking his meals at the Champion House.

The first of Charles Koehler's family to feel it was son Thomas, 19 years old and a ship carpenter working on the wharf opposite the tavern.[8] A sharp headache directly behind the eyes, pain shooting from temple to temple. Debilitating backache, intense thirst, sudden lethargy, and malaise. Chills alternating with high fever. The young man's illness progressed rapidly. After a brief respite, the early symptoms would have given way to nausea, vomiting, and bloody or tar-like stools. Hallucinations typically came next, along with increasingly halting and incoherent speech, then delirium. Blood flowing uncontrollably from his nose. Then there was the jaundice—yellowing skin and yellow, bloodshot eyes—that gave the disease its name. Finally would come the horrifying symptom that announced an imminently fatal outcome: huge quantities of black vomit.

That same day, Wednesday, July 20, a German immigrant couple who ran the Red Bank Ferry House at South Street Wharf became ill, as did the second mate of the ship docked between the *Mandarin* and the *Effort*. (Also that same day, the *Mandarin* moved down a few hundred feet to the pier above Almond Street.) Six patients in two days. A week later, all six lay dead.[9]

On Thursday July 21, four more neighborhood residents fell ill. Fanny Martin, the Koehlers' 22-year-old maidservant, fell ill that day and was dead five days later. Thomas's 17-year-old brother, J. M., and 9-year-old sister, Pauline, also fell ill that Thursday. Another resident sickened on Friday, then two more on Saturday—including Captain Campbell—all within two blocks of South Street Wharf, and all with the symptoms of yellow fever. Three of these seven sick people progressed to the stage of black vomit and died, including Frederick Kellogg, the *Mandarin*'s mate. The captain survived, as did J. M. and Pauline Koehler. At this point, even Campbell and Dr. Stokes, who had seen no danger in allowing the *Mandarin* up, could not deny that an extremely virulent illness had spread rapidly in the immediate vicinity of the ship after the discharge of its cargo. After just a few days, the death toll was already at nine.[10]

One day passed without any new illnesses, but ten more people were seized with the same set of symptoms in the week of July 25—all in the same riverfront area. Seven of them died. On Tuesday the twenty-sixth, the Board of Health ordered the *Mandarin* sent down to the cove below the Navy Yard (about a mile south of South Street Wharf) and later back to the Lazaretto to be more fully disinfected. Its bilgewater was to be completely pumped out and replaced with fresh water. Ever mindful of the importance of managing the public's fears, the board noted that the bark's removal would place it "out of sight of the citizens" and put the city "beyond the reach of . . . infection" from it. Noting the filthy condition of the area around South Street Wharf and calling it "a nuisance prejudicial to health," the board also ordered the entire vicinity "thoroughly cleansed and whitewashed" and all cellars drained, cleaned, and disinfected with a chloride solution. A full week's respite followed—the entire city now on high alert, but with no new cases.[11] Had the board acted in time to prevent an all-out epidemic?

It had not.

The reprieve ended with the illness of 22-year-old Mary Williams, who took sick on North Front Street in Northern Liberties, nearly a mile and a half north of South Street Wharf. The next patient, a 20-year-old carpenter named John Williams (no relation to Mary), lived on Almond Street west of Front Street—only 200 or 300 yards from South Street Wharf, but much farther west than any of the previous cases. The disease seemed to have suddenly burst out of the narrow bounds of the originally infected district.

Dr. Wilson Jewell, an 1824 medical graduate of the University of Pennsylvania and fellow of the College of Physicians of Philadelphia, practiced in Philadelphia his entire career and served on the Board of Health in all but two of the twenty years following 1848, including several years as its president. Tall, portly, and unfailingly dignified in his bearing, Jewell exuded authority. But he was no dogmatic localist—in his early years on the board, he pressed for strict quarantine enforcement on several occasions. Jewell tracked the spread of the outbreak in detail as it was happening. Puzzled by the two Williamses, he eventually traced Mary Williams to a boardinghouse on Swanson Street in the deadly zone, where she had lived until August 3 with one of the previous victims. Jewell's interview with John Williams's doctor revealed that it was the young man's custom, in the oppressive heat of summer, to visit Almond Street Wharf in the evening in search of "cool river air." There, Jewell concluded, at the very place recently vacated by the *Mandarin*, John Williams instead found not relief but sickness and finally death.[12]

Jewell's detective work, the removal of the *Mandarin*, and the Board of Health's aggressive cleanup unfortunately did little to stop the fever's spread. Residents who had anywhere else to go fled the area, but the remainder of August saw thirty-eight more cases in the area of South Street Wharf (figure 7), and September brought only an acceleration of the epidemic. Factories near the infected district shut down because their employees were afraid to show up for work. By the time the cold weather arrived in mid-October, 170 Philadelphians had sickened with yellow fever, and an astonishing three-quarters of them (128) had died. Dr. Stokes treated eight yellow fever patients in the Lazaretto hospital that year, and lost only two of them.[13]

Wilson Jewell traced 147 out of 170 cases directly to a small radius around the wharves where the *Mandarin* had lain, between Lombard and Mead Streets. What he learned about each patient's whereabouts led him to conclude that contagion was not a factor in the fever's spread. But what spread it, then? Jewell had also shown that the *Mandarin* was at the South Street Wharf for six days before anyone fell ill, and that 90 percent of the cases occurred after the bark had left the area. Moreover, there had been no illness on board the *Mandarin* between July 9 (when the second of the two sailors died en route to Philadelphia) and July 21, when mate Frederick Kellogg's first symptoms occurred.[14] How, then, could the *Mandarin* be responsible for the epidemic?

Jewell identified the culprit as a localized contamination of the air that could in certain conditions (such as the hot, wet cargo hold or bilgewater of a seagoing vessel from the West Indies) be transported over long distances. Unloading the *Mandarin*'s cargo on July 16, Jewell argued, liberated the "noxious emanations" that had been "latent" in its hold and brought them into contact with "other elements of decomposition existing on shore and in the docks." The lethal combination not only "poisoned the atmosphere of the immediate neighborhood" but persisted there long after the bark departed, its virulence kept alive by the area's continuing heat, damp, and filth.[15]

Jewell's 1853 report on the South Street Wharf epidemic demonstrated an awareness that quarantine could be crucial, but also that it was only one ingredient in an effective recipe for disease prevention.[16] Charles and Forrest Koehler disagreed.

Sometime during that nightmarish week when Thomas, J. M., and Pauline Koehler and Fanny Martin were bedridden and feverish, and the tavern was deserted, Charles Koehler and his oldest son, Forrest, discovered that their family's ordeal could be traced back to the Lazaretto physician's decision to allow the *Mandarin* up on July 13, after only a cursory detention. They were furious. They did not wait to find out whether their loved ones would turn out to be isolated cases or part of a full-scale epidemic; to them, the damage was already done. The carelessness of a common functionary on Tinicum Island, who had probably acquired

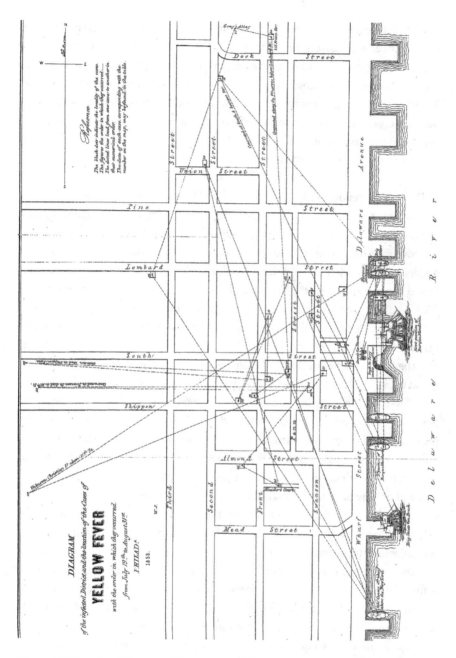

Figure 7. Wilson Jewell's map of the cases in the 1853 yellow fever outbreak near South Street Wharf, purporting to show that each case resulted from close proximity to the contaminated air imported by the bark *Mandarin*. From Philadelphia Board of Health Annual Report, 1853.

his appointment through political machinations rather than through professional competence, was costing this family everything that mattered to them. Why bother having such an elaborate state health law if the officers sworn to enforce it could violate it with impunity? Charles and Forrest Koehler were out for blood. Twenty-three-year-old Forrest was a lawyer, and he immediately took up his pen. If his emotions could have transferred to the ink, it would have burned the page. The newspapers were first; later, if necessary, the authorities could be contacted directly. Someone was going to pay.

In Dr. Jewell's report, he stopped short of saying that Lazaretto physician Stokes should have detained the *Mandarin* for longer than a day, or that quarantine master Van Dusen had failed to thoroughly disinfect the vessel or pump out its bilgewater. But he did not need to say so; the unstated conclusion was apparent. And residents of Philadelphia and the township of Southwark—in this case, the infected district straddled the boundary between the two—did not wait for a report from the Board of Health before reaching their own conclusions. The press got hold of the story on July 27, eight days after Joseph Sharp's first chills and fever and one day after the board ordered the *Mandarin* back to the Lazaretto. It was also the day that Charles Koehler's son Thomas died. The *Public Ledger* reported "great complaint among the residents" about the "apparent neglect of the Quarantine Physician" in allowing the vessel up to the city without proper "cleansing and fumigation." As the deaths continued to mount in those first two weeks, the press reported increasing alarm and "public indignation against the quarantine officers" in the neighborhood. Southwark's Board of Commissioners passed a resolution condemning "the authorities at the Lazaretto" and calling for the removal of "any person who may have neglected his duty."[17]

Stokes and Van Dusen tried to defend themselves in a letter to the *Public Ledger*. The two men were jointly implicated, because it was the quarantine master's responsibility to oversee disinfection operations, and the Lazaretto physician had decision-making authority on all matters related to quarantine. They denied claims that Captain Campbell and Frederick Kellogg were sick when the *Mandarin* left the Lazaretto, and they enumerated the precautions they had taken during the vessel's brief quarantine ("an entire day," in the words of Stokes and Van Dusen). While the two quarantine officers expressed "regret" that disease had broken out in the city, they rejected any notion that "human foresight could have anticipated or prevented it."[18]

But the city needed someone to blame for the return of yellow fever after such a long absence, and Stokes and Van Dusen fit the bill. Charles Koehler in particular needed someone to blame, and he soon became the public face of the distraught South Street Wharf neighborhood.

Charles had an eager and aggressive spokesman in his oldest son, the lawyer. Maybe the young attorney saw an opportunity to make a name for himself in the profession by pressing the case against Stokes and Van Dusen publicly. Surely Forrest's and his father's grief and anger were at work too. Forrest jumped right into the fray, firing off a response to the *Public Ledger* the same day that Stokes and Van Dusen's letter appeared. Calling their defense "exceedingly lame," the younger Koehler accused the officers of "gross neglect and dereliction of duty." He disputed their claim that all aboard were healthy when the *Mandarin* was at the Lazaretto, and pressed the point that a crew member had died of fever just three days before it arrived at the station. Describing the vessel's condition when it came into port as "most filthy and offensive," Forrest scoffed at the notion that one day was enough time for thorough disinfection. But his key argument was a lawyerly one, which left little room for rebuttal: if the *Mandarin* had been fully "cleansed and fumigated" when initially detained, as Stokes and Van Dusen claimed, then why did the Board of Health order it sent back down to the Lazaretto on July 26 "to have that done which the doctor and his assistant say had been done?" If they had *not* disinfected the ship, they were guilty of negligence. If they *had*, they had obviously done a poor job of it, which "would seem to make the negligence . . . more gross and palpable."[19]

The board issued a statement defending Stokes and Van Dusen and expressing full confidence in their performance of their duties. The two accused officers answered Forrest Koehler by disputing his timeline of the captain's and mate's illnesses. They dismissed his letter as having been written "under the influence of a powerful excitement, a condition of mind not very favorable to a true exposition."[20]

The Koehlers were not amused. Had Forrest written under a "powerful excitement"? Perhaps he had, Forrest granted:

> With the conviction on my mind that the sickness and suffering of many of the members of my father's family, the death of a dear and promising brother, with all the hopes of life bright about him—the loss of an excellent domestic in the blossom of her days, and the breaking up of that father's business and the dispersion of his household, were the consequences of [Stokes's and Van Dusen's]

gross and criminal negligence . . . it would be strange indeed to find *me* as cool and calm as *they* would like to appear.

Seizing back the offensive, the young lawyer hinted that the sad story might have future chapters yet to be written. A more lengthy reply to Stokes and Van Dusen, he said, was unnecessary, "as the causes of complaint as to the official misconduct of these gentlemen may be investigated in other quarters, and lead to more definite results than can be reached by newspaper discussion."[21] No official action had yet been taken or announced; Forrest's insinuation suggests that after two weeks of terror and grief, the Koehlers may have turned their anger into action behind the scenes, lobbying judicial authorities to prosecute the quarantine officers.

As the epidemic continued its ravages, the press joined in the call for criminal accountability. "There is great culpability somewhere, and the public ought to know where the blame truly rests," pronounced the *Ledger*. If quarantine laws were not going to be strictly enforced, the paper continued, the Lazaretto "had better be abolished." The Philadelphia County grand jury began to investigate the matter in early September. On the twenty-third of the month, it came back with an indictment against Stokes and Van Dusen for misconduct in office.[22]

On April 3, 1854, as the clerk of Philadelphia's Court of Quarter Sessions read out the state's case against them in *Commonwealth v. Stokes and Van Dusen*, quarantine physician Stokes and quarantine master Van Dusen must have replayed in their minds for the thousandth time the events of that fateful day at the Lazaretto station on Tinicum Island the previous summer. No doubt both men fervently wished the decision, and the outcome, had been different.

Both quarantine officers pleaded not guilty, and challenged the jurisdiction of the Philadelphia authorities, inasmuch as the alleged misconduct occurred at the Lazaretto in Delaware County. Judge Oswald Thompson rebuffed that challenge, ruling that since the *effect* of the defendants' alleged negligence occurred in Philadelphia County, his court had proper jurisdiction. District attorney William Reed charged that Stokes and Van Dusen, knowing that a sailor had died of a malignant fever just a few days earlier, failed in their duty by permitting the *Mandarin* up to the port only "partially purified," in a condition to spread disease in the city. The defendants argued that they had performed all the legally prescribed duties of their offices and had taken all precautions to ensure that the bark was in a healthy condition before allowing it to leave quarantine.[23]

The prosecution zeroed in on the state of the bilgewater, claiming that it was "not properly changed" at the Lazaretto and still "in a state to engender malignant diseases" when the vessel proceeded up to port. Stokes and Van Dusen countered that they had "changed and sweetened" the bilgewater "as much as it was possible to do in a vessel of her construction, laden as she was with sugar and molasses," and that it had become "so offensive" only after the *Mandarin* had arrived in port.[24] They did not mention the countless times Lazaretto physicians had ordered cargo unloaded precisely because thorough disinfection could not be accomplished in a full cargo hold.

Had the bilgewater in fact been flushed out and replaced with clean water at the Lazaretto? There is no evidence that Dr. Wilson Jewell was called as a witness; as a member of the Board of Health he would certainly have done whatever he could to avoid testifying against the quarantine officers and embarrassing the board. His report on the epidemic, however, which thoroughly investigated the bilgewater question, had been presented to the College of Physicians and published serially in the College's *Transactions* in October 1853 and January 1854. Had prosecutor Reed known about the Jewell report, he could well have used it to show that the vessel could not possibly have been "pumped clean" at the Lazaretto, and that Stokes's responsibility was therefore to detain it for as long as necessary to do a thorough job of cleaning and fumigating it.

In the report, Jewell quoted Stokes's original statement to the board on his handling of the *Mandarin*, which detailed all precautions taken without ever mentioning the bilgewater. Jewell also interviewed a well-respected shipwright, who examined the *Mandarin* carefully and pronounced its bilge pumps defective. Their intakes were located more than twelve inches above the keel, "whereas they ought to be at least eight inches lower." As a result, the bilgewater could never be fully flushed out, no matter how often or how long the pumps were activated. Jewell cited the shipwright's assessment to show that the *Mandarin*'s hold had become "impure" *after* being "pumped clean" at the Lazaretto.[25]

It is not hard to imagine Dr. Stokes standing in the courthouse at Sixth and Chestnut Streets, across from Independence Hall, wishing he could still keep that cursed *Mandarin* in quarantine. But he had followed the rules. How could he be held accountable for the horrible chain of events that happened later, after the bark arrived at South Street Wharf? He had worked hard to get where he was, through years of medical school, service to his community, and endless political meetings. Whatever well-placed connections he had were the product of his own hard work. He had a wife and two young children to support.

And now it could all be undone by this capricious prosecution brought about by the tavernkeeper Koehler and his hot-headed lawyer son, neither of whom seemed able to grieve stoically. Both of them were almost certainly in the court that day, staring the doctor down. Their loss was unfortunate, certainly, and regrettable, without a doubt, Stokes might have mused. But to whip the newspapers into a frenzy over some supposed "gross and criminal negligence"? That was going too far. The references to "a dear and promising brother, with all the hopes of life bright about him" and "an excellent domestic in the blossom of her days" were shamefully sentimental.[26] Thomas Jefferson Perkins Stokes might well have believed that it could only be misguided and vengeful to hold someone criminally responsible for something that, under the circumstances, he could not reasonably have foreseen. And he could only hope that the jury would see past such crude appeals and leave the business of quarantine to the duly appointed officials.

After two days of arguments, the case went to the jury. Judge Thompson instructed jurors to consider only two questions: (1) Did the defendants' alleged actions fall within their official duties? and (2) Had they performed those duties? If the Koehlers were present for the verdict the next morning, they were surely surprised and dismayed: Stokes and Van Dusen were acquitted. There would be no satisfaction for the bereaved family, nor for their many neighbors who lost loved ones in the 1853 epidemic. There was only a grim relief for the two quarantine officers, and perhaps for the Board of Health as well, which was spared further embarrassment. One week later Stokes petitioned the Board of Health to pay his legal fees. The board declined, citing the Lazaretto physician's status as a state officer appointed by the governor, and rejecting the notion that it bore any responsibility for an "error of judgment" he may have committed.[27]

The Lazaretto was a victim of its own success. The quarantine-plus-cleanliness strategy that emerged from the Caldwell-Donaldson compromise had endured for half a century, keeping yellow fever away for thirty consecutive years before the *Mandarin's* ill-fated voyage. The predictable result was complacency—perhaps on Dr. Stokes's part, but certainly on the part of ordinary Philadelphians. An outbreak claiming 128 lives would have been almost an afterthought in the days of Benjamin Rush and William Currie, but in 1853—even in a much larger city—it provoked public outrage.

The long absence of yellow fever had given rise to a new public expectation.

Most often grave consequences did not follow a decision to allow a ship to proceed to the city from the Lazaretto. But because they occasionally did, the dreadful memory of past epidemics and the high stakes of this everyday judgment call weighed on every doctor who ever held Stokes's job. Philadelphians wanted the security of quarantine, even if they did not want to be quarantined themselves.

Stokes stayed on at Tinicum Island through the 1854 season as he continued to feel the sting of what seemed to him an unjustified assault on his character. In an effort to clear his name (and perhaps cleanse his conscience), he began writing three books on yellow fever. One volume, he confided to his political patron James Buchanan, was to be an authoritative account of the 1853 epidemic that would vindicate him. In June 1855, Stokes sent his friend the text of a grateful dedication and asked permission to include it in one of the yellow fever books. Buchanan, then serving as minister plenipotentiary in London and considering a run for the White House, gave his consent, but only on the "absolutely required" condition that Stokes delete the phrase "and destined to the high office of Chief Magistrate [US president]." Buchanan considered that his chances of winning would be improved if he avoided appearing to actively seek the office, and sure enough, he went on to win the presidency in 1856. His loyal friend Dr. Stokes, however, never got to see him take the oath of office. Only 40 years old, Stokes died at his Spruce Street home on February 17, 1857, his yellow fever books unfinished.[28] No cause of death was publicly disclosed.

The South Street Wharf epidemic reminded Philadelphians that the question of quarantine was timely and consequential rather than a quaint vestige of a distant era. Those who were detained at the Lazaretto or whose business dealings were affected by quarantine found the practice as bothersome and burdensome as ever. Medical partisans of the exclusively local origin of disease continued to denounce it as a misguided waste of resources. The *Public Ledger*'s editor captured a common sentiment when he called on the authorities to either enforce quarantine fully or abolish it.[29] Inconsistent half-measures satisfied no one.

Dr. Wilson Jewell had chronicled the 1853 epidemic, and he wanted to do something about the maddening, capriciously enforced quarantine laws and regulations in America's port cities. As it turned out, he would use the hoary question of quarantine, with its medieval heritage, as a springboard for creating a modern discipline of public health.

In US ports, merchants faced unpredictable and costly delays that had no basis in the protection of public health. Ports with lax enforcement could benefit unfairly from increased commercial traffic at the expense of their more conscientious rival cities, which then had a financial interest in spreading rumors about incipient epidemics in the ports with lax enforcement. The whole messy business offended Wilson Jewell's sense of rationality and efficiency. In the second half of the nineteenth century, after the tumultuous revolutions across Europe, when the railroad and the telegraph and other technological marvels were shrinking the world and expanding people's sense of possibility, a question as important as quarantine ought to be resolved scientifically, definitively, and uniformly.[30]

What began as a recurring frustration on the Board of Health when witnessing the everyday headaches caused by quarantine grew into a mission: reform America's patchwork health laws by creating a uniform national code that would apply at all ports. Jewell found that the origins of quarantine were bound up with the "false doctrine" of contagion. (He seems not to have recognized that for half a century at his city's Lazaretto, quarantine decisions had often been driven by fears of contaminated cargo and "infection" rather than contagion.) Far from *preventing* epidemics, Jewell claimed, the enforced shipboard isolation that followed from fear of contagion paradoxically *caused* them, as exhausted and malnourished people were crowded together for extended periods in an increasingly foul atmosphere. The existing quarantine laws of his day, he told the Philadelphia County Medical Society, unquestionably confronted commerce with "unnecessary interruptions and unreasonable embarrassments" and amounted to "a vexatious system of taxation upon the merchant and the mariner." It was finally time, in Jewell's view, to bring public policy into line with "the prevailing opinions of the best informed medical men of the present age," all of whom repudiated the notion of contagion. Convinced by his study that a complete repeal of quarantine laws would be unwise, Jewell redoubled his determination to modernize them from top to bottom.[31]

Only a nationwide effort would do. In the fall of 1856, Philadelphia's board approved Jewell's plan to coordinate with the boards of health of other large port cities. Health boards in Boston, New York, Baltimore, and New Orleans unanimously embraced Jewell's proposal for a conference the following spring in Philadelphia. Health authorities across the country, it seemed, shared the same frustrations and considered a joint initiative overdue. Jewell extended the invitation more widely, and on May 13, 1857, seventy-five delegates from ten cities assembled in the old Supreme Court room of Independence Hall for the National Quarantine Convention. Representatives from boards of health, boards of trade, and state and county medical societies attended.[32] This convention agreed on resolutions emphasizing ventilation and disinfection of certain vessels and cargoes, recommending that detention be limited to the medical care of sick passengers and sailors.

Next, Jewell came to the daunting but also thrilling realization that his mission demanded a national network of public health authorities who would meet regularly to discuss and debate the latest developments in medical science and public policy. There was now at stake nothing less than a new nationwide regime of public health. Henceforth known as the National Quarantine and Sanitary Convention, the group would meet annually and would expand its scope beyond quarantine to "sanitary reform" and public health in general. More cities representing more states joined each year through the late 1850s.[33]

Each year, a chorus of scornful and vitriolic complaints rang out—quarantine was "oppressive," "exceedingly faulty," "tyrannical," "absurd," "a commercial curse," and a "barbarity." The whole matter of quarantine was "simply a relic of superstition and ignorance," Dr. John McNulty of New York thundered in 1859, adding that "it has been the means of producing more deaths, ten to one, than it has ever saved lives." Enforcing quarantine at the entrance to New York's harbor, McNulty argued by way of analogy, made as much sense as building "an immense Fire Department at the High Bridge" to protect the city against fire. All agreed that quarantine rested on the erroneous premise of contagion, which had proved itself time and time again incapable of explaining the spread of epidemics. All agreed that to prevent epidemics, local health authorities ought to focus above all on fighting filth and overcrowding.[34]

Still, surprisingly, abolition was out of the question. Only one delegate ever proposed doing away with quarantine entirely. Despite the rhetorical emphasis on contagion and superstition, the convention delegates shared a tacit understanding that the basis of quarantine went beyond fear of contagion per se. No one who had ever inspected a ship laden with decomposing hides or filthy rags, or sloshing with putrid bilgewater, wanted vessels like that to sail directly into port and expose crowded urban neighborhoods to their infection. And there was also the simple fact, raised at the 1859 convention by the respected New York sanitary reformer John Griscom, that quarantine stations routinely received patients with deadly diseases. Griscom noted that the quarantine hospital in New York harbor had seen cases of yellow fever every year, but that there had not been a full-fledged epidemic in the city since 1822. Would the city have been as safe, he asked, if every vessel had been allowed directly into port without inspection or detention? In effect, every year that passed with yellow fever at the station but not in the city proved the value of quarantine.[35]

To a twenty-first-century reader, the proceedings of the quarantine conventions sound hopelessly anecdotal rather than scientific. One after another, the delegates rose to tell the story of a single patient or a single family or a single city block that either escaped or fell victim to one particular outbreak, thereby demonstrating one quality or another of yellow fever or contaminated air or human susceptibility. The delegates reasoned outward from the particular circumstances of individual patients to the means by which disease could be transmitted and, by extension, prevented.

This reasoning seems unscientific today because it differs so starkly from biomedical science, in which laboratory experiments prove that specific bacteria or viruses cause specific diseases—always, everywhere, no matter what—and that they enter the human body only in certain ways (inhaled droplets, food, water, mosquito bites, etc.). But the cumulative anecdotes of the quarantine conventions represent the timeless essence of epidemiology: empirical observation and correlation.[36] Many of the delegates had read most of the published medical literature on yellow fever, which consisted of highly detailed reports of every known outbreak in the world. The science consisted of compiling, comparing, and correlating the accounts, to determine which factors consistently appeared in connection with yellow fever epidemics. Prevention followed logically from the identification of those factors. It was not an *experimental* science, but it was evidence based, methodical, rigorous, and practical.

In New York in 1859 the National Quarantine and Sanitary Convention committees charged with preparing a uniform national health code presented their reports. One year later, the Code of Marine Hygiene was approved by delegates meeting in Boston. The code included general provisions along with some specific to yellow fever, cholera, typhus, and smallpox. It represented the "almost unanimous" conviction of the assembled authorities that, in the case of yellow fever at least, "foul merchandise, clothing, and baggage" were far more likely to spread disease than "the body of the sick afflicted therewith." If yellow fever had occurred during a voyage, the vessel, cargo, and baggage were to be "detained until thoroughly expurgated," any sick landed and treated, and healthy passengers and crew allowed to proceed freely. For all vessels, regardless of the health of passengers and crew, the code prescribed different treatments for three distinct categories of cargo. Subject to mandatory quarantine would be "bedding, personal baggage and dunnage, rags, paper, paper-rags, hides, skins, feathers, hair, and all other remains of animals, woolens, and silks." Cotton, linen, hemp, and cattle would be detainable at the discretion of the officer in charge. All other cargo would be exempt from quarantine. (Coffee was not mentioned.)[37]

The 1860 code marked a triumph of national coordination over intercity rivalries. Its framers had taken a big step toward the recognition of public health as a

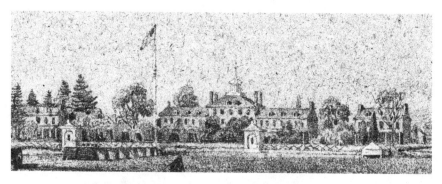

Figure 8. Detail of the Lazaretto seen from the Delaware River in 1856, on the eve of the first National Quarantine Convention in Philadelphia. Drawing by James F. Queen, 1856. Courtesy of the Library of Congress.

public priority, and toward a nationwide health infrastructure. By downplaying the danger of healthy passengers and highlighting the risk posed by foul cargoes, the code also ratified what had become standard practice over the years at Philadelphia's Lazaretto, where healthy passengers were only occasionally detained, and cargo routinely received more attention. The adoption of the code might well have led to uniform enforcement and greater national coordination in matters of public health.

The 1861 convention was scheduled for the last week of May in Cincinnati. Six weeks before it was to be convened, however, the bombardment of Fort Sumter put a temporary end to the union and a permanent end to the National Quarantine and Sanitary Conventions. The 1860 code was a dead letter. Wilson Jewell's vision of a national system of public health science and policy died at Fort Sumter as well. He did not live long enough to see it resurrected eleven years later, when ten men met in New York to form the American Public Health Association. Four of them, including the president, Stephen Smith, were alumni of the quarantine conventions.[38]

After what seemed to be a very public failure of quarantine in 1853 and the successful mobilization of nationwide antiquarantine sentiment on the eve of the Civil War, operations at Philadelphia's Lazaretto continued much as before. The city's quarantine was unpopular but also, seemingly, indispensable.

Less than a decade later, it would face its darkest hour (figure 8).

Chapter Fourteen

The Darkest Hour, 1870

"Exceedingly heavy" explosions of thunder woke Philadelphians on the night of August 10, 1870. Lightning struck houses, barns, and a pair of horses pulling a fire engine in East Falls. The press welcomed the thunderstorm's thorough drenching, which washed away the filth that had accumulated in the streets and gutters and chased away the "noisome odors" that had plagued the city. In the view of the *Philadelphia Inquirer*, the storm was a sanitary blessing: "To the health of the city the storm was equal to an army of physicians," the newspaper exulted. "It has cured more and saved more human beings than the whole medical profession could have done in so short a time."[1]

August's torrential rains came on the heels of a prolonged drought that had significantly lowered the water levels in the Schuylkill and Delaware Rivers. Those rivers did not overflow their banks, but many tributary streams and creeks did, including Darby Creek next to the Lazaretto in Delaware County.[2]

But the quarantine station was awash in tears. Death seemed to be stalking its staff at every turn.

Memories of the Civil War were still fresh, and still painful. The slaughter of Antietam, Shiloh, the Wilderness, and elsewhere had forged a new American attitude toward death. Numb incomprehension now stood in for hopeful acceptance of the Good Death, which for so long had promised meaning and redemption. "Individuals found themselves in a new and different moral universe," as one historian has put it, "one in which unimaginable destruction had become daily experience."[3]

In 1870, the country was still trying to patch itself together after the butchery of that war. The radical phase of the great social experiment that was Reconstruction was at its peak: the Fifteenth Amendment enfranchising Black men

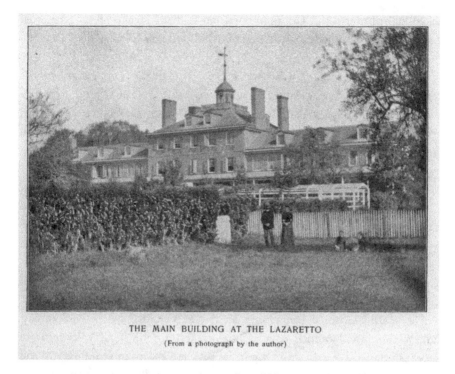

THE MAIN BUILDING AT THE LAZARETTO
(From a photograph by the author)

Figure 9. The Lazaretto's main building in the late 1880s. Photograph in Henry Leffmann, *Under the Yellow Flag* (Philadelphia: G. F. Fell et Societas, 1896).

had just been ratified (though it would be another half century before women won the right to vote). The engines of the nation's industrial might were firing up in earnest. Headlines that summer announced that France and Prussia were preparing for war.

None of these dramatic changes was likely to affect the Lazaretto. And so, as May turned to June and quarantine operations began on Tinicum Island, no one there had any reason to believe that this year at the station would be any more eventful than 1869, when only six patients had been treated in the hospital all season. (All of them recovered.) After all, the outbreak that followed Dr. Stokes's blunder in 1853 was the only time yellow fever had revisited Philadelphia in a half century (figure 9).

But on June 29, 1870, another sweltering day in the heat wave that held Philadelphia in its grip, the brig *Home* arrived from Black River, Jamaica. A bargeman who had worked on the water for nearly six decades said the *Home* was the filthiest vessel he had ever seen.[4] Lazaretto physician William Thompson later reported that "language was inadequate to describe the condition" of the vessel.

The *Home* spelled trouble.

Even in more temperate weather, the Lazaretto's tidal river frontage, with its rank vegetation, often resembled a lowland marsh. The *Home* came to in the inner channel opposite the main building, where Thompson and quarantine master Robert Gartside boarded the vessel for inspection. It carried a cargo of logwood (a product used in dye making) and thirteen bales of what were variously described as foul rags or clean sailcloth clippings.

Thompson soon learned that the brig's captain, John Phillips, had died at sea. The mate and crew, hoping to avoid quarantine, insisted that he had succumbed to a heart attack. J. P. Ellingsworth, the *Home*'s cook, appeared a bit frail, but otherwise the crew seemed healthy despite the vessel's foul condition. All aboard swore that there had been no prevalent illness in Jamaica at the time of departure. Thompson suspected otherwise and ordered the *Home* detained, unloaded, and disinfected. He reported to the Board of Health by the next morning's mail.

The board confirmed Thompson's decision at its daily meeting on Saturday, June 30. But just as caution seemed to be the watchword, small leaks began to appear in the dike of quarantine vigilance. Maybe Thompson and the board had become complacent after so many years without a yellow fever epidemic. Or maybe hindsight makes perfectly reasonable decisions seem reckless. It didn't help that the mate had persuaded the rest of the crew to lie about Captain Phillips's illness and about the presence of yellow fever in Jamaica. Whatever the case, Thompson allowed the *Home*'s river pilot Stephen Bennett to leave the Lazaretto, on the condition that he proceed directly to the Delaware breakwater at Cape Henlopen, where the pilots met seagoing vessels headed upriver. When Bennett reached Wilmington, though, he felt sick. Turning around, he proceeded all the way to Philadelphia. The day after the *Home*'s arrival, second mate George Griffiths took advantage of porous security at the Lazaretto and escaped to his house in the city, near the corner of Swanson and Christian Streets. Five days later, both Bennett and Griffiths were dead. While they were absent, sailor Joseph Elliott of the *Home* fell ill and was admitted to the Lazaretto hospital, where he later recovered. The board voted on Tuesday, July 2, to allow the *Home*'s remaining crew to come up to the city if the Lazaretto physician deemed it safe. Thompson preferred caution and kept the crew for a few more days. He likely had not yet learned of Bennett's and Griffiths's deaths when he incautiously freed the rest of the *Home*'s crew from the Lazaretto on July 7.

Released from quarantine, Frenchman Olivier Pierre went to a sailors' boarding-house at 511 Swanson Street, near South, where he fell ill a few days later. He then moved to another boardinghouse at the other end of Swanson Street, between Queen and Christian. He wasn't admitted to the municipal hospital until July 19. On July 11, three barges arrived to discharge the brig's cargo, with twelve steve-dores aboard. Two days later, the Board of Health voted to allow the barges and stevedores up to the city, as long as the Lazaretto physician deemed it safe. Again opting for caution, however, Thompson ordered barges and crew to remain at the station for the time being.

The captain of the stevedores and the crew of one of the barges, with a load of the *Home*'s logwood, defied the doctor's order and came up to the city, landing at the logwood wharf on Windmill Island in the Delaware just opposite the city's southern riverfront neighborhoods. On Friday, July 15, around the time that the sailor Pierre fell ill in the city, the *Home* was moved to the US Customs House wharf next to the Lazaretto for the unloading of the remainder of its cargo and for disinfection. The *Home* had been at the Lazaretto for seventeen days. In that time, there had been four new illnesses and two deaths. In hindsight, there might still have been time to limit the damage with a full lockdown quarantine, but even that might not have been enough to prevent what came next.

On July 16 and 17, four stevedores and barge crew members who had unloaded the *Home* fell ill and were admitted to the Lazaretto hospital. So far, everyone who had come down with the symptoms of yellow fever had been aboard or in direct contact with the *Home*. But on July 22, when the son of barge captain Thomas Doggett died in the Lazaretto hospital, innkeeper Jacob Pepper's servant and mother-in-law fell ill at his house behind the U.S. Customs station next to the Laz-aretto. Head nurse Fanny Gartrell came down with a fever on July 23 and felt very weak. She was ordered to rest, but (as one newspaper later put it) "her good-ness of heart would not allow her to remain idle, and she soon was tending to the ills of others."[5] There was precedent for the Lazaretto physician and Board of Health declaring the federal customs property under quarantine jurisdiction, and under the circumstances, they would have been justified in including Pepper's house as well. Neither Thompson nor the board apparently saw any reason for de-claring such an emergency. Captain Doggett's wife, also hospitalized at the sta-tion, died the next day.

Four days followed with no new cases and no deaths. Dr. Thompson, his staff, and the Board of Health had reason to hope that the storm had passed. But then Pepper's mother-in-law, Mrs. Ennis, died on Thursday, July 28. Lazaretto matron

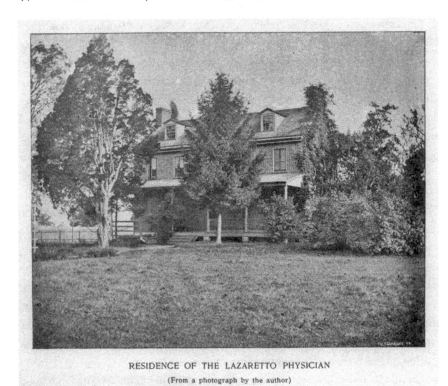

RESIDENCE OF THE LAZARETTO PHYSICIAN
(From a photograph by the author)

Figure 10. The Lazaretto physician's house in the late 1880s. Photograph in Henry Leffmann, *Under the Yellow Flag* (Philadelphia: G. F. Fell et Societas, 1896).

Eve Kugler, wife of the steward Lewis Kugler and effectively co-superintendent of the station's facilities, helped prepare Ennis's body for burial. Washing, dressing, handling the newly lifeless corpse—what task could be sadder, more selfless, or more pious than preparing a body for burial amid a disease outbreak? On Friday, Pepper's servant died; on Saturday, several friends and relatives came to the island to attend Ennis's funeral. On Sunday, Jacob Pepper took sick; and on Monday, August 1, Eve Kugler did, too. What had been a slow trickle of cases limited to those who had boarded the *Home* was turning into a steadier flow that had widened to include Lazaretto staff and neighbors (figure 10).

The station, which had withstood the ship-fever nightmares of many floating cemeteries over the years, was in a state of turmoil and on the verge of collapse. On those stormy days of August 10 and 11, the Lazaretto physician, the quarantine master, and the head nurse died, one after the other. Not since 1808 had a

Lazaretto physician died while serving at the station,* and never before had so many staff and neighbors on the island been stricken.[6] The surviving employees were in terrified disarray and at times turned to outright mutiny. Replacement doctors and nurses were hurriedly recruited with no planning or coordination.[7] The pestilence had even escaped past the fence and into the few houses that stood nearby. That year, yellow fever sickened twenty-nine and killed eighteen in the Lazaretto and its immediate vicinity. Philadelphia's papers fueled city residents' alarm with headlines that screamed, "Pestilence—Terrible Danger Menacing Philadelphia" and "The Black-Vomit at Our Doors."[8] Was this a return to the bad old days?

The Lazaretto epidemic of 1870 was the most minutely documented yellow fever outbreak in Philadelphia's history. The shock of the disease's reappearance for only the second time since 1820 forced the Board of Health to investigate and explain the disaster, and because most of the outbreak occurred on premises controlled by the board, information was easier to come by than it had been in other epidemics. By 1870, too, one of the board's senior members was Dr. René La Roche, an internationally recognized authority on yellow fever who had published a 1,400-page treatise on the disease in 1855 and who was eager for another opportunity to prove that it was not contagious. The board published three detailed reports on the epidemic: one by Dr. H. Earnest Goodman, the port physician who pitched in to help at the Lazaretto during the crisis; one by Dr. J. Howard Taylor, who took over as Lazaretto physician from Dr. Thompson in the middle of the outbreak; and one by La Roche, who closely followed the events as a member of the Board of Health.

In addition to the twenty-nine cases and eighteen deaths at the Lazaretto, seventeen cases (thirteen fatal) occurred in the vicinity of Swanson Street near the wharves, but the city was spared a full-fledged epidemic.[9] A long-term casualty of the 1870 epidemic may have been the Lazaretto itself: the outbreak galvanized public opinion in Delaware County in favor of closing the station and building a new one farther downriver. That outcome, however, was more than twenty years away. The immediate result of the 1870 calamity was a wave of shock and grief unmatched in the Lazaretto's history. In this epidemic, death and chaos shattered the fragile sense of security that had sustained the quarantine station for seventy years.

---

* Dr. James Hall died in 1801; Dr. Nathan Dorsey died in 1806; and Dr. George Buchanan died in 1808.

The first two weeks of August 1870 were the bleakest and most harrowing days in the Lazaretto's history. The total number of patients in the hospital never approached the ship-fever days of 1804 or 1847, but never before had an epidemic felled the station's employees in such numbers so quickly. (The Tinicum station's first three physicians had died while on duty there in 1801, 1806, and 1808, but those deaths, from unreported causes, did not appear to be part of larger disease outbreaks.) Dr. Thompson fell ill on Tuesday, August 2; just as Earnest Goodman, the board's replacement physician, arrived the next day, nurse Fanny Gartrell, who had enjoyed a brief recovery, fell ill again. On Thursday, it was Thompson's daughter Lizzie's turn, followed by his wife, Rebecca, on Friday. On Saturday, August 6, quarantine master Robert Gartside fell ill, along with the Pepper family's housekeeper and a family friend who had attended Mrs. Ennis's funeral. Jacob Pepper died on Sunday.

It seemed that no one was safe. The dread of wondering who would be next vied with the anguish of losing trusted friends, co-workers, and loved ones forever. Eve Kugler died on Monday the eighth, William Thompson and Fanny Gartrell on Wednesday the tenth, and Robert Gartside on Friday the twelfth. In five days, yellow fever had claimed four of the Lazaretto's five highest-ranking employees. Only steward Lewis Kugler remained, and he was now a grief-stricken widower.

Robert Gartside was an ordinary civil servant, not a hero. He wasn't even the fourth most prominent Gartside in the county: In Henry Ashmead's 1884 *History of Delaware County, Pennsylvania*, Robert's father and three of his younger brothers each merited a full-page portrait and biographical entry. They owned textile mills in Chester that employed 124 people in the 1880s. They served on many business and civic boards, and one even had a public school named after him.[10] Robert Gartside may not have done anything heroic, but he was appointed quarantine master to protect the people of Philadelphia. He showed up and did his job in the face of uncertainty and at no small personal risk. When he was first appointed, in 1861, a schooner arrived in Philadelphia with smallpox aboard on April 1, two months before the opening of quarantine season. It was sent to the Lazaretto, and Gartside was called in to disinfect the vessel and "attend to the sick" at the hospital.[11] He must have been blindsided by this unusual request, outside his normally prescribed duties and schedule, but he did it. And even beyond the quality of his work, his loss was deeply felt by friends, family, and colleagues. Gartside's friends Thomas Cooper and D. A. Vernon, editors of the *Delaware County American*, occasionally made favorable mention of the quarantine master in their newspaper, even praising his wife's planked shad just two months before the 1870 outbreak. When he died, Cooper and Vernon departed from the solemn tone of the formulaic nineteenth-century obituary to share the depth of their shock and grief. They quoted Shakespeare and lamented that they had been led to believe that their friend's illness was only a mild case: "It is indeed difficult to believe, and most painful to know, that he whom we met, it seems, but a few days ago in the full blush and glow of health and strength, with his beaming genial smile, warm, cordial and hearty manner, has passed into the final 'bourne,' and that 'the places which knew him shall know him no more forever.'"[12] Their sadness was frank and raw. The sudden and devastating loss of this unexceptional man reminds us of the strong personal ties that bind members of a community together and that damage the social fabric when they are so abruptly sundered. Epidemics simply amplify this damage.

Seamen George Griffiths and Olivier Pierre, who left the brig at the Lazaretto, took sick at boardinghouses along Swanson Street near the wharves in Southwark, where river pilot Stephen Bennett also ended up. These cases occurred in early to mid-July; only Pierre recovered. A month later, just as the Lazaretto staff were being carried off one by one, a new cluster of cases began to appear around Swanson Street. The first was night customs inspector Alexander Campbell, who showed signs of yellow fever on August 8 and died four days later. Exactly a month after Campbell fell ill, the seventeenth and last case of the Swanson Street outbreak occurred; its thirteenth and last death occurred a week after that, on September 15.

William F. Carpenter was hired as a nurse at the height of the emergency in early August, when hands were scarce, to attend to the gardener William Dillmore. Carpenter got sick with yellow fever and suffered in the Lazaretto hospital for a full month. Described as "old, fat, feeble" and "broken in health," he nevertheless found the strength to beat the disease. Carpenter's discharge (recorded as "cured") on September 24 marked the end of the Lazaretto epidemic.

That same day, in a filthy and overcrowded tenement on Penn Street, a 32-year-old Irish immigrant named Michael Dowlin also arose from his sickbed. At the end of a long, ruthlessly hot summer, in late September the temperature was still lingering in the eighties.[13] The familiar stew of mud, garbage, manure, and other urban offal continued to ripen in the narrow alleyways. But the epidemic had burned itself out. Two days later, 19-year-old Mary Ann Stanley returned to her home two blocks from Dowlin's at Swanson and South, after having spent

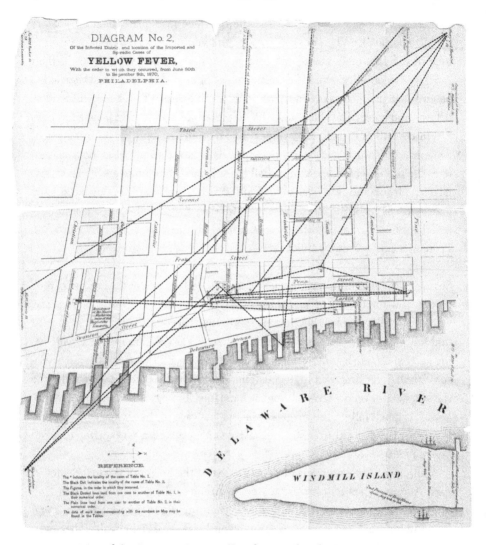

Figure 11. Map of the Swanson Street yellow fever outbreak in 1870, connecting each case in the city (including patients at two hospitals in the upper right corner of the map) to the Lazaretto or to the brig *Home*. Image modified to show dotted lines more clearly. From Philadelphia Board of Health Annual Report, 1870.

nearly three weeks battling yellow fever in the municipal hospital. Dowlin and Stanley were the last two cases in the Swanson Street outbreak (figure 11). Eighty-nine days after the foul brig from Jamaica had stopped at the Lazaretto for inspection, the long parade of sickness and death had finally ended.

The combined death toll of the Lazaretto and Swanson Street outbreaks was thirty-one. Only fifteen patients recovered. Everyone connected with the Lazaretto was forced to confront the mortal risk associated with the work there, and to reflect on and commemorate the sacrifice of their fallen colleagues. The toll taken on the city's morale and the Board of Health's reputation is harder to calculate.

Day after day, year after year, behind-the-scenes labor by unseen and unsung men and women made the Lazaretto work. When patients or staff needed to be fed, when laundry needed to be washed, when bodies needed to be prepared for burial, it was usually women like 52-year-old matron Eve Kugler who did the work or otherwise made sure it got done. If the laborious unloading and disinfection of vessels and cargoes contributed to the retreat of yellow fever from Philadelphia, then it was in part thanks to the work of quarantine masters like Robert Gartside. And the "care cure"—food, drink, clean clothing and bedding, and supportive treatment—depended on the thankless and unpleasant physical work of nurses like Fanny Gartrell.

As the body count began to rise, those running the Lazaretto, including substitute doctors Goodman and Taylor, must have sensed the futility of their efforts, but they threw themselves unquestioningly into the breach, even when the cost was impossibly high. Three women in particular distinguished themselves for their dependability and dedication to duty—their integrity, in other words—during the 1870 epidemic. Two of them paid for their dedication with their lives.

Matron Kugler and her husband, Lewis, had served at the Lazaretto for at least five years when the yellow fever struck. Dr. Taylor's report was unusually effusive in her regard, and his eulogy for "this estimable lady" was quoted and seconded in La Roche's account of the epidemic:

> Zealous in good works, kind, attentive and self-sacrificing to a fault, where sickness and trouble existed, she gave her time and services freely both day and night, as well to her afflicted neighbors as to the wants of the patients in the hospital; and it may be truly said of her that she was always found at the post of danger, never shrinking from any duty wherein it was possible to relieve suffering, or to assist at the last sad rites preceding sepulture. Her many excellent qualities and unvarying kindness will long be held in grateful remembrance by those whose privilege it was to know her under circumstances which called forth the exercise of those virtues which so preeminently marked her life.[14]

Nurse Fanny Gartrell had cared for patients at the Lazaretto for thirteen years. Among them were sixty-two yellow fever patients, fifty-one of whom survived. Nursing, then as now, was intimate, dirty, often backbreaking work. Much of it was endless drudgery: dust, clean, wash, and repeat. After the clothing and the linens, there were the soiled dressings and poultice cloths. Nurses carried heavy wooden trays of food and drink and medicines up and down stairs. Patients' even heavier bodies also needed to be lifted and turned in bed. What nurses today call "body work" included how to apply blisters and care for the irritated skin afterward, and how to administer douches and enemas. It also involved cleaning sweat, blood, urine, feces, and vomit off patients' bodies. Lazaretto physicians had nurses collect the black vomit of yellow fever patients in tumblers for inspection, with the predictable result that hands and clothes ended up covered in vomit. Nurses often needed to know how to prepare specially prescribed diets and a variety of poultices or compresses, and they also needed to master the self-control that would allow them to suppress their fear of contagion and their sheer disgust provoked by intimate contact. When patients screamed at them or demanded constant attention, nurses were expected to swallow hard and continue working. They often slept in the same crowded rooms with their patients.[15]

Fanny Gartrell left no record of how she felt about her work, but she kept doing it until she couldn't do it anymore.

The final heroine of the 1870 epidemic survived her illness, which she contracted while working at the Lazaretto not as a hired employee, but as a concerned then grieving visitor turned impromptu volunteer. It was another sweltering 92-degree day when Mary Riddle of Philadelphia arrived at the Lazaretto on August 7. Mrs. Riddle had come to visit her friend Eve Kugler, whom she had visited several times before at the station. This time, she found utter chaos. Discipline had broken down entirely. No fewer than four physicians (Goodman, Taylor, and the Chester doctors J. F. M. Forwood and William B. Ulrich) came and went from day to day, quarreling among themselves about the proper treatment of yellow fever. The board scrambled to find emergency nurses, but even the higher wages they offered succeeded in recruiting only a few old or infirm candidates (including D. C. McGuinn and Carpenter, who soon became patients themselves). The remaining healthy employees were terrified and demoralized.[16]

Fifty-year-old Mary Riddle—her occupation listed on the census as "Keeping House"—lived with her 17-year-old daughter, Bessie, and her 13-year-old son,

Robert, in a rowhouse on 12th Street near Pine in central Philadelphia. "An elegant and accomplished lady" (in one newspaper's words), she was the widow of Robert Riddle, a Pittsburgh banker and newspaper publisher who served a term as mayor of that city in the 1850s and was involved in the founding of the Republican Party. Robert died of "inflammatory rheumatism" in 1858, and Mary then moved with her six children to Philadelphia. The four oldest had grown up and moved away by the time Mary learned of her friend Eve Kugler's illness in August 1870.[17]

Mary may have intended to nurse her friend when she left the city for the Lazaretto on August 7, the day after the *Home* returned there from its brief and ill-advised trip to Windmill Island. Perhaps she had learned of the growing number of yellow fever cases there and thought the staff might need help, or perhaps she simply wanted to pay a visit to a sick friend. Whatever the case, Eve died the very next day.[18] At a time when most bereaved friends might have been immobilized by grief, or by the terrifying prospect of a rapidly snowballing epidemic, Mary Riddle instead leapt into action.

With no official authority, she took control of the frightened and rebellious staff and delegated responsibility for the tedious but critical work of administering, cleaning, and feeding a hospital in crisis. When a job needed to be done and no one else was available, she did it herself. She personally cooked for more than thirty people. When the Lazaretto's gardener, William Dillmore, took sick on the day Eve Kugler died, Mary Riddle nursed him. She kept up this regimen for a week—one of the deadliest weeks in the history of the Lazaretto, with an average of one death every day—until Dillmore died. She returned to the city, only to fall ill herself three days later. Her case proved to be a mild one, however, and she recovered.[19]

The press, desperate to extract a morsel of uplifting news from the dismal disarray of the Lazaretto epidemic, eventually got wind of the story. The *Philadelphia Sunday Dispatch* and the *Delaware County American* hailed Mary Riddle as "a heroine at the Lazaretto," praising her "courage" and "devotion." Her noble self-sacrifice, like that of Eve Kugler and Fanny Gartrell, fit neatly within the prescribed feminine virtues of the age. She departed from the Victorian script in assuming a leadership role when she took control of the Lazaretto's daily operations, but this act of self-assertion was only temporary. "It is eminently proper that women should record the doings and the sufferings of sister women in the cause of humanity," wrote the "Woman Department" of the *Dispatch*. The paper challenged its male readers to match Mary Riddle's courage: "You may boast of your acts of heroism, and of your deeds of daring; but it requires a nobler heroism, a more sublime courage than any man is possessed of, to risk life at the sick-bed of strangers, leaving, with full faith, dear and dependent ones in the merciful hands of God."[20]

In these three women—the kind, devout, and self-sacrificing Eve Kugler; Fanny Gartrell, singled out by Dr. Taylor in his report for "a conscientiousness which secured to her the confidence of the various medical officers at the station, and the uninterrupted approval of the Board of Health"; and Mary Riddle, whose bond of friendship, respect, mutual obligation, and love linked her to Eve Kugler and her circle—the desolating Lazaretto epidemic of 1870 had found, if not heroes, at least figures worthy of respect and admiration.[21]

Reading through La Roche's, Goodman's, and Taylor's reports, trying to piece together the progress of the 1870 epidemic, day by day, it's hard to resist reinterpreting the outbreak based on the science of viruses, mosquitoes, and incubation periods. How did it *really* spread? What was the *true* explanation? But these are the wrong questions if we want to understand why things happened the way they did at the time. How was the epidemic experienced by the patients, nurses, doctors, and terrified onlookers? Why did the various people involved do what they did before, during, and after the outbreak? What did the ordeal mean in the larger context of local and national life at the time? None of these questions can be answered if we see the story through the lens of the virus-and-mosquito theory of yellow fever. If a future historian were to try to tell the story of our lives from the perspective of a worldview that hasn't been dreamed of yet, would that history tell the truth?

A different approach may better capture what happened in 1870 and why: telling the story in three different voices, taking three different perspectives, each voice representing a different theory about the causes and spread of yellow fever as of 1870: one contagionist, one localist, and one based on imported contamination.[22] All three would be considered unscientific nonsense today, but each of the three explanations fits the observed facts of the epidemic reasonably well, and each was internally consistent and coherent. None of the three could predict when or where the next outbreak would strike—even the science of viruses and mosquitoes can't do that—but all three could have predicted the kind of environment and circumstances in which it would happen. Telling the same story three ways shows that for these purposes, multiple competing scientific doctrines can all be valid, even when later scientific developments prove all of them wrong. Taking these bygone perspectives seriously helps us see why quarantine as practiced at the Lazaretto made sense.

∽∾∾

1870: CONTAGION

In the contagionists' view, yellow fever is often spread directly from person to person, and has always arrived in Philadelphia aboard ships sailing from the West Indies and the Spanish Main. The illustrious William Currie was right about this terrible disease, and the so-called experts today who deny that it is contagious would do well to heed his wisdom. "Many inconveniencies and evils arise from the dread of contagion when it does not exist," Dr. Currie admitted in 1800, but he added that "still greater inconveniencies and injuries are the consequence of believing that there is no danger in visiting and attending the sick, when the disease *is* contagious."[23] This epidemic once again proved him right. The whole episode unfolded as a chain of person-to-person transmissions, either through direct contact or indirectly through personal effects that had absorbed the disease poison from a sick person's body. Currie emphasized the danger of indirect contagion or fomite transmission in his writings on yellow fever. When transported even over long distances in confined air, porous materials that had absorbed "the atmosphere that surrounds the sick" could produce the "same effect as an immediate communication with the sick themselves."[24]

The deaths at the Lazaretto and in the neighborhood of Swanson Street in the city should be blamed on the imprudence of the quarantine authorities, who failed to strictly isolate the brig's crew and their effects at the Lazaretto. The patient at the origin of the epidemic was J. P. Ellingsworth, the *Home*'s cook and steward, who fell ill at sea around June 10. He must have contracted the disease from someone on land shortly before the brig's departure from Black River on June 3. John Phillips, the *Home*'s captain, was the next case; his symptoms arose at sea around June 16 or 17 after he had acquired the disease either from someone in Jamaica or, more likely, from his cook, Ellingsworth. Phillips succumbed and was given a watery funeral on June 24 or 25, when the vessel was still quite a distance from Philadelphia. Upon arrival at the Lazaretto on June 29, Dr. Thompson found Ellingsworth "just about recovered."

Meanwhile, as the *Home* neared the Lazaretto, the cook transmitted the disease to Stephen Bennett, the Delaware River pilot, and to his shipmates George Griffiths (who "absconded" to the Swanson Street neighborhood shortly after arriving at the Lazaretto), Joseph Elliott, and Olivier Pierre. Thompson allowed the remaining healthy *Home* crew members, including Pierre, to leave the Lazaretto on July 7. Pierre fell ill the next day at a boardinghouse on Swanson Street. A gap in the chain of transmission follows the seamen's departure, as the next recorded cases did not occur until July 17 at the Lazaretto. This delay can be explained by an unusually lengthy incubation period or by an intervening case among the Lazaretto employees or visitors that went undiagnosed—perhaps one of the bargemen engaged in the unloading and disinfection of the brig. Alternatively, personal effects left behind by one of the *Home* patients may have retained the yellow fever poison and spread the disease a week or more later.

In either case, the disease was transmitted next to the crew of the three barges that arrived at the Lazaretto on July 11 to unload the *Home*'s cargo. Three stevedores and a cook fell ill around July 17 and were admitted to the Lazaretto hospital, where two of them later died. Either they or, more likely, the undiagnosed intermediate case had contact with members of Jacob Pepper's household next door to the Lazaretto. Several members of that family took sick around July 20. On July 24, the captain of one of the cargo barges was admitted to the station's hospital, having probably taken sick after contact with the other infected stevedores.

Soon thereafter, Jacob Pepper contracted the disease from his servant or his mother-in-law, and the mother-in-law's funeral spread the illness to at least two of the mourners. The first week of August saw the rate of transmission accelerate, as Dr. Thompson fell ill along with his wife and daughter. At this point, so many potential sources of contagion were active within these two adjacent properties that establishing clear chains of transmission is impossible. Mary Riddle, who arrived from Philadelphia to attend to her friend Eve Kugler, also helped nurse the Lazaretto's gardener, William Dillmore, and she too took the contagion at the Lazaretto. Dillmore's brother-in-law William Hess helped with the gardening duties at the Lazaretto for ten days in late July, and he contracted the disease as well. The melancholy succession of fatalities among Lazaretto employees in mid-August marked the beginning of the end of the Lazaretto outbreak. Five more people in the Lazaretto or its vicinity fell ill in the last week of August; most of their cases were mild, but one was fatal. D. C. McGuinn had been hired at the height of the crisis to nurse Robert Gartside. On September 8, 1870, this most dangerous occupation took McGuinn's life, thus bringing an end to the chain of contagion that had desolated the quarantine station.

There may be some who infer from the clustering of yellow fever cases around the Lazaretto and in the city along Swanson and Penn Streets between Pine and Christian that they were dealing with two distinct outbreaks of strictly local origin. Nothing could be further from the truth. What Dr. Goodman called "the Swanson Street Epidemic of 1870" was in fact nothing more than an extension of the Lazaretto epidemic by means of direct contagion. Griffiths had taken the contagion while at sea, and took sick on Swanson Street a few days after leaving quarantine on June 30. Pierre bedded down in boardinghouses on Swanson Street. By mid-July—even if they had not moved from their beds once ill—Griffiths and Pierre alone had sown yellow fever along the entire length of Swanson Street.

Alexander Campbell had suffered diarrhea for several weeks, and it is possible that Pierre transmitted the disease to him. No obvious contact between the two men can be determined, as they seem to have been no closer than half a mile from each other during Pierre's illness. A more likely explanation is an undiagnosed case on Swanson Street, someone who acquired the fever from Pierre and transmitted it to Campbell, who frequented a tavern on Swanson shortly before his illness. Fifteen of the remaining sixteen cases in this outbreak occurred within the roughly four city blocks of the wharf district along Swanson, Larkin, and Penn Streets between Pine and Mead. The bustle and crowding of this neighborhood is tailor-made for contagion.

The contagious nature of the Lazaretto outbreak and its Swanson Street offshoot is clearly demonstrated by the chains of contact linking the patients. It is well known that a period of variable duration elapses between the act of transmission and the appearance of yellow fever symptoms in the new case. In most of the 1870 cases, this incubation interval appears to have lasted no more than a week. This delay caused some authorities to erroneously deny contagion. Moreover, one must avoid being misled by circumstances in which those attending closely to a yellow fever patient do not appear to acquire the disease. Contagion need not be "permanent and always existing" to be a real threat, Dr. Currie reminded us years ago. It often "arises occasionally in certain climates and situations," and to deny it because some escape its clutches is a dangerous fallacy—one that is unfortunately all too common today among the aristocracy of the medical profession.[25]

1870: LOCAL ORIGIN

In the localist's view, yellow fever didn't come from the brig *Home*—it came from home. This disease originated locally, as it always has. Contagionism is nothing but superstitious bunk. It is a relic of the Dark Ages, and in this scientific era, all respected medical authorities concur in rejecting it. More than a century of carefully documented experience with yellow fever epidemics in the West Indies and in North America have taught us the same lesson over and over: this late-summer scourge is strictly of local origin and arises in crowded, filthy neighborhoods or low-lying wetlands during prolonged hot weather, especially after heavy rains.

The Lazaretto site on Tinicum Island has been plagued from the beginning by the encroachment of a wide marsh on its own riverfront. The Delaware is a tidal river at Tinicum, and the island is prone to marsh formation. The Board of Health itself acknowledged that this marsh "renders the site . . . unhealthy" and "has caused sickness to prevail among the officers and men stationed there." It blames the US Customs wharf next to the Lazaretto's western edge, which extends a considerable distance into the river and was built without sluices or channels to allow tidal flow to wash the shore. The resulting alluvial deposits from the ebb tide have created the marsh along the front of the Lazaretto. Others blame the board for sinking a hulk to serve as a boathouse on the eastern edge of the riverfront. It has blocked the tidal flow from cleansing the shore, and it collects deposits from the flood tide in front of the Lazaretto.[26]

The marsh is known to produce malarial emanations, and visitors and residents alike have remarked on the "effluvia" that arise from its "rank vegetation" at low tide on hot late-summer days. When one adds to these more or less permanent dangers the extreme circumstances that prevailed in 1870, the cause of the epidemic is no mystery. The Board of Health's experts acknowledged that after the flooding spring rains of 1870 and "the most intensely hot weather" that had been seen in more than eighty years, "everything seemed combined to make up this sad history."[27]

The Swanson Street outbreak is just as easy to explain. This neighborhood is the heart of the city's overcrowded, filthy wharfside district. Its boarding-houses and taverns teem with the dissolute sort who neglect cleanliness and always seem to provide fodder for epidemics. In fact, this area is immediately adjacent to the South Street Wharf, the epicenter of the 1853 yellow fever epidemic that was blamed on the decision to allow the bark *Mandarin* to proceed to the city.[28]

The Board of Health's official record of yellow fever cases in the vicinity of Swanson Street in 1870 includes notations such as "Lived filthily," "House dirty and overcrowded," and (in three cases) "Locality filthy; house over-crowded." When port physician Goodman visited Swanson Street, he found the conditions there "unfavorable for health" and blamed the outbreak on the "state of the weather, its excessive continued heat . . . [and] the neglected, filthy condition of . . . this locality." Only the sanitary measures ordered by the board, including street cleaning, privy disinfection, and burial of the victims put an end to this outbreak.[29] When the highly unusual weather and the distinctive physical characteristics of the two localities are taken into consideration, there can be little doubt that local conditions generated both outbreaks of yellow fever in 1870.

1870: IMPORTED CONTAMINATION

Yellow fever is not, strictly speaking, contagious. It *can* arise locally from filth under certain weather conditions, but it can also be imported from the tropics in the unventilated cargo holds of vessels coming from infected ports. One expert on this disease, whose authority is unrivaled in the entire world, is a Philadelphian, member of the Board of Health, and longtime fellow of the College of Physicians, Dr. René La Roche. His two-volume 1855 treatise, *Yellow Fever, Considered in Its Historical, Pathological, Etiological, and Therapeutical Relations*, is the most detailed and exhaustive compendium of knowledge about this disease ever assembled.[30] It compiles evidence from scores of epidemics over two centuries in a definitive and systematic refutation of the contagionist doctrine. It is the last word on the subject—or it would be, if new epidemics weren't continuing to offer us new information. The Lazaretto epidemic of 1870 was especially well reported and studied, as many cases occurred at the quarantine station under the aegis of the Board of Health. The reports were filed with the Board of Health by physicians acting on its behalf: the port physician Dr. Goodman, who investigated the Swanson Street outbreak; Dr. Taylor, who replaced Dr. Thompson as Lazaretto physician; and Dr. La Roche, whose expertise is unquestioned.

Few errors are more damaging to the health of our city—indeed, our entire country—than that of ascribing to our periodic epidemic diseases the property of contagion. This superstitious belief sows needless panic among the credulous masses, leads caregivers to abandon their patients, and diverts attention from the true sanitary imperative: public and private cleanliness. In the utter absence of that cardinal virtue can be found the origin and cause of the 1870 yellow fever epidemic aboard the brig Home.

Physicians tell us that in many cases, the "morbific fermentative agent" of what they call "zymotic diseases" consists of microscopic organized biological entities. In other words, the disease-causing principle is a tiny living being. Whether this is the case for yellow fever or not matters little as a practical concern. Whatever the precise nature of the agent, the febrile poison likely saturated the air in the port of Black River, Jamaica, when the Home departed for Philadelphia, and it permeated the vessel and its hold. It is also possible that the poison was generated aboard during the voyage, as the vessel was indescribably filthy when it arrived at the Lazaretto. It is not uncommon for cases of this disease to appear during an ocean journey without any apparent connection to illnesses at the port of departure.[31] Thus the Home's cook, Mr. Ellingsworth, and Captain Phillips sickened at sea from exposure to the shipborne poison, and the captain became the first fatality of the Lazaretto epidemic before even reaching the station.

The contamination took longer to affect three of their crewmates (Elliott, Pierre, and Griffiths), who fell ill (along with the pilot Mr. Bennett) after arriving in Philadelphia. The outbreak accelerated and intensified, however, only after the critical moment when the Home's cargo hatches were opened on July 13 or 14. Indeed, Dr. Goodman identified this as the time when "the epidemic may be said to have fairly commenced," and Dr. La Roche found that the disease "became more rife and assumed a disposition to spread" from that moment forward. This is no surprise, as yellow fever often makes its initial appearance and takes a more severe form near the main hatchway and pumps of a vessel. Filth accumulates and the heat is most intense at those locations. Furthermore, during the unloading of the cargo on July 15, more than 500 pounds of filthy rags were found stowed in the Home's cabin. Dr. Thompson ordered them burned, but whether the poison originated in

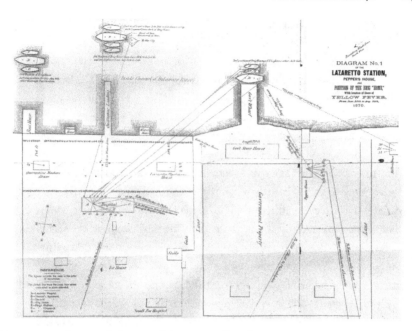

Figure 12. René La Roche's map of the 1870 yellow fever outbreak at the Lazaretto, purporting to show that each new case was closely downwind from the brig *Home* at the time of infection. From Philadelphia Board of Health Annual Report, 1870.

the rags or in the cargo hold, the stevedores had already been exposed to the infection—that is, to the contaminated air.[32]

From the July 16 to July 24, at least one person fell ill at the Lazaretto every day. Dr. La Roche's exhaustive research has uncovered many instances in which "morbific effluvia wafted ashore" from an infected ship and, "through the agency of the wind," sickened even people who had no direct contact with the vessel itself. This appears to have been the case at the Lazaretto. "Appears" is perhaps putting it too weakly, and here is where immense erudition met sheer genius in Dr. La Roche's report. The circumstances of the Lazaretto outbreak presented the author with an abundance of detailed information about each case and about the day-to-day movements of the patients and the *Home.* The doctor transformed this profusion of anecdotal narration into a single eloquent image: a map of the epidemic (figure 12).[33]

The brilliance of the doctor's map lies in its superimposition of time on space. The successive positions of the *Home* are indicated at the corresponding map locations, as are the positions of the barges alongside the brig during the unloading of cargo. Each patient is indicated by a number, which represents his or her position in the overall sequence of cases; the numbers are displayed at the location where the patient spent most of his or her time shortly before experiencing symptoms. An inconspicuous arrow accompanied by five small words in the upper right corner of the map unlocks the entire mystery quietly, without fanfare: "Prevailing Winds from South West." Only the translation from text to map could show it: virtually every patient had been downwind and within 200 yards of the *Home* shortly before falling ill. (The Pepper house and the Miller house next door stood south-by-southeast and southeast of the brig, respectively; the winds may have temporarily shifted for a day or two, or those patients may have been infected while on the Lazaretto property, as some of them were known to spend time there.) This simple illustration closes the case.

And what of the Swanson Street cases? Any putative connection between the Swanson Street cases and the Lazaretto or the *Home* is, on careful investigation, simply untenable. On the other hand, the area in question is notoriously unclean, its courts and alleys "narrow, damp, close-crowded, ill-ventilated, and filthy," in the words of Dr. La Roche's report. Its residents are "reckless, improvident, and intemperate." At the time of the outbreak in early August, the alleys and gutters were "in a most filthy state, devoid of everything like proper paving, filled with decomposing rubbish and animal and vegetable refuse from which issued . . . an insufferable stench." The average daily high temperature in the city during July and early August was between 85 and 87 degrees. After the unusually wet spring, the same conditions that had prevailed during the city's many previous epidemics in the wharfside districts were once again present. The conclusion is inescapable: the Swanson Street outbreak was strictly local in origin and unconnected to the Lazaretto epidemic.[34]

⌒∞⌒

During the yellow fever outbreak of 1870, nobody knew that it would be the last one in Philadelphia's history. It might just as well have been the first in a new wave of assaults, or the herald of a shift in the disease's ravages toward smaller communities. Residents of Delaware County took notice with alarm, as did Philadelphians. The death toll this time had been fairly modest, but all wondered what would happen next time. Very few people alive in the 1870s remembered the devastating epidemics of the 1790s, but 1870 soon weighed heavily on many minds, as a potential harbinger of disasters to come, and as a cautionary tale urging continued vigilance.

Chapter Fifteen

Quarantine, a Political Minefield

When central Pennsylvania lawyer and Civil War hero James A. Beaver won the governorship in 1886, he earned more than just the opportunity to preside over the political machinery of the nation's second-largest state. He also won the power of patronage—the spoils of victory. Dozens of positions all over the state were filled by gubernatorial appointment, from cabinet secretaries to judges and county sheriffs, from mine inspectors and railroad inspectors to the members of the Board of Fisheries and the keeper of the Harrisburg arsenal. Every job came with a salary, and every appointment came with a flurry of applications, jockeying for the governor's attention, and behind-the-scenes negotiations.

If governor-elect Beaver had only paid attention to the parade of past Lazaretto physicians, he would have known that the post could be a political minefield. James Mease was the first doctor appointed as resident physician at the old quarantine station on State Island, in 1795. His willingness to seek waivers, exemptions, and relaxations of quarantine regulations for ships at the station kept him in hot water with the Board of Health, and when yellow fever returned in 1797, some in the press pointed the finger at Mease for allowing sickly vessels up to the port. His decision to allow the brig *Pilgrim* from Port-au-Prince, Saint-Domingue (now Haiti), to bypass quarantine at State Island and sail past the city to Burlington, New Jersey, did not help matters. Critics began to allege that, like his teacher Benjamin Rush, the doctor did not even *believe* in quarantine. Mease's denials failed to convince the board, which maneuvered to oust him from the job before the 1798 quarantine season. Mease responded by publicly denouncing the quarantine laws and proclaiming his conviction that yellow fever always originated locally.[1]

James Hall, the first physician at the Lazaretto on Tinicum Island, died after less than a full quarantine season in 1801. Michael Leib, Governor Thomas McKean's choice to succeed Hall, opted to serve in the House of Representatives in Washington rather than to accept the post. Next up was Nathan Dorsey, who served until he too died of unknown causes, in 1806. McKean's next choice for the sensitive quarantine job was his son-in-law, George Buchanan of Maryland. The appointment ignited a partisan blaze that threatened to bring down the imperious governor. McKean, who tapped more than a dozen relatives to serve in state office, had been feuding with the Leib faction of the Democratic-Republican Party and had alienated many former supporters of every political stripe through his punitive use of executive powers.

Leib's ally William Duane, editor of the *Aurora*, wryly asked why, instead of Buchanan, a Pennsylvania doctor could not be found for the job, and then answered his own question: because "there were none of them the governor's relations—people talk of Bonaparte providing for his relations!" "The reins of empire drop from King Tom's hands in a couple of short years," Duane continued, "and he must make hay while the sun shines." The *Philadelphia Gazette* thundered, "The governor, in thus providing for his family, contrary to the wish and expectation of the community, does no more than evince the supreme contempt in which he holds public opinion!!!" Duane and Leib set out to impeach McKean on six counts, including the Lazaretto appointment, but the governor, mounting a lawyerly defense and maneuvering behind the scenes, managed to survive—by just a few votes. When after just two years on Tinicum Island, George Buchanan became the third consecutive Lazaretto physician to die while on duty at the station, the job may no longer have been seen as such a desirable patronage appointment.[2]

Joel Sutherland lasted only one quarantine season as Lazaretto physician, but it was not illness that did him in. It was an acute case of candor complicated by indiscretion on the part of a young man in a hurry. In 1812, 20 years old and fresh out of the University of Pennsylvania medical school, Sutherland simultaneously joined the American war effort as an assistant surgeon (later promoted to lieutenant colonel) and embarked on a political career. He was elected to the Pennsylvania House of Representatives the following year, then to the state senate in 1816, when he was also appointed Lazaretto physician by Governor Simon Snyder. Snyder had built a broad Democratic coalition on a combination of ideology and patronage, only to see it gradually splinter apart. Rival factions plotted as the 1816 federal and 1817 statewide elections approached.[3] Sutherland could not resist political intrigue, and even the relative isolation of Tinicum Island and his quarantine duties did not keep him from diving into the bruising partisan scrum.

The young doctor wanted to use the split between the radical "old school" Democrats led by Leib and Duane and the pragmatic "new school" led by *Democratic Press* editor John Binns to advance his own career. More than sixteen months before the gubernatorial election (in which Snyder was barred from running for reelection), Sutherland hatched a plan to gain appointment from the next governor as adjutant-general of the state militia under an arrangement involving hints of financial chicanery and in which Sutherland would rally a band of young activists to organize the campaign of the candidate-to-be. But whom should he back?

In a letter to his friend Joseph McCoy on June 27, 1816, the doctor laid out his plan in brutally frank terms. The wealthy and popular Nathaniel Boileau, Governor Snyder's secretary of the commonwealth, was a logical choice, but the young Sutherland considered him "but a child in politics" who was "not half enough acquainted with the underhand work that marks the bold and discerning politician," and worried that he was too "avaricious" to go along with the plan. State treasurer William Findlay, on the other hand, had acquired a reputation for building valuable political relationships through lavish entertainment, and Sutherland saw him as more likely than Boileau to go along with Sutherland's scheme because Findlay himself was "so full of schemes and notions that he is literally running over with them." "You may think me a damned strange creature," Sutherland confided to McCoy, "to be vacillating between Boileau and Findlay—but as you and I and all politicians are men of principle in proportion to our interest, I have written to you undisguisedly upon this matter." Undisguisedly indeed! Sutherland even suggested that he and McCoy might support a pro-Leib ticket with McCoy's name on it.[4]

Signing the letter "Your friend, J. B. Sutherland," Sutherland sent it by the Lazaretto mail service to the Board of Health office on Fifth Street in the city. After folding it in the typical manner for postal delivery, he addressed it to "Jos. McCoy, Esq., New Market, Philadelphia." The only thing Sutherland forgot to do was *seal it.* The mail coach from Tinicum Island through Kingsessing, across Gray's Ferry, and through Passyunk to Fifth Street was like a 12-mile-long lit fuse. As soon as Sutherland's letter arrived at the Health Office, an unidentified employee intercepted it and—instantly grasping its potential impact—took it to John Binns at the *Democratic Press.* Binns did not publish it but circulated copies of it to party power brokers. They in turn kept it quiet—or, at least, out of the press—for nine months, through the presidential election of 1816 and into the following spring, when the letter finally appeared in Duane's *Aurora.*[5]

Sutherland had done the unforgivable. He had admitted publicly what the insiders knew (and many outsiders suspected) was going on privately. He had exposed democracy—and "the Democracy," as the Democratic-Republican Party was often called in print—as an idealistic façade fronting for a venal game of raw influence and gain. And he had embarrassed some very powerful people. Shock waves rippled in concentric bursts of indignation throughout the country. "A disgusting scene of villainy," cried Duane in the *Aurora*, denouncing the letter as part of a campaign being carried out by a "clan of calumniators and corruptionists." Fifty miles northwest, in Reading, a newspaper printed the letter with this rueful comment: "Who can read it and not blush at the degraded state into which Pennsylvania has fallen?" In the nation's capital, the *National Register* published the letter with regret: "We are really sorry to observe that he thinks *public principle is bottomed on private interests*. We are far from believing that to be the fact." Elsewhere, the letter was a "scoundrel's creed," "alien to freedom, purity, honour, and patriotism," "infamous, demoralizing, and corrupting," and a cause for "the bosom of every patriot to swell with indignation." Protests echoed even as late as 1845, when New York journalist and political agitator William Lyon Mackenzie considered the letter an embarrassing advertisement for the "Sutherland principle," by which "a rapacious band of midnight conspirators for public office" managed to "blind, deceive, and plunder the millions."[6]

Everyone involved in the sordid affair was tainted—even Duane and Leib, with whom Sutherland and McCoy had been flirting. The young doctor was forced to resign in disgrace from the post of Lazaretto physician after just a year at the station. His fast-track political career appeared to have ended ignominiously at age 25. His name had become synonymous with shameless political corruption.

How could he have been anything but a pariah?

It took Sutherland a few years to climb the ladder, and he gave up medicine to study law, but he went on to serve five terms in Congress. The unforgivable was forgiven: he was elected to the county assembly from his home district of Southwark only one year after the purloined letter affair, and for the next few years, he also served on the Southwark District Commission. He was even chosen twice as the district's representative on the Board of Health. In 1826, when he was serving as judge overseeing the election of constables and inspectors in Southwark, Sutherland was arrested and charged with opening and reading voters' ballots before placing them in the ballot box. He did not contest the allegations and paid a fifty-dollar fine.[7] That same year he was elected to Congress for the first time. Even after defecting to the Whig Party and being defeated for reelection in 1836 and

1838, he continued his own brand of public service in various appointed positions.[8] There was always a place for a smart, shameless man with sharp elbows who knew how to play the game.

So, as James Beaver considered candidates for Lazaretto physician in 1887, he must have been aware that he could easily take a wrong step. The stakes were higher than they were for, say, the Board of Fisheries. The governor-elect received recommendations on behalf of seven applicants, but his choice should have been easy, because one dossier stood out from the rest. Other applicants had one or two letters of endorsement in their files, but this one had more than twenty. And not from just anyone, either: a United States senator, two congressmen, one former congressman, department store titan John Wanamaker, one of the owners of the colossal Cramp Shipyards, newspaper publishers, lawyers, doctors, and a Who's Who of Philadelphia merchants. All praised the would-be Lazaretto physician lavishly and urged his appointment, which they assured Beaver would be greeted warmly by the city's business community.[9] Civil War hero General H. G. Sickel, who had been president of the Board of Health during this candidate's previous tenure at Tinicum Island, marveled that the doctor's "six years service at the station was without a single word of complaint from importers or shipowners, which is more than can be said of any of his predecessors in my twenty-one years continuous connection with the Board of Health."[10] Few knew—or perhaps, few remembered, because who remembers the fire that did not break out?—his greatest achievement: saving Philadelphia from a disastrous reprise of the 1870 Lazaretto epidemic. At a time when the quarantine station was under attack, and its future very much at risk, he was the only one with the experience, skill, and judgment to save it.

Governor-elect Beaver had pledged to give preference to qualified veterans in his appointments. Like Beaver, the candidate was a Civil War veteran, having volunteered in the fall of 1861 and served through the rest of the war as a regimental surgeon. Since the war, the doctor had worked tirelessly in the service of Republican interests in Montgomery County and beyond. His backers described him as a "staunch" and "earnest and patriotic" Republican, whose "fidelity to the country in the late war and . . . devotion to the . . . party" were well known. In the decade after the war's end, he worked to turn the small settlement of Hatboro, north of Philadelphia, into an incorporated town, and alongside his medical practice, he founded a weekly newspaper there. The *Hatboro Public Spirit* soon became an influential Republican mouthpiece in Montgomery County.[11]

Beaver's allies among Philadelphia's mercantile elite were less interested in the doctor's partisan activities than in his stance toward the flow of commerce in the port. After all, the Lazaretto physician faced many decisions every day that could do mischief to merchants' bottom lines. But this doctor's supporters assured the governor-elect that his appointment would give the city's business community "general satisfaction," and that they anticipated no cause for complaint if he were to assume the duties on Tinicum Island. The doctor's recommenders also praised his skill as a clinician: his medical education was from the prestigious University of Pennsylvania, and he had traveled to the regions of Cuba where yellow fever was endemic to learn more about the disease and its treatment.[12]

If all this were not enough to qualify one applicant for the job of Lazaretto physician, there was the fact that *he had already served in the post for six quarantine seasons*, from 1878 through 1883. The candidate in question was William T. Robinson, who had guided the Lazaretto through the 1879 *Shasta* crisis described in the introduction.

Never was there a more professionally or politically qualified candidate for Lazaretto physician than Robinson. It is hard to imagine that any of the decisions facing Governor Beaver when he took office on January 18, 1887, were easier than this one. But as the quarantine season did not start until June 1, he took his time with the appointment, waiting until late May to announce it.

Nine springs earlier, when W. T. Robinson had relocated his family to Tinicum Island, he had known perfectly well that he owed his job to politics. Governor John Hartranft had named him Lazaretto physician in 1878 in recognition of his work on behalf of the Republican Party in Montgomery County. But Robinson was not the kind of man to go through the motions and collect his paycheck while hatching political schemes. He felt called to public service and was proud of his war service, proud of the newspaper he had founded, and proud of his most recent appointment. He would take his demanding job at the Lazaretto seriously, as he labored alongside the demoralized ghosts of T. J. P. Stokes and William Thompson, each of whom had suffered the consequences of a single lapse.

Beginning in the early 1880s, laboratory scientists identified specific microorganisms that caused particular diseases. One after another, the disease dominoes fell: malaria, typhoid fever, tuberculosis, diphtheria, cholera. These microorganisms could be cultured in a lab, observed, and—at least in theory—neutralized. Robinson followed breakthroughs in the germ theory of disease with the divided attention of a busy doctor and newspaper publisher. Like most physicians at the time, he does not appear to have changed his medical practice in response. In any case, diphtheria antitoxin was the only important new medicine to come out of the bacteriological laboratories, and it did not become widely available until 1895. Furthermore, not being a surgeon, Robinson would not have seen his practice altered by the new antiseptic or aseptic surgical techniques. But he did pay special attention to research on diseases he encountered regularly at the Lazaretto, including one Brazilian study in 1883 that claimed to have found disease-causing germs in the soil of cemeteries where people who died with yellow fever were buried. Robinson expressed enthusiasm about the power of bacteriology eventually to improve public health, and he reserved special scorn for those who stood in the way of medical progress—including the "prejudiced and ignorant . . . cranks" who resisted mandatory smallpox vaccination.[13]

In fact, Robinson had long embraced a progressive agenda reaching beyond public health. In 1860, just a year out of medical school, as a fledgling doctor trying to establish a practice in Montgomery County just north of Philadelphia, he took a public stand that could have damaged his career prospects. Ten years earlier, a group of Quaker reformers had founded the first medical school for women in the world, the Woman's Medical College, in Philadelphia. Many conservative doctors, not appreciating the competition of the school's graduates in the marketplace, expressed a conviction that women were constitutionally unfit to practice medicine. Agitating against the recognition of female physicians, the Philadelphia County Medical Society circulated a resolution among other county, state, and national medical organizations. The resolution advocating the exclusion of women from medicine came before the Montgomery County Medical Society on May 26, 1860, and its Philadelphia sponsors were preparing to take it to the statewide society the following month.[14]

For young Dr. Robinson, who had recently joined the Montgomery County society, the prudent course of action would have been to go along with the majority of the profession, or perhaps to steer clear of the matter. But Robinson stuck to his principles and joined with six of his colleagues to defeat the Philadelphia resolution. The Montgomery County delegation went on to lead the opposition to the resolution at the statewide meeting in June—in vain—and continued to do so for eleven more years, until finally the Pennsylvania Medical Society recognized women as equal members of the profession in 1871.[15]

More frustrating than conservative physicians and more dangerous than opponents of mandatory vaccination was the one obstacle to progress that perennially bedeviled Robinson: the South. During his years at the Lazaretto, the doctor complained about "the careless, neglectful ways" of southern health officers, who routinely failed to give bills of health (which certified the absence of epidemic disease at the port of origin) to vessels sailing for Philadelphia. When a representative of the short-lived National Board of Health toured Philadelphia's public health facilities, Robinson boasted that the visitor had never seen "a more complete or effective quarantine than the one he witnessed here." Philadelphia did not need a National Board of Health, Robinson groused. With "northern forethought and foresight," the city had "put the most enlightened theories into successful practice," and it was protecting itself just fine. Only because the southern states were "so poorly protected and so poorly governed," and because their cities "cannot and will not protect themselves," did the federal government find it necessary to create the national board. Even then, "blind opposition" from the South based on the principle of states' rights nearly torpedoed the new agency. It was not until southern congressmen realized that the board would be employing only southern men and spending money only in southern states, Robinson maintained, that the states' rights opposition melted away.[16]

Six or seven decades earlier, Benjamin Rush and his disciples had used quarantine as a polemical weapon to stand for backwardness, ignorance, and superstition—the antithesis of enlightened science and civilization. Now Robinson was using quarantine—Philadelphia's modern, efficient quarantine, with a steam tug and telegraph and pier-side disinfection tank—as the emblem distinguishing northern science and civilization from southern backwardness and inertia. For a moment, at least, he had redeemed quarantine and the Lazaretto from the scorn that the Enlightenment generations had heaped on them.

Robinson was a careful, understated writer, even in his political editorials. Only when the subject was the South did his tone turn acerbic or, very rarely, downright vitriolic. One such occasion came in the summer of 1880, when Robinson was on duty at the Lazaretto. The Democratic Party nominated General Winfield Scott Hancock, the hero of Gettysburg, as its candidate for president. A native of Montgomery County, Hancock was beloved by many Republicans for his bravery on the battlefield and his personal integrity. He had earned the trust of Democrats by showing leniency toward former Confederates when he oversaw the government of Texas and Louisiana in the early years of Reconstruction.[17]

Some Republican leaders flirted with supporting Hancock in the 1880 general election, but Robinson was having none of it. A Hancock presidency would mean a cabinet full of southern Democrats. "No man in his party stands higher in the opinions of Republicans than General Hancock," Robinson admitted. But, he thundered, "does anyone suppose for one moment that the people of this country are about to lie down and allow [the] fag-end of [a] treasonable, liberty-hating generation of slave dealers to place their traitorous feet upon the northern neck?" Even a photocopy of a decades-old microfilm version of Robinson's newspaper seems to glow with the embers of his rage.[18]

The war had been over for fifteen years, but some wounds never fully heal. Robinson's grudge was personal, it turns out. He had a history with the "traitors." A few months after the bombardment of Fort Sumter, the young doctor had put his medical practice on hold and enlisted in the 104th Regiment of Pennsylvania Volunteers at the rank of assistant surgeon. He helped prevent the spread of typhoid fever and smallpox when those diseases broke out in camp in Washington, then proved his worth at the siege of Yorktown and the battles of Williamsburg, Seven Pines, and White Oak Swamp, earning promotion to regimental surgeon. In the summer of 1864, when Sherman was preparing to sack Atlanta, the 104th Pennsylvania was sent to attack Charleston, both to divert attention away from Atlanta and to prevent the reinforcement of Lee's army in Richmond. While tending to sick soldiers on John's Island, 8 miles southwest of Charleston, Robinson did not hear the announcement of a change in the route of march and became separated from his unit. Seeing him alone, South Carolina rebels immediately captured him. It was Independence Day.[19]

Confederate forces kept Robinson in the Charleston jail before moving him to a stockade in Macon, Georgia. Released as part of a prisoner exchange, he returned to his unit about three months later.[20] Most of the soldiers in the 104th Pennsylvania went home when their three-year enlistment terms expired in October 1864, but Robinson stayed with the regiment as it threaded itself into the noose that was gradually tightening around the neck of Lee's army in Virginia. The doctor continued to care for the sick and wounded of the 104th for more than four months after the surrender at Appomattox, finally mustering out in Norfolk at the end of August 1865 (figure 13).

Maybe Robinson's experience as a prisoner of war embittered him toward the South. Maybe his most deeply felt moral principles were simply offended by a society based on the ownership and violent subjugation of fellow human beings. Maybe the daily experience of tending to the sick, the wounded, and the dying—giving them their quinine and whiskey, cleaning and salving their wounds, mopping their brows or holding their hands through their delirium, closing their eyes and covering their bodies when the end mercifully came—maybe that experience gradually seeped into his soul and left a poisonous residue there. Of the 1,049 men who broke

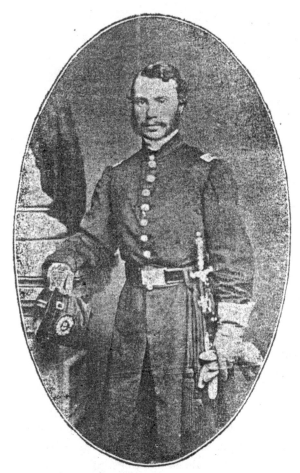

WILLIAM T. ROBINSON, M. D.

Figure 13. William T. Robinson in his Civil War uniform, undated photograph. Courtesy of the Old York Road Historical Society.

camp with the 104th Pennsylvania in November 1861, 70 died of battle wounds and 115 more of disease—and its death rate of 18 percent made the regiment luckier than most.[21] Hundreds more from the 104th were nursed back to health, or at least to life. William T. Robinson treated most of those men, witnessing and sharing their suffering. How could that pain *not* leave a lasting imprint?

For the polite, courtly Dr. Robinson, the newspaper publisher and Lazaretto physician who rarely complained publicly and made a point of downplaying political slights, the years between 1864 and 1880 merely allowed his resentful scorn toward the ex-secessionists to ferment and fester. A Hancock presidency, with traitors and slave dealers in the cabinet? The mere prospect was an outrage, an insult to the memory of his fallen comrades.

Apart from writing newspaper editorials, the best thing Robinson could do in 1880 to avoid a Hancock presidency was to show the world how a quarantine based on "northern forethought and foresight" and "enlightened theories" should be run. Since his arrival in 1878, he had already made operational and personnel changes at the Lazaretto "in accordance with the spirit of the age"—that is, to usher in a modern, efficient quarantine service that could keep up with the rapidly expanding commercial traffic of Philadelphia's port.[22]

Robinson's quarantine master, Dr. C. C. V. Crawford, had his own wartime memories; most vivid among them, likely, was being wounded at the Battle of Fort Stevens in Washington by a bullet likely intended for President Lincoln, who was standing next to him at the time.[23] At the Lazaretto, Robinson and Crawford needed to be dressed and fed and ready to go by the time the bargemen's first bell rang to signal the sighting of a vessel sailing or steaming upriver that needed to be visited promptly. If the clanging shortly after sunrise woke the doctor up, then his day was already off to a bad start. Boarding the station's steam tug *Visitor* as early as 5:30 a.m. was not uncommon (figure 14).

When the *Visitor* tied up alongside the arriving vessel, Robinson and Crawford would climb up a ladder tossed over the side the vessel. Once on board, they were greeted by the captain, who was never happy to see them. Nevertheless, chilly civility was the norm at quarantine. Robinson ran through the battery of questions: port of origin, health of the city of departure, number of passengers and crew, illness during the voyage, nature of cargo, and so on. There were forms to fill out (including reports to the Board of Health), permits to proceed to the port, and certificates reporting the results of the inspection. If the vessel arrived with a clean bill of health—a sworn and sealed statement from a consul or other local official that no epidemic disease prevailed at the port of origin when the vessel sailed—matters would be relatively straightforward. If the captain could show only a "foul" bill (reporting disease) or had no bill to show, then his and Robinson's headaches multiplied. Meanwhile, Crawford inspected the decks, hold, and cargo for filth, decay, or other potential harbingers of disease as well as concealed sick passengers or seamen. He ordered a sailor to pump out the bilgewater and if necessary to flush it with river water until it ran clear and odorless. Robinson looked over the crew and passengers for signs of illness. In 96 percent of vessels in a typical

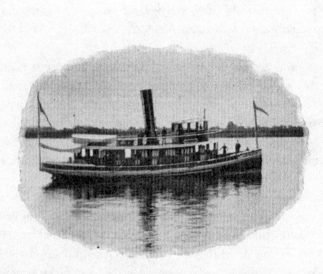

THE "VISITOR" IN THE INSIDE CHANNEL AT THE LAZARETTO
(From a photograph by the author)

Figure 14. The steam-powered tug *Visitor* in the late 1880s. Photograph in Henry Leffmann, *Under the Yellow Flag* (Philadelphia: G. F. Fell et Societas, 1896).

year during Robinson's tenure on Tinicum Island, the final product of the questions, the inspections, and the report writing was a permit to proceed. But reports of outbreaks at the port of origin, a worrisome illness aboard, a filthy ship, or even suspicious behavior by the captain or crew—any one of these warning signs could trigger a detention at the Lazaretto lasting from a couple of days to several weeks.[24]

Then it was on to the next schooner, bark, brig, or steamship. Lumber from Savannah, sugar from Barbados, immigrants from eastern Europe via Hamburg, one after another, every ten or fifteen minutes at the busiest times. Climb the ladder, interview the captain, examine the passengers and crew, inspect the hold and cargo, pump the bilgewater, fill out the forms, climb back down, and start over again with the next. Break for a midday meal if you have a chance, but even that respite could be interrupted by the clanging of the watch bell and another visit via the *Visitor*. On a slow day, there might be three or four vessels; on a busy day, ten or fifteen.[25] The ladder climbing alone could be taxing. And if ever Robinson was tempted to cut corners in his inspections, he had only to remind himself of what had happened to his predecessors when they let down their guard. "The place is hardly a bed of roses," Robinson wrote. "No one of this station eats the bread of idleness and the work does not cease between sunrise and sunset." To say nothing of the "great mental strain" of the job: Lazaretto physicians were always likely to be damned if they did, and damned if they didn't.[26]

But there was more to William T. Robinson than work, stress, and the quest for efficiency. He was acutely aware of his place—in the political and bureaucratic hierarchy, in the long line of quarantine officials who had served at the Lazaretto, and in his physical surroundings. When preparing the station for the opening of quarantine season, Robinson was just as likely to stop and admire its lawns and its roses as to fret about staffing and supplies. He regularly treated the readers of his weekly newspaper—which somehow, despite the demands of his job, he continued to edit from Tinicum Island—to his extended reveries about the everyday beauty in the world that was too often taken for granted. At the beginning of his second quarantine season, he described the scene on the island:

> At daylight on Sunday morning everybody in the station was astir, and at sunrise the yellow flag with its gigantic initial letter Q was run up to the top of the tall flagstaff. The station was in fine condition, its buildings tidy and in complete order without, and in a perfect state of cleanliness within. The wooden buildings and fences were as bright as whitewash could make them, and the lawns and grassplots as smooth shaven as lawn mowers and good care could produce. Their bright green shone in the morning sunlight, while the roses of the garden were just opening in their varied beauty to the eye.
>
> The evening before on a stiff southerly breeze, a fine procession of white sailed ships from abroad had scurried by the station, as if to shun the delay which might be their fate on the morrow, and as darkness fell, the moonlight clear and full enabled them to reach the city on the swelling tide.[27]

Robinson's occasionally lyrical tone betrays a sensibility that runs deeper than politics, deeper than science, and deeper than modern efficiency. There is a hint of this sensibility in one surviving photograph of him. Most portrait photographs of bourgeois men in the second half of the nineteenth century show intractably serious, almost expressionless faces. Robinson fairly beams, with a glint in his eye that suggests some private joke or pleasure (figure 15).

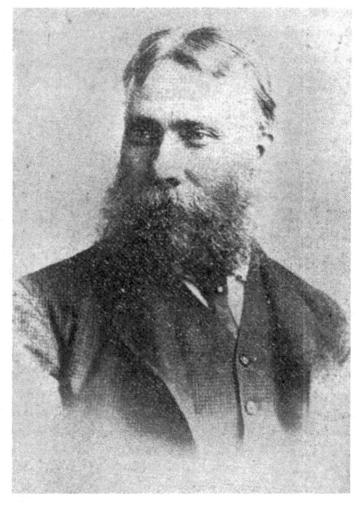

Figure 15. William T. Robinson, undated photograph. Courtesy of the Old York Road Historical Society.

His painterly eye showed itself frequently in his "Letters from the Lazaretto" column, as when he noted that both yellow fever and the bobolinks that feed on the island's marsh grasses usually arrive in late summer: "Yellow fever and reed birds are still scarce at quarantine," he wrote one year in late July. "The season for reed birds [bobolinks] is still a month distant. A fine crop of reeds in bloom is forming into grain along the margin of the river banks. Like a wide green satin ribbon of exquisite shade it is wondrously beautiful to the eye."[28]

And there was even a hint of melancholy when quarantine season ended: "At sundown the colors came down. The boats were housed. The big bell, the regulator and time keeper of the establishment, was covered and muffled for the winter to come. All official business came to an end as the *Visitor* . . . left the wharf. Dull quiet fell upon the quarantine. Scarcely a mosquito thought to hum; all was quiet." Robinson added, as if to remind himself, "Everybody is glad when the season comes to an end."[29]

What Robinson understood better than anyone was that a quarantine physician needed to be more than just vigilant and medically competent. The job required one to have the *perspective* to understand the human and economic stakes, the *discernment* to know a mountain from a molehill, and the *skill* to reconcile parties with conflicting interests and to reassure patients suffering from terrifying diseases.

In contrast to his predecessors George Lehman in 1817 and Joshua Jones in 1847, Robinson treated only about eight or nine patients per year at the Lazaretto hospital from 1878 through 1883. They were all men, mostly sailors, from Scandinavia, Germany, the British Isles, the West Indies, Canada, and the northeastern United States. Every quarantine season, Robinson inspected between 500 and 1,000 vessels arriving from all over the world. Many still plied the lucrative West Indian trade, and the specter of yellow fever continued to haunt the city and its Lazaretto throughout Robinson's tenure. He treated seventeen cases of the dreaded "yellow jack" during his six seasons on the island, more than any other disease.

In 1882 Robinson noted matter-of-factly in his newspaper, "The patients are getting well in the fine hospital here. They all get well for that matter. I have been here five years, and only one patient with yellow fever, or any other disease, has died in the hospital. [That] one was moribund when I took him off the ship, insensible, and it was impossible to save him."[30] He did not write about his general therapeutic philosophy or his treatment regimen for any specific disease. Apparently readers of the *Hatboro Public Spirit* were more interested in Pennsylvania Republican infighting than in the relative advisability of emetics or tonics for malignant fevers. Robinson may have followed the teachings of his Penn professor George B. Wood, who in 1856 advocated the moderate use of mercury in yellow fever to induce "ptyalism," or excessive salivation. Echoing his colleague Samuel Jackson's conclusions in the report on Philadelphia's 1820 yellow fever epidemic, Wood claimed that "whenever mercurial ptyalism can be fairly induced in yellow fever, the patient recovers." "As patients almost always get well who come under the influence of mercury," he added confidently, "the medicine certainly cannot be accused of producing any serious mischief."[31]

Administering small amounts of mercury is a far cry from the "heroic" deple-tion practiced by Rush and his followers around 1800, but even moderate use of harsh drugs like mercury was falling from favor by the late 1870s, when Robinson first saw yellow fever patients at the Lazaretto. He may have been more likely to take guidance from Alfred Stillé, another Penn graduate and professor, whose trea-tise on yellow fever was published in 1879. Stillé scolded the inexperienced phy-sicians who instinctively leapt to fight an aggressive, malignant disease like yellow fever with aggressive measures: "If they are men of a teachable spirit, they soon learn prudence in the school of experience, and reserve their cups and lancets, their pills and potions, their blisters and sedatives, and douches and sali-vants, for some field in which there is more hope of their doing good, and less fear of doing mischief than in yellow fever."[32]

Stillé prescribed rest, comfort, and gentle treatment: bedrest with enough cov-ers to ensure mild perspiration; warm mustard foot baths; cool, acidulated drinks given in moderate quantities; half an ounce of castor oil or a soap-suds enema if the patient was constipated; and quinine for relief of muscle and back pains, as well as to promote sleep. (Other doctors around this time prescribed quinine primarily as a fever reducer and as a tonic when bodily strength was much depleted. Quinine was also widely used and effective against malaria.) When the patient began to improve, Stillé insisted on still more restraint: "Nothing is required to be done but to maintain the bodily and mental rest of the patient, and to administer food ap-propriate to his condition, such as delicate animal broths . . . in small quantities at a time." Indeed, one newspaper account from Robinson's time on Tinicum Island reported that "the usual course [at the Lazaretto hospital] for yellow fever is beef tea, lemonade, lime juice, ice water and plenty of quinine."[33] What Stillé proposed was a version of William Wood Gerhard's 1830s approach to typhus treatment: pro-tect the patient from the worst manifestations of the symptoms and provide the rest, comfort, and nourishment that will allow the body to withstand them while the disease runs its course. It was the "care cure" again.* Or, essentially, nursing.

W. T. Robinson alluded publicly to his treatment practices at the Lazaretto only once. The patient was Patrick Kelly, a 20-year-old British sailor aboard the brig

---

* *Care cure* is my designation (also discussed in chapter 12) for the therapeutic value of basic nursing care, symptom management, and meeting simple bodily needs such as food, clothing, and rest. It was not a term that Robinson or anyone else used in the nineteenth century, although I argue that the underlying concept was widely understood.

Julia Blake in late July 1883. Robinson had a bad feeling about the ship before he even boarded it. It was sailing from Havana with a cargo of iron, bones, and hoofs loaded in bags on deck. Robinson noted, "Swarms of flies and creeping things hovered over the bags of hoofs and crept over the piles of bones." The usual boarding-house runners who attach their small boats astern of arriving vessels to hawk their services were, this time, keeping their distance. Robinson's experienced eye—it was his sixth season at the Lazaretto—told him the *Julia Blake* was trouble. Once he climbed aboard, he ordered the captain to muster his crew amidships. When they assembled, one was missing; the captain said he "had a cold or something" and was recuperating in the forecastle. Robinson gingerly picked his way over the bags of hoofs until he found young Patrick Kelly hiding in his bunk. "His yellow skin, his blood-shot eyes, glaring from the dark from his narrow, low-roofed bunk," Robinson reported, "soon showed me he had yellow fever." And this was no mild case: "The floor of his little cell had been just wiped up to remove the stains of his black vomit. A cursory examination was enough."[34]

Black vomit meant a late-stage, terminal case. Robinson must have been feeling a stew of emotions—alarm, pity, disgust, fatigue, with perhaps a dose of fear mixed in—but he kept them all to himself, as he told readers of the *Public Spirit*. "I had little hope of him, but of course I treated him as I always do, as if I expected him to recover. I have seen many bad cases come to, under careful management." He immediately transported Kelly to the Lazaretto hospital and "arranged his medication and his diet with the nurse, who watched him and waited on him carefully."[35]

What medication? What kind of diet? Robinson did not say, although a regimen of beef broth, ice water, citrus juice, and "plenty of quinine" was most likely. His offhand references to "careful management"—indicating alleviation of symptoms rather than aggressive treatment—as well as diet and the nurse's watchful attention to the patient's needs all suggest that he took the importance of the "care cure" for granted.

Kelly rallied, vomited less frequently, regained his senses, and was able to answer questions rationally. But, as Robinson expected, the recovery was but a brief pause in the young man's death spiral. Within hours the fever and chills had returned, the jaundice worsened, and delirium set in. "In a moment, he threw up his arms above his head, straightened himself out and was slipping towards the floor. The nurse seized him around the waist with both arms. He was heavy. I helped to lay him in his bed. His jaws locked, his eyes closed—in five minutes he was dead." Kelly was only the second of seventeen yellow fever patients—and the second of fifty patients overall—to die under Robinson's treatment at the Lazaretto. The other, like Kelly, arrived at the station in the final, black-vomiting stage of the illness. Even if some of the other cases were mild ones, an 88 percent survival rate for yellow fever in any nineteenth-century hospital would have been an enviable achievement.[36]

Robinson's stolid, imperturbable optimism was not a *consequence* of his cure rate. It was part of his treatment regimen, and likely one of the reasons behind his success. The ability to hide one's emotions, to face setbacks and hopeless cases and improbable triumphs with the same impassive demeanor, was the cardinal virtue of physicians, which the great William Osler called "*aequanimitas*" (or "equanimity") in his landmark commencement address to the University of Pennsylvania's medical graduates a few years later. "Imperturbability," Osler told the fledgling doctors, "means coolness and presence of mind under all circumstances, calmness amid storm, clearness of judgment in moments of grave peril." "The physician who has the misfortune to be without it," he added, "who betrays indecision and worry, and who shows that he is flustered . . . in ordinary emergencies, rapidly loses the confidence of his patients."[37] And, in the case of a Lazaretto physician, of the general public.

Robinson displayed *aequanimitas* in full measure in his dealings with the Board of Health, Pennsylvania politicians, and the growing number of Delaware County residents who were not happy to have the Lazaretto as a neighbor. It was the trait that served him best in his confrontation with Mayor Jonathan Forwood of Chester in 1879.

When Robert Pattison defeated James Beaver in the 1882 governor's race, it marked the first time in a quarter century that a Democrat had ascended to Pennsylvania's highest office. Pattison thought enough of Robinson's record to keep him on as Lazaretto physician for the 1883 season. A year later, however, the governor yielded to the temptation of patronage and replaced Robinson with a Democratic loyalist, Dr. Francis Wilson. At the next election, in 1886, Beaver claimed his revenge, and it was time to put a Republican back on Tinicum Island. Robinson was the candidate whose dossier outshone all others on Governor Beaver's desk. But by late May 1887 the quarantine season was about to start, and the governor had still not filled the position. With all of Robinson's political connections, his military service, and his universally praised record during six difficult years in the post, what was Beaver waiting for?

The answer: a chance to pay back a minor political favor. On May 26, 1887, less than a week before the opening of the quarantine season, the governor appointed a little-known physician named Henry Brusstar from the small town of Birdsboro in Berks County to succeed Wilson as Lazaretto physician.

Reaction to the appointment was swift.

"Republicans in Rage," the *Philadelphia Inquirer* trumpeted. No one claimed that Brusstar was appointed because of his qualifications for the job. The word in Republican circles was that Beaver, at the urging of state party chairman Thomas Cooper, was repaying the doctor for a vote he had cast at the state party convention the previous year. The slate of candidates proposed by Cooper and other party leaders that year had triggered a rebellion among many delegations, including the one from Berks County. Brusstar had promised to support an alternative slate but then defied his county delegation at the last minute and voted for the party leaders' official candidate for lieutenant governor, William Dailey, who won the nomination by just a handful of votes. Cooper did not forget Brusstar's sudden change of heart. Other Berks County Republicans were incensed at the news of the doctor's appointment and wondered whether Cooper had promised him a job in exchange for his vote at the convention.[38]

Robinson had no comment. He may have wept with disappointment, or seethed with rage, or displaced his frustration in outbursts of ill temper toward his family or co-workers. But it was not in his nature to react publicly. No commentary in the *Public Spirit*, no letter to the governor, no statements to the press. He just swallowed whatever sense of unfairness he felt and soldiered on.

Hic Jacet
The Mortal Remains of
Dr. W. T. Robinson
Born 1838—Died 1900.
Educated in Public Schools of Philad[a] and University of Penn. He served his country four years as Surgeon of the 104th P. V. Bucks County Regiment in the field. Practiced medicine ten years in Hatboro. Was six years Lazaretto Physician for City of Philad[a] and eight years in the medical service of the Board of Health of that city with the approval of the Department and his colleagues.[39]

As a young man, Robinson had almost singlehandedly brought about the incorporation of the borough of Hatboro. He had devoted two-thirds of his adult life to the newspaper he founded, the name of which—the *Public Spirit*—expressed his guiding principle. Yet what seemed to be his life's work was nowhere to be found in his epitaph. Education, defense of his country on the battlefield, medical practice, and public service as Lazaretto physician and medical inspector—these were his proudest achievements. They were what he wanted posterity to know about his life and work. They were his place in history.

History was never far from Robinson's mind, and it would not be surprising if he had planned his epitaph carefully. "This ancient and honorable station, which has been the efficient office of quarantine since 1800," he wrote at the start of the 1883 quarantine season, "looks as well to-day as ever, during its 83 years of establishment." Later that summer, the brig *Julia Blake* brought Patrick Kelly, in the late stages of yellow fever, to the Lazaretto, but it also carried an unusual cargo that sent Robinson into one of his lyrical reveries: cracked church bells. A Havana merchant collected them, then shipped them once a year to be melted down in Philadelphia. Robinson could not help musing about the centuries of life and death the bells had commemorated. "The curious old bells made in old Spain and in Italy, with legends of the scriptures and adornments of crosses and other sacred signs, wonderfully sweet tones in their rolling music, presented by pious hands from noble Hidalgos and stately ladies, frightened, despairing misers, and repentant, profligate prodigals, have rung out their last thunders and tuned their last music." He imagined the bells as once-noble dignitaries reduced to a pathetic state: "Ruined and broken bells whose chimes are dead and long since silent, dethroned princes and prelates of the church, cast down from their high places, their bones groveling in the dust, with the dust of bull-fighting champions, in a yellow fever ship." The doctor added that he could not see the bells "without thinking over their curious history."[40]

In such moments, Robinson felt the romance and the tragedy of history. Just as he did when he gazed out from the main building at the Lazaretto and admired the well-kept lawns, the order and symmetry of the station's buildings, or the reeds in bloom at the river's edge, he felt a kind of sublime transcendence in which past, present, and future blended in a landscape or in an object. Although he knew better than anyone that he owed his job to politics, he felt bound by a sense of duty and considered himself the steward of a long and honorable tradition of public servants at the quarantine station. He felt the weight of his predecessors' dilemmas and decisions when facing his own.

Better than any Lazaretto physician before or after him, W. T. Robinson understood the *art* of quarantine as public policy, usually uneventful but always with high stakes. The sangfroid and political savvy that allowed him to weather what could have been a disaster in 1879 with the *Shasta* served him well throughout his career. But even more rare than his skill was his outlook on life. He saw the world through the double face of Janus, the god of beginnings, transitions, and duality: he embraced a future of progress and improvement while studying, cherishing, and feeling in his bones the importance of the past.[41]

Robinson was even the Lazaretto's first historian. During his tenure on Tinicum Island, between visiting vessels from sunrise to sunset, corresponding with the Board of Health several times a day, and treating patients in the hospital, he somehow found time to research and write a history of quarantine in Philadelphia. The board gave him permission to borrow its minute books (apparently only at the Lazaretto, and only during the quarantine season), and he gathered up enough documentation to open his chronicle in the year 1700, with the response to the city's first incursion of yellow fever. He began writing early in the 1881 quarantine season, and the first serialized chapter appeared in the *Hatboro Public Spirit* on June 11. By the time the season ended, Robinson had published thirteen chapters and brought his story up to 1800; that is where he restarted the narrative when he began writing again the next season. The physician-historian worked his way through the tumultuous first half of the nineteenth century, with its outbreaks of fever and of fear, its changing health laws and political controversies. He relished the evocative details of Lazaretto life, including the repair of the mustering horn that at one time roused the bargemen at dawn to prepare to board vessels and the conch shell horn that called them in to dinner.

By the end of the 1883 season, Robinson's history had grown to thirty-nine chapters, covering Philadelphia's maritime quarantine up to the year 1849, a time when the Lazaretto was struggling to cope with the Irish famine migration and the onslaught of disease it brought with it. But there the story ended abruptly. The reason? Politics, of course. In the spring of 1884, when Governor Pattison replaced Robinson with the Democrat Wilson as Lazaretto physician, the departing doctor no longer had access to the Board of Health's records, and his history of quarantine was fated to remain unfinished.

Chapter Sixteen

The Final Days, 1888–1895

None of W. T. Robinson's successors carried out their responsibilities with Robinson's calm resolve. Nor did they possess the kind of political acumen that served him so well. As the Lazaretto increasingly came under attack from politicians, nearby residents, landowners, and the press, the officers on the front line either shrank from the battle or gave ammunition to their opponents.

Philadelphia's industry and population mushroomed in the post–Civil War years, and Delaware County shared in the region's expansion, its population nearly doubling between 1870 and 1890. Ridley Township, which enveloped Tinicum on the north and west, quadrupled in population over those same years, from just over 1,000 to more than 4,500.[1] Settlement and the demand for settlement were pressing in on the site that in 1799 had been chosen for its utter isolation.

Chester politicians called the Lazaretto a "pesthouse." And a pesthouse in their midst now not only spelled danger to those living and working near it, but was also a barrier to local development. By the early 1890s, the murmur of voices in Delaware County calling for the Lazaretto's closure swelled to a chorus. After the catastrophic Lower Mississippi Valley yellow fever epidemic of 1878, the federal government heeded calls for it to take control of quarantine operations nationwide, and in the mid-1880s the US Marine Hospital Service opened its own maritime inspection and quarantine station at the breakwater that protected the mouth of Delaware Bay.[2]

The year 1888 was a bad one for the Lazaretto's public image. There was no deadly epidemic at the station or even any close calls, but there was plenty of petty squabbling and name calling. Even the scandal-mongering press grew weary and vaguely embarrassed. The trouble began as soon as the quarantine season opened, although in hindsight there were warning signs even earlier, in February, when the

Board of Health found it necessary to remind the Lazaretto steward Robert Carns that the law forbade him from leaving the grounds of the station during the season, except on "important occasions," and even then only with prior written permission from the board. And it was not even a week after the big yellow Q flag had been hoisted up the flagpole to inaugurate the quarantine season before the board ordered an investigation into "the alleged want of harmony and insubordination" among Lazaretto officers.[3]

Governor Beaver's Lazaretto physician, Dr. Henry Brusstar, complained that the steward frequently departed the station without warning, leaving the rest of the staff either to procure needed supplies themselves or to do without. Carns countered that his job required him to leave the station periodically, that he never left when there were patients with contagious diseases in the hospital, and that on the specific occasion cited by Brusstar, he had been obeying an order to appear before the Board of Health. President William Ford, in presenting his findings on these matters to the board (recently again reduced from twelve to five members), recommended stricter oversight of permissions to leave the station. His colleagues were not satisfied. One demanded that Brusstar and Carns be questioned under oath, so that "one would be apt to tell something about the other," and the board could get to the bottom of the problem. A weary Ford ventured that as long as all officers performed their duties adequately, it should not matter that they were not the best of friends. The meeting resolved nothing, but newspapers fed their eager readers juicy quotes from the volley of accusations between board members:

"Steward Carns never did an hour's duty at the station last summer. When a patient arrived he was not on hand to receive him and the nurse had to do it. Dr. Brusstar has written to me charging the steward with neglect of duty."

"Dr. Brusstar is not fit for his place; he has violated the rules himself and then charged Carns with doing so, and these charges have been proved to be unfounded."

"You kept quarantine open two months later last year to punish Dr. Brusstar."[4]

Three weeks later they were back at it. "That Same Old Row—The Troubles at the Lazaretto Revived," the *Inquirer*'s headline smirked. When Carns's cook quit, and he hired a woman who lived outside the station to replace her, Brusstar called the hire a violation of quarantine regulations and refused to allow the new cook inside the gates. And Brusstar could not resist a swipe at what he considered the board's habitual penny pinching. The doctor was visiting a vessel near Thurlow, downriver from Chester, and knew that by the time he got back to the Lazaretto, the board would have adjourned for the day. He had no choice but to telegraph his report from Thurlow. His report the next day concluded, "I wanted to pay for the message, but the operator could not make the change. I enclose the 45 cents."[5]

On one occasion Brusstar prevented Carns from going to the city because Brusstar feared that a seaman who was in the hospital with diarrhea might have cholera. The *Inquirer*'s succinct headline a week later? "Dr. Brusstar Again." This time the board attacked the doctor from opposite sides simultaneously. The diarrhea patient, a crew member from the American Line steamship *Lord Clive* from Liverpool, had died in the Lazaretto hospital; Brusstar listed cholera as the cause. One member accused Brusstar of taking the sailor off the ship, where he was under a doctor's care and in isolation, just to have an excuse to refuse all permissions for staff to leave the Lazaretto to celebrate the Fourth of July. Another pointed out that after admitting the patient, Brusstar allowed the ship to proceed to the city— which would be "a gross dereliction of duty" if he suspected cholera.[6]

As the board ordered another investigation, the press began to mix exasperated commentary in with its blow-by-blow reporting. The *Inquirer* adopted a diplomatic stance: "Without wishing to reflect on either Dr. Brusstar or the Board of Health, we may be permitted to remark that the sooner they part company the better for the public's peace of mind. Their dispositions evidently are not congenial and the oft-repeated story of their squabbles has ceased to be either edifying or profitable."[7] (The story, of course, was profitable enough for the newspaper that it continued to cover it.)

By late July—still less than halfway through the quarantine season—the already poisoned relationship had deteriorated even further. Board members routinely mocked Brusstar and called him "grossly incompetent," whereupon the *Inquirer* openly called for his dismissal from "a post which is certainly too important to be filled by an incompetent man."[8] Lazaretto physicians had been maltreated in the press before, but without the support of the board, it is hard to imagine how Brusstar could carry out his duties effectively in the face of public ridicule. He held onto the job only because Governor Beaver apparently did not take advice from Philadelphia's Board of Health, and because that board, riven by internal strife, could not present a unified front.

As the 1888 season rolled on, Brusstar found himself in the middle of a dispute between Carns and the crew of the Lazaretto's steam tug about allegedly rotten meat the steward had served. Yet another investigation by the board. "Clean the whole place out" and "Fumigate it," critics in the press howled. "The feud among the officers at quarantine is growing as tiresome as the McCoy-Hatfield feud in Kentucky." Chester mayor Joseph Coates complained that the same steam tug that carried yellow fever patients from their vessels to the Lazaretto regularly ferried staff from the station to his city for errands and recreation. He threatened his own quarantine if the practice continued. The chief officer of the US Marine Hospital Service's station at the Delaware breakwater accused Brusstar of retaining in his own files the federal health certificates issued to vessels at the breakwater—documents that were supposed to be submitted to federal customs officers at the Port of Philadelphia.[9] Ordinary workplace disagreements that in more experienced hands would be handled quietly, without any public fuss, turned into loud embarrassments. Who would trust these men to protect the city from an epidemic? Brusstar, Carns, the Board of Health—all available evidence painted them as petty and vindictive at best, and inept at worst.

Sensing disarray in Philadelphia and on Tinicum Island, the Delaware County "land jobbers" and politicians intensified their campaign to close the Lazaretto. Leading them were Ward Bliss, an ambitious young state representative and publisher of the *Delaware County Republican* newspaper, and Dr. Jonathan L. Forwood, the former Chester mayor who in 1879 had threatened to use Gatling guns and cannons to prevent the *Shasta*'s logwood from entering his city. Forwood had founded the *Delaware County Democrat* just after the Civil War, but he switched parties in the late 1880s and became an active Republican organizer as well as president of the Chester Board of Trade.[10]

Bliss and Forwood began in the spring of 1889 to recruit allies and organize events to publicize the cause of shuttering the Lazaretto.[11] Over the next four years, in the back rooms of Harrisburg, in public meetings, and in the press, their campaign hammered relentlessly at a few key allegations: the Lazaretto was a danger to neighboring communities; it did not protect Chester, Wilmington, and other downriver towns; and it was little more than an "expensive toy" for the Philadelphia Board of Health, serving as a destination for leisure junkets and banquets for board members and guests such as city officials and former board members. (These allegations appear to be a reference to the board's practice of visiting the Lazaretto twice a year, at the beginning and end of quarantine season, to inspect the facilities and take inventory of the property. Each outing ended with the ceremonial raising or lowering of the yellow flag and a banquet [figure 16].) Just after Christmas in 1890, the Chester Board of Trade managed to get ninety people who supported

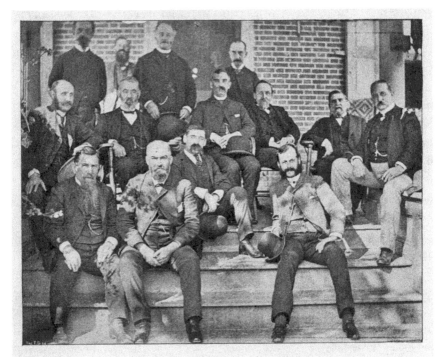

"AFTER DINNER," LAZARETTO, SEPTEMBER 30, 1886
(From a photograph by the author)

Figure 16. Lazaretto officers and Board of Health members relaxing on the portico after the banquet commemorating the end of the quarantine season, September 30, 1886. Photograph in Henry Leffmann, *Under the Yellow Flag* (Philadelphia: G. F. Fell et Societas, 1896).

removal of the Lazaretto out in freezing temperatures to rally at Miller's Hotel, at the very gates of the Lazaretto. Forwood brandished "well signed" petitions demanding that the legislators in Harrisburg close the station down. Less than two months later, Bliss introduced a bill that would do exactly that. In an interview with the *Inquirer* in early February 1891, he claimed that at least two members of the recently established state Board of Health were on his side, as were numerous Philadelphia-area physicians known for their expertise in sanitary matters. Residents of the growing settlements between Chester and Tinicum Island (including Eddystone and Ridley Park) joined the cause, and one newspaper reported that "the Reading and Pennsylvania Railroads [which stood to profit from increased development in the area] have enlisted under the flag that isn't yellow" (a reference to the yellow flag of quarantine that flew at the Lazaretto). Bliss charged that "rules of the station are openly violated during the season," "money is openly squandered," and "the place is used as a high-tone club house." Forwood and Bliss had momentum on their side, and they would give no quarter.[12]

"Caught napping" by the Bliss bill, according to the *Philadelphia Press*, the city's Board of Health and civic leaders promptly "woke up" to the growing possibility that their 90-year-old quarantine system would soon be defunct. The board repeatedly and emphatically denied that it used the Lazaretto for junkets and recreation, countering that it was one of the most efficient quarantine stations in the country, that it posed no threat to its neighbors, and that its removal would endanger a city of more than a million people while benefiting only a few land speculators in Delaware County. The board wrote dismissively to the state legislature that the "country surrounding the Lazaretto is most sparsely populated, the nearest town being two miles distant." Advocates for removal, on the other hand, claimed that 41,000 people lived within 3 miles of the station, and that "every available piece of land is occupied."[13]

Philadelphia's Board of Trade and its Maritime Exchange, plus every other major commercial and shipping organization, joined in protest to stop the Bliss bill. After meeting at the Maritime Exchange, they sent a joint statement to the governor, lieutenant governor, and all members of the Pennsylvania Senate and House of Representatives calling the Lazaretto's location "judicious and efficient." The *Inquirer* lined up with other city newspapers defending the status quo, attributing the anti-Lazaretto campaign to the "intense selfishness" of "real estate speculators" and concluding that "the people who are put in imaginary peril by the present station are only a handful compared with those who would be placed in real jeopardy by its removal."[14]

Bliss and the other members of the legislative committee considering his bill met with city officials at Mayor Edwin Fitler's office on February 21. The *Inquirer* christened the goings-on "The Lazaretto War." Board of Health president Ford began by calmly laying out the case for keeping the quarantine station on Tinicum Island. Bliss stood to respond, his voice rising with excitement. "The people of Philadelphia are with us," he insisted, "and if the expression of the people prevailed it would be removed." He claimed to have petitions with Philadelphia signers, and he maintained that the only people holding out against progress were the city officials who depended on the revenue from incoming vessels' health fees and therefore had a vested interest in the status quo. At this Mayor Fitler rose, his face flushed with anger. If Bliss wanted Philadelphia signatures, he would give him "thousands" in favor of keeping the Lazaretto. He hotly denied that opposition to the bill came from bureaucratic self-interest. "We officials are here not to consult our personal interests but to watch the interests of the people, and we propose to do our duty." "The fire fairly shot out of the mayor's eye," wrote one reporter present at the meeting. It didn't help Fitler's blood pressure when someone else at the meeting reported that landowners were selling property near the Lazaretto with the promise that "the buildings were to be removed and a fine hotel erected there." The mayor could only stammer, "No, it is not right, and the people should rise up against it."[15]

Quarantine master Robert Newhard was another interested party who was irked by the Chester campaign against the Lazaretto. When the *Philadelphia Press* reported allegations that the station was a "plaything" for the Board of Health, and that bargemen and other staff routinely took the quarantine tug on leisure outings, it added one more charge to the list: "Some of the Chester opponents of the station have said that there were evening dances at quarantine, but inquiries failed to confirm this." Newhard shot back to the newspaper that if it wanted confirmation, it could simply have asked him: "There is no rule forbidding the families of the officers and employees of the station dancing. Your correspondent failed to find that they had dances. Well, we had dances, and quite frequently, but no one took part in them excepting residents inside of the station."[16]

It did not take long for cracks to appear in Philadelphia's unified front. The Bliss bill had proceeded to a second reading before the full House of Representatives when the city's newspapers began to call for removal of the Lazaretto. The *Times* mocked those who defended the Tinicum Lazaretto as "reminiscent and venerable gentlemen who . . . cherish half-century-old memories of 'fishin' for catties down at the Lazarett.'" The paper reassured such nostalgics that "it is not contemplated to remove the river or any portion of it, nor any of the surviving catfish remaining therein; it is believed that even the ancient and now decayed wharf, where erst they got their youthful panties wet, will be allowed to remain."[17]

Around the same time, the *Inquirer*, too, had a change of heart. The paper acknowledged that the Lazaretto posed little danger to its vicinity, but still called it "an eyesore and constant menace" for the mere possibility of contagious disease that it represented in the public eye. Moreover, the nearly century-old brick buildings had been built "according to the old and mistaken notions of hospitals" and

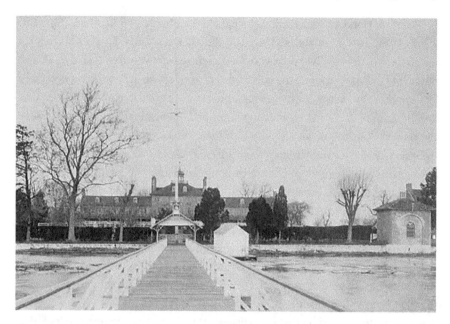

Figure 17. The Lazaretto seen from the pier, ca. 1890, lantern slide image. Reproduced with permission of the Historical Society of Pennsylvania.

were "doubtless to this day full of disease germs." The new bacteriological science of health demanded wood-frame buildings, open to as much air and light as possible, that could be "burned to the ground" to prevent the spread of a disease outbreak "with but little loss." But the *Inquirer's* bottom line was more psychological than microbiological: "The quarantine buildings always carry an unpleasant suggestion, if not danger," and therefore ought to be demolished (figure 17).[18]

The Lazaretto originally functioned as a theater of vigilance, in which stately, imposing public buildings helped make the city's commitment to public health visibly and tangibly real. By 1891, the same buildings *provoked* the popular dread they had been created to soothe. The only question that mattered, the *Chester Times* maintained, was whether the continued existence of the Lazaretto on Tinicum Island "brings a feeling of apprehension to thousands of people." "As long as the station remains, there is that feeling of fear on the part of the people and it is the duty of the Legislature, as the people's servants, to respect that feeling and to take every means in their power to remove anything which menaces them."[19] The question of actual danger was irrelevant; the people's fear of the Lazaretto, even if baseless, constituted grounds for removal.

The state House of Representatives passed the Bliss bill on April 22, 1891. Two weeks later, at the Senate hearing, the Philadelphia and Chester contingents squared off in debate. Two physicians led their respective sides: Board of Health president Ford spoke against the bill, while Forwood spoke in favor. Ford, described by a reporter as "aristocratic looking and gray, with mustache and imperial of Second Empire cut" (that is, sporting fancy and old-fashioned facial hair), called the removal campaign "an effort to humiliate the second city in the country in the interests of the rural building enterprises and land schemers." He denied that anyone had ever "caught a disease directly from any patient in the hospital." When it was his turn, Forwood "grew very emphatic and red in the face" and denounced the Lazaretto "pesthouse" as "an outrage . . . being perpetrated upon the people of Chester." One senator asked Forwood why the Chester Board of Health had taken a stand in favor of keeping the station in Tinicum. "Well," the doctor replied, "the Chester Board of Health went up to the Lazaretto, where they were wined and dined, after which they came back home and signed a resolution that had been written for them." At this, Ford "sprang to his feet" with a furious denial: Chester's board had asked to inspect the quarantine facility, and its Philadelphia counterpart had granted the request. "A lunch was served," Ford added flatly. He insisted that the Chester board's resolution came as a surprise to him and to his Philadelphia colleagues.[20]

Just as Forwood and Bliss prepared to celebrate their victory, the bill's path to final approval took a surprising detour. A week after the Senate hearing, both houses of the legislature passed a resolution appointing a five-member commission to negotiate with the federal government, Delaware, and New Jersey with the goal of finding an appropriate site for a new quarantine facility farther downriver than Tinicum. The Senate then promptly killed the Bliss bill. Some Harrisburg observers called this a defeat for the removal campaign, but it may instead have been a savvy strategic retreat. As eager as they were to push through to victory, Forwood and Bliss recognized that their biggest obstacle was the absence of an alternative site that could perform all the functions of the Tinicum Lazaretto. Many lawmakers considered it rash to close the existing station when there was nothing ready to replace it. Forwood and Bliss must have reasoned that with a new site lined up, their bill would be all but unstoppable.[21]

As the Bliss bill stalled in the spring of 1891, Democratic governor Robert Pattison (who both preceded and succeeded James Beaver in the office) appointed Edwin Herbst, another unknown physician from a small town in Berks County, to replace the much-abused Henry Brusstar as Lazaretto physician. A year later, Herbst was leading a station operating under a kind of temporarily suspended death sentence. When he looked toward the city from Tinicum Island, he saw a feuding and mistrustful Board of Health, which had lost much of its credibility in the eyes of Philadelphians. When he turned downriver toward the sea, he heard rumblings of something far more ominous: cholera. It cannot have been a comforting position for the 34-year-old doctor.

Philadelphia had experience with cholera, as did nearly every other US city, and recent advances in bacteriology had gone far to clarify the science of the disease, but unfortunately neither experience nor the laboratory taught clear lessons about how to prevent it. German microbiologist Dr. Robert Koch's identification of the cholera germ, known as the *comma bacillus*, in 1884 had confirmed the hypothesis that emerged from Dr. John Snow's 1854 epidemiological studies in London: cholera spread through microorganisms in contaminated urban water supplies. But Koch's discovery did not mean that the disease could not also spread in other ways. In fact, now that the germ could be seen microscopically in patients' feces, in fecally contaminated water, and in food that had come into contact with contaminated water, anxious observers trained their sights on clothing and other objects that might have been touched by feces or by tainted water or food— especially when those objects belonged to poor people or foreigners. And even though no one could point to a quarantine that had successfully prevented the entry of cholera, everyone agreed that Herbst and the rest of the Lazaretto staff needed to heighten their vigilance as the disease spread via rail lines from Afghanistan to Russia in the summer of 1892, reaching Moscow in July.[22]

On Tinicum Island, the first three quarters of the 1892 season passed mostly quietly, but there were warning signs that Dr. Herbst and the Board of Health did not always see eye to eye. When the steamship *Indiana* arrived from Liverpool in early July with a case of smallpox aboard, two physicians from the federal quarantine station at the Delaware breakwater came up to the Lazaretto to insist that the vessel be detained until twenty-one days had elapsed since the patient's first symptoms. Herbst isolated the patient in the hospital and declared the steamer safe to proceed to the city as soon as it could be fumigated. Not trusting Herbst, board president Ford went down to investigate for himself and ordered all passengers vaccinated, regardless of prior vaccination status, and the vessel detained. Two days later, Herbst asked the board for permission to release the *Indiana*. Two days after that, the board decided that it resented the federal intrusion more than it mistrusted the Lazaretto physician and approved the release, subject to Herbst's determination that no further cases had appeared among the passengers. As soon as the ship arrived in port, a passenger was found to have a mild case of smallpox. The board rebuked Herbst sharply in a public statement: "The eruption had been out for at least three days preceding and could easily have been detected if looked for. The vessel was detained for the purpose of detecting just such cases. During these three days, the Lazaretto physician daily and urgently recommended the release of the vessel and criticized the board for exercising its lawful prerogative."[23] No major outbreak followed, but the handling of the *Indiana* did not bode well with the threat of cholera looming.

Imported rags for paper manufacturing continued to be a staple of Philadelphia's maritime commerce. As cholera marched through eastern Europe in late July and early August, the call to bar all rags collected from infected areas—or even all rags from any foreign port—grew louder. One of the leading sources of imported rags was the German port of Hamburg, which was also one of the busiest departure points for the unprecedented "third wave" of immigration to the United States from eastern Europe that had begun around 1880 and was in full force in 1892.[24] The news that cholera had broken out in Hamburg in mid-August struck health authorities in American ports like a thunderbolt.

In the Lazaretto's early days, it would have taken several weeks for Philadelphia officials to learn about an overseas epidemic, and they would not find out whether any ships were headed their way from the affected area until such vessels arrived. But international communication had been transformed by the telegraph, which reached across the Atlantic beginning in 1866.[25] Now, as soon as the news of the 1892 cholera in Hamburg became public, Dr. Herbst and the Board of Health knew that the American Line steamship *British Princess* from Liverpool was four days out from Philadelphia with about 600 passengers, of whom 200 were reported to have transited through Hamburg.

The Lazaretto had already begun preparing for the disinfection of passengers' baggage on a much larger scale than ever before. The Board of Health dedicated a special barge for transporting baggage to the US Customs warehouse next door to the Lazaretto, where it would be fumigated by sulfur for six to eight hours. The experts felt confident that "neither germs nor spores will survive the ordeal." The board entertained the idea of separating immigrants from the cholera regions from all other passengers but in the end decided to disinfect all steerage passengers' baggage on any vessel that carried any passengers from the affected areas. It also "respectfully" requested an emergency appropriation of $50,000 from the city councils for urgent expenditures to prevent the arrival and spread of cholera.[26]

Only six years after the dedication of the Statue of Liberty, with all American ports on high alert, a crescendo of voices demanded a complete prohibition on all immigration into the United States. Nativism was nothing new in American politics, but before the third wave and especially the cholera scare of 1892, the institution of quarantine had not been directly implicated in the restriction of immigration. The confluence of the new flood of migrants from southern and eastern Europe, the expanded federal role in quarantine affairs, and the specter of epidemic cholera turned the Lazaretto into an arena of xenophobic discrimination for the first time in its history. John Huggard, chairman of the state board appointed to investigate alternative sites to replace the Lazaretto, told a reporter at the time, "I favor immigration, but not of persons so uncleanly in habit as . . . the Huns, Slavs and Russians who seek entrance."[27]

The *British Princess* passed by the breakwater station early in the morning of Monday, August 29—it was required to stop there only if there was illness aboard— and arrived at the Lazaretto at 1:00 p.m. Herbst promptly reported to the board that all passengers and crew members were healthy and that there was "not a single person from Hamburg" among them, "as far as could be ascertained from inquiries among the immigrants." (It is difficult to imagine a Lazaretto physician from the heyday of yellow fever taking the passengers' word at face value when it came to such critical information.) The shipping line's official manifest, forwarded before the ship's departure from Liverpool, included 150 steerage passengers from in and around Hamburg. The credulous Dr. Herbst was unsure what to make of this discrepancy, but the health officer back in Philadelphia instructed him in no uncertain terms to get started with the disinfection of the baggage from steerage. There was plenty of it, and it would take time. Nevertheless, the newspapers assumed the *British Princess* would be headed for port as soon as the fumigation was finished—perhaps by Tuesday afternoon, August 30.[28]

They were mistaken. On Tuesday, when the baggage was unloaded, the board ordered all the interior spaces of the ship disinfected. When that was done, Herbst considered the ship safe and ready to go. On Thursday, the board sent port physician Henry Leffmann down to the Lazaretto to "have oversight" of the quarantined immigrants and to stay there until further notice. The board had long since lost whatever trust it had in Herbst. But Leffmann agreed with the Lazaretto physician that the *British Princess* no longer posed any threat and told the board so. No one claimed or even hinted that there was illness among the passengers. Faced with a consensus, the five members of the board did nothing. It was as if the anticipation of cholera's arrival and the accumulated pressure of gathering public anxiety had paralyzed them.[29] By the time they saw the newspaper headlines on Friday morning, September 2, they surely wished they had released the ship as Drs. Herbst and Leffmann had urged.

In Thursday's daily written report, Herbst let slip an anecdotal tidbit that he knew would embarrass the men who had so antagonized him. Board of Health member Dr. Peter Keyser visited the Lazaretto that day to have a look for himself at the station's preparedness. When Herbst brought Keyser and noted cholera expert Dr. Edward Shakespeare alongside the *British Princess* in a boat, a familiar face called down to Keyser from the deck railing: John Clark, a former Philadelphia councilman and a cabin passenger returning from Europe. He politely but insistently explained to the three doctors how devilishly inconvenient the ship's detention was to him. Keyser told him to grab his valise and climb down into their boat. In his report to the board, Herbst noted drily that since one passenger had been released, he did not see any reason why the others should not be as well.[30]

The press had a field day. Incompetence, cronyism, discrimination against steerage passengers—accusations and questions flew at the board from all directions. Would Keyser be punished for violating the quarantine laws? Would Clark be forced to return to the ship? Who was in charge of the city's efforts to prevent an epidemic, and why was it being bungled so badly? "So big a rumpus was kicked up over the affair," wrote the *Inquirer*, that it would take several days to clean up the mess. All agreed that the incident had "made a spectacular farce of the administration of the health laws." A furious mayor Edwin Stuart openly worried that other cities would "point the finger of scorn" at Philadelphia. Dr. Keyser defended himself, claiming that he had conferred with the city's director of public safety (whose department included the Board of Health) and some of his colleagues on the board before he went to the Lazaretto, and that they had given him authority to act on their behalf. (No one else remembered any such conversation.) Perhaps in a bid to end the embarrassing attention being paid to the affair, two members of the board offered motions to release the *British Princess* from quarantine, but both motions failed. Dr. Leffmann reported to the board that there was no danger in allowing the ship up to the city, and that the surest way to cause a disease outbreak would be to continue confining so many immigrants in its crowded steerage. With that, he promptly resigned as port physician, citing the board's lack of confidence in his judgment.[31]

After Friday's raucous, recrimination-filled board meeting, Saturday found tempers somewhat cooled. Keyser offered a conditional apology ("If I made a mistake . . ."), and the other four board members firmly but diplomatically reminded him that yes, he had made a mistake. The board then unanimously voted to send the health officer to return the "fugitive" Clark to his ship, and to rebuke Dr. Herbst—the ever-ready scapegoat—for allowing the ex-councilman to leave the Lazaretto in the first place. But someone tipped Clark off at his Walnut Street law office, and he took a hasty "lunch" break just a few steps ahead of the health officer. Clark was last seen boarding a westbound trolley. Meanwhile, after yet another favorable report from Herbst and (in his last official act) Leff-mann, the board quietly voted to liberate the *British Princess* from its weeklong Tinicum detention.[32]

Summoned by telegram, Clark reported to the Health Office on Monday September 5. An employee of the office escorted him to the wharf where the *British Princess* had moored. An absurd legalistic ritual followed, in which the ship's first officer was summoned (in the captain's absence) and gave the health office employee "a receipt for the body of John A. Clark," at which point "they passed a social hour very pleasantly," according to a reporter, while some more paperwork was processed. Clark then left the ship and boarded a train for his country residence. In Herbst's daily report to the board on Monday, he protested that he should not be blamed for Keyser's peremptory release of Clark. Contradicting Keyser's claim that he "had no interest" in Clark, the Lazaretto physician alleged that Keyser had told him beforehand that "he had a friend, a cabin passenger, whom he was going to take back to the city with him." Herbst went on to scold the board for causing Leffmann's resignation. "Send someone in whom you have confidence to assist me, if you see proper," Herbst wrote, "but then, show confidence in him yourselves." He continued with customary sarcasm: "Invest such a man with responsibility and I will be port policeman, which is about all the free will left me, anyhow." Such a report normally would arouse indignation and anger among board members. So low had this board's relationship with Herbst sunk that this caustic report was greeted only with contemptuous laughter.[33]

The ugly waltz of mutual antagonism between Herbst and the Board of Health dragged on endlessly. Herbst (in the board's view) allowed vessels up without board approval; the board (in Herbst's view) refused to allow him to do the job he was appointed to do; and more than once his correspondence was returned to him as unacceptably "insolent and untruthful."[34]

Aggressive additional precautions in anticipation of cholera's arrival continued through September and into autumn. The Board of Health requisitioned hundreds of tents from Harrisburg for use at the Lazaretto if large numbers of passengers needed to be accommodated there. A local steamship excursion company leased the *Georgeanna* to the board, which fitted it out with a steam disinfection chamber along with facilities to accommodate 1,100 passengers and sleep 350. Desperate for dependability, the board hired Dr. W. T. Robinson, who had been working in Philadelphia as a city medical inspector, to oversee the *Georgeanna*. German-speaking watchmen and an inspector who was a Russian Jewish immigrant were hired on an emergency basis to improve communications at the Lazaretto. The authorities' preoccupation with rags and baggage intensified.[35] All hands were on deck to an extent never before seen when there was no illness present at the Lazaretto.

The federal government continued its gradual takeover of maritime quarantine by ordering all vessels carrying foreign immigrants to undergo a twenty-day quarantine before entering any US port. Only Hamburg among western European cities suffered a major cholera epidemic in 1892, but that city's importance as a commercial and emigration hub kept much of the world on high alert. With its unmatched volume of immigrant traffic, New York experienced forty-four cholera deaths in quarantine (on top of seventy-six cholera deaths at sea on New York–bound ships) but avoided a major outbreak in the city.[36]

Philadelphia's Board of Health extended the quarantine season indefinitely, until finally, two days after Christmas, the inner channel between the Lazaretto and Little Tinicum Island was a solid sheet of ice, and the Delaware River was impassable.[37] Through it all and despite it all, somehow, the unwieldy and disharmonious federal-state-municipal hybrid quarantine apparatus had managed to keep cholera out of Philadelphia. With a different cast of characters in charge, it might have been an opportunity to tout the benefits of the city's modern and efficient quarantine. But with all that squabbling and incompetence? Nobody was in a position to boast.

Viewed from the water's edge, the enduring legacy of 1892 was not America's triumph over cholera, but the conversion of maritime quarantine into a tool for restriction, confinement, and stigmatization of impoverished immigrants. Discrimination and even violence against newly arrived Americans had a long pedigree, but until the third wave of immigration and the threat of cholera, the institution of quarantine had not been mobilized as part of the machinery of xenophobia. During the cholera scare, even the elite doctors who railed against the "inhumanity" of confining passengers in the unsanitary conditions of immigrant ships during extended quarantines argued that the best course of action would be to "put an end to the perpetual menace of indiscriminate immigration."[38]

In other words, the desperate suffering of the migrants at our shores should persuade us to keep them out permanently.

The cholera alarm continued into 1893. The other shoe in the federal takeover of quarantine dropped in February, when President Benjamin Harrison signed the National Quarantine Act into law. Without abolishing state and local quarantines, the law subordinated them to a new network of facilities run by the US Marine Hospital Service. In Harrisburg a month later, Ward Bliss introduced a new version of his anti-Lazaretto bill, this one fully vetted by the Marine Hospital Service and US Surgeon General Walter Wyman. The new Bliss bill provided for the Tinicum station to remain open (under the control of a single executive officer, appointed by the governor) only until a newly organized federal quarantine was fully up and running at both the breakwater station and a new facility with extensive disinfection facilities on Reedy Island in Delaware, 30 miles downriver from Tinicum. The governor would have authority to build a small new station for inspection only—no disinfection or medical care—and to remobilize a full state quarantine "whenever the federal government should fail to maintain such a service."[39]

The rhetoric surrounding Bliss Bill II was just as overheated as it had been around its predecessor, but it was more one sided. The Lazaretto's defenders had seen the writing on the wall and found themselves fighting for a delay in the station's closure and for greater city representation in the oversight of the state quarantine. This time, Bliss's and Forwood's supporters pointed to the almost comical series of contretemps between Herbst and the Board of Health as all the evidence needed that the current system was broken and bad for business. The board met with representatives of the business community to form a unified front that accepted the outlines of the Bliss bill but would push to strengthen the city's role in the future system. Meanwhile, the local press welcomed the new legislation and bemoaned the bungling and quarreling that had marked the previous season.[40] The *Inquirer*, once a staunch voice in favor of retaining the Lazaretto, now consigned it to the dustbin of history: "The best thing the city can do . . . is to go down to the Lazaretto and touch a match to the century-old hospital. The sight of it is enough to breed disease and the smell from its germ-laden walls is enough to spread a pestilence. Down with it. It is a disgrace to modern science."[41] The stage was set for the final debates and amendments in the spring of 1893, but this time few doubted the outcome.

In view of the cholera threat, the Board of Health decided to open the quarantine season a month early, on May 1. The city had invested in new bathing and disinfection facilities as well as in cosmetic improvements to the Lazaretto buildings. When the board undertook its annual preseason inspection of the station, it took the unusual step of inviting reporters from the city's newspapers to join them. By tradition, after the inspection and property inventory at the beginning and end of each season, board members and a few invited guests sat down to a banquet in the central pavilion of the Lazaretto's main building. This time, the reporters showed less interest in cholera or disinfection than they did in entertainment. After the meal, the newspapermen performed a satirical comedy skit lampooning the Board of Health. Nothing was off-limits—the board's attention to bureaucratic and procedural minutiae, its investigations of exotic nuisances, its stinginess with permissions to enter and leave the Lazaretto, and Herbst's constant complaints were all parodied. The ritual use of disinfectants figured prominently in the skit.[42] The fact that such a comedic performance took place in the public eye (that is, with journalists present) while legislators were debating the Bliss bill could only have meant two things: one, plenty of alcohol was served; and two, the outcome in Harrisburg was a foregone conclusion.

The banquet attendees missed their train back to the city. By three hours.[43]

As if to self-sabotagingly give additional impetus to the Bliss bill just as the final vote loomed, Dr. Herbst and the Board of Health dove into yet another quarantine skirmish. First a reported case of smallpox was discovered on the ship *Lord Gough* on May 29, after Herbst had permitted it up to the port, and the board upbraided him for missing it. Herbst responded defensively, as usual, then two days later complained that scattered cases of smallpox continued to appear on the ship *Ohio*, in quarantine for a week, and that he had nowhere to put the 840 passengers, who were in greater danger of illness every day that they remained confined aboard in quarantine. Could he send the ship back to the breakwater station, he asked? The Lazaretto had prepared for large numbers of passengers on ships carrying cholera, but for some reason Herbst felt paralyzed and claimed the current law left him no options. Rather than suggest ways of accommodating most or all of the *Ohio*'s passengers, the board contented itself with blaming Herbst for their predicament: "He is a most incompetent man in a most important position." Later, the board brought in two other doctors to examine the passengers, determine their vaccination status, revaccinate those of uncertain status, and find alternative shelter for as many as possible.[44]

In the first week of June, the new Reedy Island station was nearly finished. Governor Pattison signed the amended Bliss bill into law on June 6. A board of seven members consisting of the Philadelphia health officer and the new state quarantine physician (both appointed by the governor), as well as the secretary of the state Board of Health and additional members appointed by the governor, the mayor of Philadelphia, and the Maritime Exchange would oversee the state's Delaware River quarantine. (One newspaper reported that Pattison would appoint Herbst as quarantine physician. He did not.)[45]

In the Lazaretto's first five years of operation, there had been three yellow fever outbreaks in the city, and 1,300 to 1,400 deaths—a considerable number, but a far cry from the carnage of the 1790s. After 1805, the disease returned only three times before the Lazaretto closed in 1895, killing a total of 224 people. The annual summertime dread gradually abated.

The Bliss Act terminated the Board of Health's authority over the Lazaretto on June 30, 1893, but the station would continue to operate under the control of the state quarantine board until the end of the 1895 season, when a smaller inspection station opened at Marcus Hook on the Pennsylvania-Delaware border. Edwin Herbst resigned shortly after the passage of the new law and departed the Lazaretto before the board could appoint a replacement. As a result, for a few days, the board turned again to Dr. W. T. Robinson.[46] Although the newspapers seemingly failed to notice that the summer of 1893 marked one hundred years since the devastating 1793 yellow fever epidemic that had set into motion Philadelphia's public health infrastructure, the anniversary was surely not lost on Robinson, who returned to Tinicum Island for an anticlimactic last hurrah in mid-June.

He felt the tug of history—he must have felt it, given all the time he had spent working at the Lazaretto and researching its history. It would have been understandable if he felt a certain sadness over the fate of this institution into which he had invested so much of himself, and which he knew so intimately. He knew the Lazaretto as a flawed but benevolent institution of social progress, forged from tragedy. He heard—he must have heard, because he knew them better than anyone—the echoes of countless unsung acts of caring and even heroism over the decades. But whatever he felt, as he walked out through the Lazaretto gates one final time, he kept it to himself.

Philadelphia in the 1890s called itself "The Workshop of the World." It was a booming, bustling industrial behemoth, ceaselessly gobbling up acre after acre of former woodland and farmland to turn into factories and rowhomes. Immigrants from southern and eastern Europe were flooding into the city by the tens of thousands to toil in the likes of the Cramp Shipyards and the Baldwin Locomotive Works. A time traveler visiting from the Philadelphia of Edward Garrigues and William Donaldson and Charles Caldwell might have thought themselves transported to another planet, so radically had the city transformed itself. Meanwhile, the Lazaretto looked much the same in the 1890s as it had in 1801. When Dr. Robinson said goodbye to the station on Tinicum Island for the last time, little had changed in its physical appearance since Garrigues had opened it for the first time nearly a century earlier. The city's growth and expansion were fed largely through the Lazaretto, where goods and immigrants passed inspection, but the station endured through the decades as a proudly unchanging reminder of a bygone age—an island, incongruous, strangely out of time, as it remains today. It is as if this site is reminding us that (in the words of William Faulkner) "The past is never dead. It's not even past." It tells us, too, as Albert Camus did in his novel *The Plague*, that what may appear to be our victories over epidemics will always turn out to be temporary at best. There will always be more plagues.[47]

Chapter Seventeen

Afterlives

A personal confession: I did not set out to write this book because I found the history of quarantine in Philadelphia a particularly fascinating or important topic. (That realization came later.) I began this work because the physical site of the Lazaretto grabbed hold of me and would not let go. In January 2006, when I first saw it, it was a grand but decaying relic, silently standing watch at the edge of the broad-shouldered, stolid Delaware. It was the incongruity of the site that intrigued me: the weirdly bucolic riverfront setting just a mile from the roaring jets of Philadelphia International Airport and half a mile from the impatient thrum of Interstate 95, the lazy pace of the river, the wildness of Little Tinicum Island, the stately architecture, the telltale signs of physical deterioration, and most of all the *scale* of it all. This place was obviously a Very Big Deal at some point in the past. But why, and how? What went on there? Why so big, and why so stately? Those questions would not leave me alone. Only years later, in dusty archives and library reading rooms, would I meet the likes of Edward Garrigues and Charles Caldwell, Mary Ann Ganges and Tobias Smith, T. J. P. Stokes and W. T. Robinson, Fanny Gartrell and Mary Riddle. But at that first wide-eyed glance, I had a feeling there were stories in those bricks.

That tantalizing incongruity, guarding secrets but revealing just enough to spark curiosity, set me off on an adventure that continues to this day. When I learned about the controversy over the construction of a new fire station on the site, I jumped into the fray with an op-ed pleading for preservation without new construction, and I joined forces with other historic preservation advocates opposing the plan. When the lawsuit over that construction was settled and the Lazaretto Preservation Association of Tinicum Township was established, I was asked to join its board, where I still sit today. Over time I became the self-appointed evangelist of the Lazaretto, giving tours, organizing events, speaking to any audience that would listen, and writing for academic and nonacademic audiences alike, continually trying to spread the word about this unmatched historic treasure—always with the help of many students, friends, and fellow volunteers. This book is my latest attempt, but I am sure it will not be my last.

In the early 1890s, accusations that the Lazaretto had become little more than a destination for leisure junkets and entertainment helped seal its fate. After its closure, that is precisely what the site became, in the first of several afterlives. Finally, though, in the early twenty-first century, it faced what seemed to be its final demise: it was to be torn down to make way for an airport parking garage. And yet, Lazarus-like—as if inspired by those many patients with yellow fever and typhus who came back to life there—the Lazaretto survived to see and speak to a new century.

It was not even three years after the yellow flag was lowered for the last time on Tinicum Island in 1895 that the Lazaretto found a new purpose. Matters of life and death gave way to entertainment and recreation.

Beginning in 1898, the Athletic Club of Philadelphia (which counted many wealthy and influential men as members) used the site of the former quarantine station as its summer home. Members enjoyed a retreat from the city's heat and congestion to the place they dubbed the Orchard for cycling, baseball, lawn tennis, lawn bowling, quoits, and other activities (figures 18, 19, and 20). Two Tinicum Island specialties—shad and reed birds—were served up as dinners and suppers, often accompanied by "quantities of liquid refreshment . . . to aid the digestion."[1]

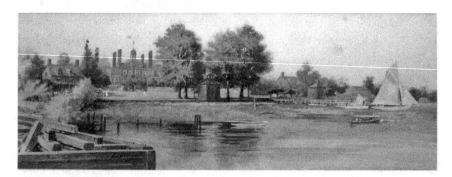

Figure 18. The Orchard, summer home of the Athletic Club of Philadelphia. Watercolor by Frank Taylor, ca. late 1890s. Courtesy of Arader Galleries, Philadelphia, PA.

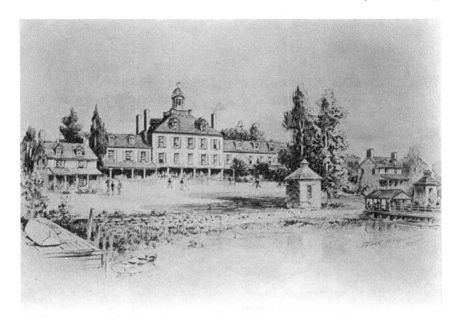

Figure 19. Lawn tennis and other games at the Orchard. Drawing by Frank Taylor, ca. late 1890s. Courtesy of Historic American Buildings Survey, Library of Congress.

A rare winter excursion to the island in 1900 provided the occasion for a true Orchard blowout. The city's movers and shakers began gathering in the afternoon, and "the popping of corks and the puffs of smoke rising continually to the ceiling" continued until past midnight, as reported in the *Philadelphia Inquirer*.[2] The after-dinner entertainment seems to have been custom made to flatter the vanities and prejudices of the urban elite. Interspersed with the banjo players, jugglers, and dancing girls were several blackface comedians; Dave Jenkins, "the colored Irish comedian"; Benny Reinhold, "the Hebrew impersonator"; and Blanche Lawrence, a singer of "coon songs." (The "coon song" craze of the Tin Pan Alley era used exaggerated vernacular and prevailing stereotypes of African Americans to en-tertain audiences while implicitly bolstering rationalizations for segregation and subordination.) For the members of the Athletic Club, casual, light-hearted big-otry was all part of a rollicking evening's festivities at the Orchard. When the smoker finally ended, the hour was so late that a special train had to be arranged for the returning guests.[3]

The leisure pursuits of Philadelphia's upper crust drove the next chapter of the Lazaretto's history, too, which soon took a surprising turn back toward the

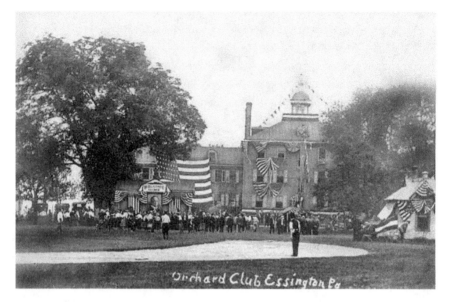

Figure 20. "Welcome Home" celebration at the Orchard for Philadelphia recorder of deeds William S. Vare (later a state senator and US congressman), returning from a European vacation, 1908. Courtesy of Tinicum Township Historical Society.

protection of public safety. In 1915 Philadelphia banker, stockbroker, and socialite Robert Glendinning purchased a "flying boat" from the Curtiss Aeroplane Company; his "hydroaeroplane" was one of the first generation of what were later renamed *seaplanes*. Glendinning's well-publicized short flights from the Corinthian Yacht Club next to the Lazaretto in Tinicum to the League Island Navy Yard in South Philadelphia tested out both his aircraft's capabilities and the landing conditions in the Delaware at the Navy Yard. Before long he and some well-connected friends in the Aero Club of Pennsylvania were encouraging wealthy men of the city to take up aviation as a sport. In late 1915, their minds on the war in Europe that seemingly had no end in sight, they reasoned that a corps of flying men could serve as an "aeroplane reserve" for coastal defense if the conflict ever enveloped the United States.[4]

In early 1916, Philadelphia City Council voted to lease the Lazaretto property to Glendinning and his partners for the establishment of the Philadelphia School of Aviation, a nonprofit institution dedicated to "national preparedness." The buildings were unused at the time, and there was ample room on the site for hangars. Furthermore, the inner channel of the Delaware between the Lazaretto and Little Tinicum Island usually provided calmer water conditions for takeoff and landing than could be found elsewhere on the river. The school opened for instruction in May, with a fleet consisting of three Curtiss flying boats. A year later, when the United States entered the war, the school was temporarily renamed Chandler Field and placed under the control of US military authorities. For seven months, hundreds of pilot trainees flocked to Tinicum. Rich men's playthings had quickly become "positive necessities" for national defense.[5]

Twenty-four-year-old Chicago native Frank Mills was one of the first two instructors at the Philadelphia School of Aviation. Mills had worked on the Panama Canal and received pilot training at the Glenn Curtiss Flying School in San Diego. His tenure on Tinicum would be nearly as long as the Lazaretto's: he and his three sons operated the seaplane base, flight school, and marina on the Lazaretto site continuously until 2000 (figures 21 and 22).[6] The family's decision to finally close up shop that year ended another chapter of the site's long, tumultuous history and left a void on the riverfront and in the community. Two centuries after the opening of the Tinicum Lazaretto, the bustle and thrum of quarantine, of sports, of entertainment, and of "flying boats" gave way to silence and slow decay.

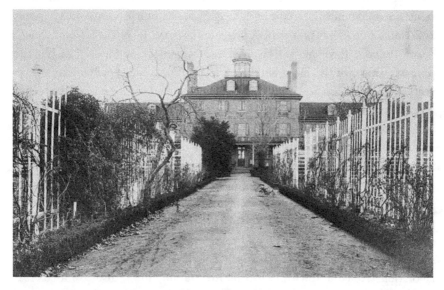

Figure 21. The Lazaretto's main building, part of the Philadelphia Seaplane Base, 1936. Courtesy of Historic American Buildings Survey, Library of Congress.

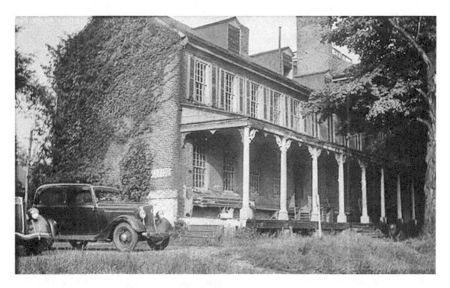

Figure 22. Southwest corner of the main building, 1936. Courtesy of Historic American Buildings Survey, Library of Congress.

In June 2000, a developer bought the Lazaretto property from the Mills family for a little more than two million dollars with a plan to demolish all remaining structures and build an airport parking garage. Historic preservation advocates and Tinicum residents protested. A few months later, the Board of Commissioners of Tinicum Township got involved and began looking for ways to buy the property and save the main building and the four smaller outbuildings. Five years elapsed before a deal was worked out, and by then the agendas of the preservationists and the township had diverged. The township saw the five acres of unbuilt space on the property as the ideal location for a much-needed new fire station, with a potentially revenue-generating banquet hall (and large parking lot) attached. Many preservationists believed the plan represented an assault on the historical integrity of the site (figures 23, 24, and 25).[7]

After the conflict came to a head in 2006—through angry private and public polemics, a lawsuit, and the creation of a nonprofit preservation board with representatives from the township and preservation organizations—the new fire station was built, and rancorous conflict eventually turned to productive collaboration. Tinicum Township had its fire station, and it also had a colossal (roughly 16,000 square feet) two-century-old building on its hands that needed

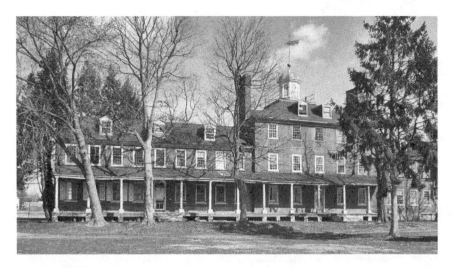

Figure 23. The main building, ca. 2005, during the debate over the preservation of the site and the construction of the new Tinicum fire station. Photo by Doug Heller.

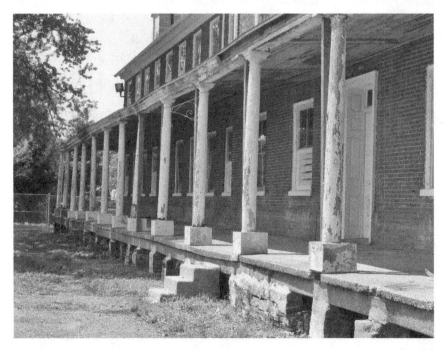

Figure 24. The main building's portico in 2006. Photo by David Barnes.

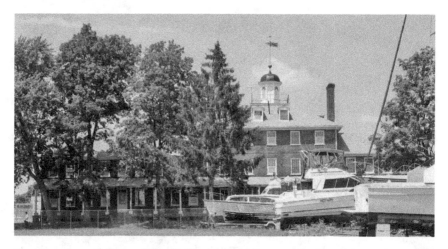

Figure 25. Boat storage in front of the main building, 2006. Photo by David Barnes.

millions of dollars of work to be restored for any kind of use. The township had raised grant money for Lazaretto restoration, and additional grant money for construction of a new municipal administration building. When it decided to move the township offices into the Lazaretto's main building, the two pools of money could be combined. Additional funding from Philadelphia International Airport (half of which is in Tinicum Township) allowed the restoration work to begin in 2016.[8]

The long-awaited and long-delayed restoration of the Lazaretto's main building was finally completed at the end of February 2020, when the township's offices moved in and opened for business in the old quarantine station. In a colossal irony that was lost on no one, this triumph of historic preservation was interrupted just two weeks later by . . . the demands of a new quarantine. COVID-19 had taken the place of yellow fever as the urgent health threat, but instead of requiring that the Lazaretto open early or stay open beyond its normal closing date, this epidemic forced the site to shut down. When the building reopened in 2021, the Lazaretto's nonprofit board was seeking to raise funds for historical exhibits and programming (figure 26).[9]

The bedrock dilemma that created the Lazaretto, of course, is with us still: How can we make ourselves safe from epidemics while still carrying on with our lives? Threatened by a deadly, rapidly spreading, and incurable disease, people need to do *something*. Nineteenth-century Philadelphians fumigated cargo to stop the

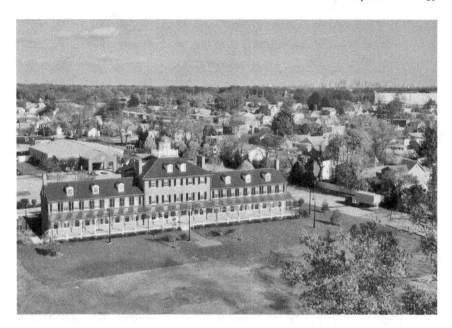

Figure 26. The newly restored main building in 2020, with the Philadelphia skyline in the distance. Photo by David Barnes.

spread of yellow fever; twenty-first-century Philadelphians wiped down groceries with disinfectant solutions to ward off COVID-19. In neither instance did they do it because it was *proved* to be effective; they did it because it was something they could do, and because it enacted their cooperation in a common enterprise of collective self-defense.

For nearly a century at the Lazaretto on Tinicum Island, each new outbreak of disease, each new epidemic, brought back the specter of all the previous epidemics. In early 2020, as COVID-19's potential for devastation became clear, comparisons with the terrible 1918 influenza pandemic were inevitably made. But as readers of this book will recognize, comparisons with yellow fever or typhus at the Lazaretto quarantine station and in Philadelphia's streets are apt, as well:

- A disease of unknown origin was spreading; its precise means of spread was unclear; no treatments were effective in curing it.
- If something was not done to stop the spread of the virus soon, many people would die because of it.
- Hospitals set apart designated beds and wings to isolate people sick with the virus—no visitors allowed.

- To avoid infection with the virus, many people, if they could or if they were ordered to, stayed inside their homes; some packed up house and moved away from densely populated areas.
- Some places closed their borders—no nonresidents allowed. Others restricted entry by travelers from specified areas.
- Politicians sparred over whether preserving commerce or public health was more important, while scientists disagreed among themselves over the source of the virus and how best and how aggressively to slow its spread.
- Previously "invisible" people working to deliver food and services and health care were suddenly acknowledged as essential to the successful functioning of a community.
- People were enmeshed in vital social fabrics that were traumatically torn by unexpected deaths, widespread mourning, and unresolved loss.

In 2020, individual cities and states mostly abandoned the idea of enforced quarantine for COVID-19 on the grounds that it was a draconian measure, but many of them recommended two-week self-isolation after potential exposure to the virus or after returning from a place known to have a high rate of infection. In March 2020, Philadelphia, for example, recommended "quarantine" for its residents under certain circumstances: "Quarantine separates people who know they were exposed to someone with COVID-19 coronavirus, or who recently traveled to a location where the disease was spreading rapidly. Quarantines are for people who do not show symptoms, but should be kept separate because they have a higher-than-average likelihood of having been exposed to the disease. People in quarantine do not leave quarantine for at least 14 days."[10] In a sense, people all over the world spent at least part of the COVID-19 pandemic in their own personal lazarettos.

But what most people experienced during COVID-19 was not quarantine in the traditional sense of the word; it was a form of semi-voluntary self-separation. Quarantine is enforced confinement in isolation. It is a place in space and time—an *away* place and a *marking time* space—where those in charge decide who can go and who must remain and for how long. *That* kind of quarantine has driven the narrative of this book. That kind of quarantine happened, in its ideal form, on an island away from the city.

The Lazaretto stories told here will not save lives or prevent future epidemics. But close attention to the *people* who lived those stories—their values, their hopes and fears, and their agendas both selfish and selfless—can teach us valuable lessons.

If we can see past his insufferable vanity, Charles Caldwell can teach us the importance of carefully targeted strategic compromise. He and William Donaldson and their colleagues on the 1803 Board of Health could give us a lesson or two about social efficacy, although they would not have used that term. If we listen to Johan Christen, Rosina Gös, and the other redemptioners of the *Rebecca* and the *Hope*, we can see that immigration is not just a choice but a *business*, the implacable economic logic of which produces suffering and death as well as freedom and prosperity.

If we take seriously the knowledge and experience of those who lived before bacteriology, virology, and antibiotics, and stop treating them as ignorant charlatans, then we have much to learn from the likes of W. W. Gerhard and Joshua Jones, who helped "cure" the incurable with nursing and supportive care. Similarly, W. T. Robinson knew nothing about viruses, and he had no idea that mosquitoes spread yellow fever. Yet his forceful determination, political savvy, and optimistic calm under pressure prevented an epidemic and saved lives.

And Fanny Gartrell, Eve Kugler, and Mary Riddle, who had no degrees, wrote no books or articles, and held no office, remind us that courage and heroism often consist in what for so long was the hidden, thankless work of women: preparing meals, laundering clothing, washing sick bodies, and emptying bedpans—the daily chores of caregiving, the tasks of what we might call "essential workers."

The world will surely see many new health threats in the future. Our readiness to meet the future challenges may depend on the extent to which we cultivate another of Dr. Robinson's skills: a deep appreciation of the past and of how it has shaped us and our environment.

Did Quarantine Work?

Hindsight blinds us. Looking at past events through the lens of what people at the time could not have known keeps us from understanding why they did what they did. Historians' task is to figure out how people living in the past, in specific circumstances, saw the world and what factors influenced their decisions. It is not to judge them for not knowing what we know now. On the other hand, to be human is to be curious, and wondering how present-day biomedical knowledge might explain epidemics of the past can be irresistible.

This is what we understand in the twenty-first century about yellow fever: The yellow fever virus, first identified in 1927, is a single strand of RNA that enters the body when an infected female of the *Aedes aegypti* species of mosquito feeds on human blood.[1] Once in the bloodstream, the virus remains dormant for three to six days while migrating to the lymph nodes and the liver, where it replicates prolifically. Initial symptoms of sudden lethargy, sharp shooting headache, debilitating backache, intense thirst, and chills alternating with high fever last two to three days and are usually followed by remission. Most people recover at this stage, but in severe cases, the virus shuts down the liver and causes copious bleeding in the stomach, intestines, and other internal organs.

Liver failure leads to jaundice, as the virus continues to proliferate. Internal hemorrhaging floods the body until it inevitably becomes *external* hemorrhaging: bloody diarrhea and bleeding from the mucous membranes. Dried blood accumulating in the stomach turns the abundant vomitus dark brown or black. Internal organs shut down, one by one. Convulsions and coma signal the terminal stage of the illness. Death generally ensues from seven to ten days after the onset of symptoms. There is still no "cure"—that is, no universally effective treatment—for yellow fever.

And this is what we understand today about typhus, the other disease seen most often at the Lazaretto: Typhus is caused by a bacterium, *Rickettsia prowazekii*, spread by the human body louse. In earlier periods it was called *ship fever, famine fever, jail fever,* or *camp fever* (referring to military encampments), because it often broke out where poor, malnourished people were crowded together in unclean conditions. Fever, headache, and body aches are followed by rash, delirium, and stupor (the word *typhus* comes from the Greek for smoke, cloud, or stupor). Typhus was "incurable" until antibiotics became available in the late 1940s.[2] (This means that there was no specific, widely effective treatment, even though, as we have seen, more than nine out of ten typhus patients treated at the Lazaretto hospital survived.) Epidemic typhus killed hundreds of destitute immigrants to Philadelphia every year (not to mention many other migration destinations), and although it generated less alarm in the city than yellow fever, it convulsed the often overwhelmed Lazaretto.

Typhus fever is now referred to as *epidemic typhus* or *louse-borne typhus*, as contrasted with the disease known as endemic, murine, or flea-borne typhus, which is less severe. Epidemic typhus was first described in Europe in the late fifteenth century and killed many millions of people between the seventeenth and early nineteenth centuries in jails, in military encampments, and wherever war, political upheaval, and famine caused people to crowd together without enough food or cleaning facilities. Every part of Europe was familiar with periodic deadly typhus outbreaks in all these settings. And there was no laboratory setting more efficient for typhus generation and transmission than eighteenth- and nineteenth-century emigrant vessels from northern Europe to North America.[3]

But for all the misery and death it wrought aboard immigrant ships, typhus killed surprisingly few American city dwellers in the nineteenth century. There were deadly typhus outbreaks in boardinghouses where recent European arrivals had clustered, but even those happened only immediately after the immigrants' arrival, and there were no sustained, indigenous epidemics. This is a puzzle, given that the conditions of crowding, hunger, and lack of sanitation that fueled typhus in the Old World were commonly encountered in the New World. Why were there no homegrown typhus epidemics in the United States? One historian has suggested an intriguing answer: there is some evidence that North American lice may have been less efficient vectors of typhus transmission than their counterparts in other parts of the world.[4]

When we give in to temptation and read the Lazaretto's history in light of present-day knowledge, we are able to see that the nineteenth-century contagionists and anticontagionists were both wrong when it came to yellow fever. The disease is not contagious, and it is not spontaneously generated by local accumulations of filth. And yet both parties had solid evidence on their sides: even though the disease did not spread directly from person to person, both the mosquitoes and the virus arrived aboard ships from the tropics. And even though crowded, filthy streets did not create yellow fever, they did provide excellent conditions for mosquito breeding and for virus transmission.

A yellow fever epidemic cannot occur unless the virus, the mosquito, and the human encounter one another under very particular circumstances. *Aedes aegypti* is not endemic to the Delaware Valley region; it must be reintroduced from abroad each summer. It often finds ideal habitats in human settlements, and it can breed in containers of standing water such as cisterns or water casks. The mosquito feeds most actively in temperatures of 80 to 95 degrees Fahrenheit. Its flight range is quite limited, and it lives its entire two-to-four-week lifespan within a radius of no more than 200 yards. Therefore, a densely crowded population of susceptible (non-immune) human beings must be present to sustain transmission and survival of the virus. (Surviving an attack of yellow fever confers immunity.) The mosquito population must also be abundant, as only 60 percent of female *Aedes* are capable of transmitting the yellow fever virus. When all these conditions prevail in one place—and only then—the introduction of a single infected person or mosquito can ignite an epidemic. If a population of non-virus-carrying *Aedes* had established itself in Philadelphia in the summertime after a voyage from the tropics in a cargo hold, then the arrival in the city of one or more people who had been infected in the West Indies or on shipboard might have been enough to start an outbreak. Likely more common was the scenario in which infected mosquitoes were transported directly to the city, whether they had spread the virus to their human fellow travelers aboard the vessel or not.[5]

The incubation period between infection with the virus and the initial symptoms of yellow fever is three to six days; the *Aedes* mosquito lives for two to four weeks; it usually took between eight and twenty days to sail from most Caribbean ports to Philadelphia in the nineteenth century. The blood of a yellow fever patient is infective for between three and six days in the early stages of the illness. The period of *extrinsic incubation*, during which the virus passes through the mosquito's digestive tract and into its salivary glands, normally lasts twelve to eighteen days.[6] All of this means that for an outbreak to occur, the encounter between each potentially infective mosquito and the crowded, susceptible population must take place at a specific moment; if the weather conditions are not right or if the virus is not at the right stage of incubation, transmission will not occur.

Even so, nineteenth-century theories about yellow fever—none of which involved viruses or mosquitoes, and all of which have long since been rejected as fundamentally erroneous—actually provide adequate and plausible explanations of the disease's observed incidence. The seasonal pattern was evident: yellow fever epidemics happened exclusively in the warmer months. The quarantine season usually began on May 1 or June 1, and most epidemics began in July or August. Epidemics often began during or shortly after rainy spells. They also flourished in the most crowded (and therefore most filthy) urban neighborhoods. At the same time, they often began soon after the arrival of a ship from a place where yellow fever was endemic and made their first appearance close to that ship.

Historians and epidemiologists have judged quarantine quite harshly, dismissing it as ineffective against all manner of infectious diseases.[7] And judged by twenty-first-century standards, maritime quarantine against yellow fever, for example, seems a hopelessly misguided public health policy, since it directly targets neither the mosquito nor the virus. It was based on disease theories we now know to be wrong, so it stands to reason that the policies could not possibly have been effective.

But the question is not whether quarantine accurately targeted the specific causes of yellow fever and other diseases, nor whether it prevented every epidemic. Rather, it is whether more and worse epidemics would have happened in seaport cities if there had been no quarantine in place at all. Southern seaports from Charleston to New Orleans were generally more hostile to quarantine than northern seaports, and they continued to suffer serious attacks from yellow fever into the early twentieth century. (Their climates were also more hospitable to *Aedes* than those of their northern counterparts, of course.) A small minority of historians has dared to suggest that quarantine may have played a role in preventing yellow fever outbreaks.[8]

Did quarantine work? One of the best answers to this question came from sanitary reformer John H. Griscom, who in 1859 reminded health officials from major American port cities that, even though active cases of yellow fever arrived every year at New York's quarantine station aboard ships coming from the Caribbean Basin, the city had not seen an actual epidemic since 1822.[9] The city's track record proved the value of quarantine, in Griscom's view. And even knowing what we know now about mosquitoes and viruses, it is hard to argue with him.

Did all the elaborate displays of vigilance make any difference? Obviously, isolating the occasional smallpox patient at the Lazaretto would have helped limit the spread of that disease. Feeding and bathing patients and providing them with clean clothing and bedding certainly did the same for typhus. But neither of these benefits justified the elaborate apparatus of maritime quarantine with its considerable expense, delays, and annoyances. If the criterion is prevention of any disease outbreak whatsoever, quarantine clearly failed. (Cholera is the most obvious example: even the strictest quarantines did not seem to interrupt or even slow that disease's spread throughout its several pandemic waves in the nineteenth century.)

On the other hand, any part of the nineteenth-century quarantine ritual that prevented all the necessary conditions of a yellow fever outbreak from coming together in the same place and time would have been beneficial. While the disinfection of vessels and cargoes would not necessarily have eliminated all *Aedes* mosquitoes aboard, fumigation doubtless killed some, and other disinfection methods may have rendered breeding areas inhospitable, especially if water casks were emptied.

Even detention alone, while it exposed Lazaretto staff and residents to the shipboard mosquitoes when the vessels were close enough to shore, at least temporarily protected the far larger and more crowded urban populations from exposure. Delayed arrival of ships at the time of the late-summer peak of the yellow fever season may also have meant that temperatures were lower when the mosquitoes or infected humans were introduced into the city. Admission, treatment, and isolation of patients in the Lazaretto hospital limited their availability to mosquitoes on site, and especially kept them from the city, where they might become the final ingredient in the recipe for an outbreak.

Where typhus is concerned, quarantine probably helped limit the disease's spread, even though the role of the louse and the bacterium were not discovered until 1909 and 1916, respectively. At the Lazaretto, patients were bathed and given clean clothes and bedding, while disinfection of their clothing and belongings likely killed most lice.[10] Ultimately, legislation (and enforcement) providing minimum standards for food, water, and accommodations aboard emigrant vessels deserves the lion's share of credit for the decline of typhus among transatlantic migrants.

Quarantine also worked in a second way—one that was well understood by the members of the Board of Health in the nineteenth century. It might or might not actually prevent epidemics, but it did provide an arena for the daily reenactment of the city's resolve. The Lazaretto was, among other things, a theater of vigilance. With its rules and rituals and decision-making conventions, this unwieldy institution succeeded in demonstrating on a daily basis the power, authority, and values of the city it protected. The watchmen's spyglass, the quarantine master's ship inspections, and the daily communications between the Board of Health and the officers on Tinicum Island all continually reiterated Philadelphia's determination to protect itself while remaining a busy commercial seaport. Providing shelter, clothing, food, and medical care to sick passengers and sailors also helped meet the city's obligation to care for its least fortunate.

Drugs and other medical interventions are evaluated according to their efficacy—that is, how reliably they achieve desired health outcomes compared to placebos or other treatments. Scholars have used the term *social efficacy* to describe a different kind of effectiveness. For example, prescribing and taking certain medicines can advertise desired traits in the patient or in the healer—eagerness to return to normal social roles, embrace of tradition, social connections, specialized knowledge—whether or not the drugs "work" in the conventional biochemical sense.[11] And it's not limited to medicine. There is social efficacy in the precautions associated with twenty-first-century "homeland security" operations. We may grumble at the cumbersome procedures of airport security, but we also have come to depend on the ritual, and we feel uneasy when we see signs of laxity or inattention. Critics who have denounced what they call "security theater" as costly and ineffective may be right, strictly speaking, but they are missing a crucial point: after a traumatic catastrophe that has left permanent scars, collective gestures and rituals of security—even if they are "only" theater—are essential for a community's survival.[12]

Public health interventions too can succeed in reassuring a population regardless of the provable effect of the specific measures on particular diseases. So it was with quarantine in the nineteenth century. Its social efficacy depended on its public visibility and on the daily repetition of its inspection and detention rituals. Each disease outbreak may have undermined the social efficacy of quarantine but did not nullify it, as long as truly catastrophic epidemics were avoided. Year after year, successive Boards of Health showed that they had learned this lesson.

Acknowledging that quarantine might have helped prevent yellow fever outbreaks in the nineteenth century, however, is not the same as advocating its widespread use in the twenty-first century. Quarantine is a blunt instrument, and curtailing the free movement of goods and people should never be undertaken lightly. The Philadelphia Board of Health's flexible doctrine of "expediency" has evolved over the years into the principle of the "least restrictive alternative" in public health policy: preventive measures should be tailored to achieve desired health goals with as little infringement of individual rights as possible.[13] Even in the case of diseases for which no other effective means of prevention is known, quarantine (and other forms of enforced isolation) can be implemented so as to affect the fewest people for the shortest periods necessary to protect others from infection.

The experience of COVID-19 has shown that quarantine, travel restrictions, and other policies designed to limit the spread of infection can play an effective role in fighting disease and protecting public health. But such policies alone can never be the answer. Germs can infect anyone, but they kill people with weakened resistance to infection. Like yellow fever, typhus, and most other infectious diseases, COVID-19 tends to severely sicken and kill those whose immune systems have been battered by age, poverty, malnutrition, and something that epidemiologists have begun to understand only in the early twenty-first century: chronic stress or *allostatic load*, a state of continual immunosuppression that afflicts people deprived of job security, income security, housing security, and physical security.[14] COVID-19 and other infectious diseases generally spare or cause only moderate symptoms in populations that are younger, more prosperous, and better insulated from the debilitating effects of inequality, racial discrimination, and other everyday stressors.

Historically, the nations that have fared best against infectious diseases have been those that have enforced carefully targeted infection-control policies with public support; provided basic care to all patients, regardless of income or status; and enacted policies over extended periods that have raised the standard of living of their most marginalized citizens above a minimum threshold of security.[15] It will take some time for researchers to assess the evidence concerning COVID-19, either to confirm that this historical pattern has persisted or to propose an alternative explanation. In the meantime, we can confront the challenges of the present and the future equipped with the lessons of the past—not as pat formulas for success, but rather as deeper insights into the ways that, in times of crisis, flawed people have made difficult choices under severe constraints.

Acknowledgments

During the unusually long gestation of this book, I have been on the receiving end of countless acts of generosity and collaboration. A mere listing of names on a page seems meager payback for so much good will and hard work. Know, all of you, that my gratitude is genuine and deep, and that if I am ever in a position to repay the favor, I won't hesitate.

Alice Hausman deserves to be first on the list, because she introduced me to the Lazaretto back in 2005. Little did she know how much a casual mention of this historic site in an academic planning meeting would change my life. Thank you, Alice. Ed Morman was also at that meeting and encouraged my initial explorations.

Next up are the resourceful, energetic, and hard-working research assistants who have devoted their time to this project. (Their names should appear in superscript or hypertext throughout the notes!) Meggie Crnic, Katie Eichner, and Catherine Campbell almost deserve coauthor billing; their insights shaped the contours of this book at critical stages of its development. Jessica Martucci, Elena Grill, Caity Weaver, Kevin Varano, Greg Kurzhals, Jung Lee, Josh Belfer, Ali Block, Dan Kurland, Amanda Mauri, Eva Killenberg, Jay Falk, and Dhivya Arasappan all contributed vital bits of research. Joan Batista contributed research assistance and supported this work in many ways during its early stages.

Generous funding came from the University of Pennsylvania's School of Arts and Sciences, University Research Foundation, and Provost's Undergraduate Research Mentorship Program; the Shelby Cullom Davis Center for Historical Studies at Princeton University; and the Andrew W. Mellon Foundation, through its support of the Penn Humanities Forum (now the Wolf Humanities Center), the Penn Humanities + Urbanism + Design Initiative, and the Mellon/ACLS Scholars and Society Fellows Program. I am grateful for this support.

The dedicated group of volunteers that came together to save the Lazaretto historic site beginning in the early 2000s, when it was threatened with demolition, have helped ever since, not only with the preservation of the site, but with my research and with public outreach and events at the Lazaretto. Thank you,

John Gallery, Randy Cotton, Doug Heller (*in memoriam*), Rebecca Sell, Larry Tise, Mike Zuckerman, Shan Holt, Bill Moller, Joan Casell, Tony and Barbara Selletti, Mary Werner DeNadai, Paul Steinke, Chris Templin, Ed Rubillo, Mike Messina, Tom Giancristoforo (*in memoriam*), Peter Benton, Rod Maroney, Andy Palewski, Pat Barr, and David Schreiber. More than anyone else, Herb MacCombie and Pat McCarthy are responsible for the restoration of the Lazaretto's main building and the new vision for Tinicum Township of which it is the centerpiece. We are all in their debt.

I have been helped in my research by descendants of the *Ganges* Africans and of the immigrants and others who passed through the Lazaretto. Kelly Ganges, Rosalind Brown, John Gartrell, Richard Ganges, Jim Thomas, Patricia Organsky, and Tripp Onnen, thank you for sharing your stories and for entrusting some of your families' heritage in this site, which is a monument to suffering and resilience.

Many archivists and librarians have gone to extraordinary lengths to help me with my research. Thank you to David Baugh, Jill Rawnsley, and Joshua Blay of the Philadelphia City Archives; V. Chapman-Smith, Gail Farr, Jefferson Moak, Dona Horowitz-Behren, and Ang Reidell of the Mid-Atlantic branch of the National Archives; the staff of the Historical Society of Pennsylvania; John Costello, Marge Johnson, and Keith Lockhart of the Delaware County Historical Society; Harriet Ehrsam of the Union Library of Hatboro; Betty Smith and David Rowland of the Old York Road Historical Society; Megan Harris of Upper Darby's Arlington Cemetery; Matt Herbison, Megan Good, and John Brady of the Independence Seaport Museum; Robert Hicks of the College of Physicians of Philadelphia library and the Mütter Museum; Stacey Peeples of the Pennsylvania Hospital Archives; and J. J. Ahern of the University of Pennsylvania Archives. Anu Vedantham, David Toccafondi, Nick Okrent, and David Azzolina of Penn Libraries facilitated many research breakthroughs.

My Penn colleagues have provided invaluable support throughout the research and writing of this book. In the History and Sociology of Science Department, Rob Kohler, Ruth Schwartz Cowan, Andi Johnson, Robby Aronowitz, Susan Lindee, Beth Linker, and Jonathan Moreno deserve special thanks, as do graduate students and doctoral alumni Joanna Radin, Elaine LaFay, Jason Chernesky, Luke Messac, Jesse Smith, Alexis Broderick, Mary Mitchell, Kelly Wiles, Matt Hoffarth, Sarah Hunter-Lascoskie, Kate Dorsch, Cameron Brinitzer, Kasey Diserens, Emma Curry-Stodder, and Aislinn Pentecost-Farren.

Jim English, Kevin Platt, and the participants in the Penn Humanities Center faculty colloquium contributed excellent questions and suggestions, as did Bethany Wiggin and Rose Nagele of the Penn Program in Environmental Humanities. The faculty fellows of Penn's Humanities + Urbanism + Design initiative have my undying gratitude for fostering the most stimulating multidisciplinary collaboration I have experienced in my career. Special thanks to founders Genie Birch and David Brownlee, as well as Mary Rocco, Alisa Chiles, Andrea Goulet, Daniel Barber, Herman Beavers, Domenic Vitiello, Francesca Ammon, and Naomi Waltham-Smith. Randy Mason and Frank Matero of Penn's Program in Historic Preservation have taught me to see the Lazaretto and the entire built environment in a different light, and I wonder if Aaron Wunsch fully appreciates how much his influence has shaped this book. Participants in the Penn Faculty Writing Retreat helped me push this manuscript over what seemed like the finish line not once, but several times. Special thanks to Jennifer Moore, Ayako Kano, Janine Remillard, Betsy Rymes, Kate Mason, and Ann Greene.

I have been inspired by, and my perspectives on the Lazaretto's history have been informed by, the historical scholarship, public history interventions, pedagogical initiatives, and creative thinking of Sean Kelley, Bill and Frank Watson, Geoff Manaugh and Nicola Twilley, Simon Finger, Maria Vita, Jeff Cohen, Sam Katz, and Nathaniel Popkin. Thank you all for keeping the past alive today in so many fascinating ways.

The book took shape in part through conversations with audiences who participated in conferences or attended presentations about one aspect or another of the Lazaretto's history over the last fifteen years, including Penn's History and Sociology of Science workshop, Health and Society Scholars Program, Barbara Bates Center for the Study of the History of Nursing (special thanks to Pat D'Antonio, Julie Fairman, Cindy Connolly, and the late Jean Whelan), and Therapeutic Landscapes conference; the Consortium for the History of Science, Technology, and Medicine (thank you, Babak Ashrafi, Mike Yudell, Janet Golden, and Julia Mansfield); the Oliver Evans chapter of the Society for Industrial Archaeology (thank you, Fred Quivik, Torben Jenk, and Reese Davis); the American Association for the History of Medicine (thank you, Chris Hamlin, Allan Brandt, Conevery Bolton Valenčius, and Jason Szabo); the College of Physicians of Philadelphia (thank you, Steve Peitzman and Russell Maulitz); the University of Ottawa (thank you, Toby Gelfand); Cooper University Hospital and Cooper Medical School of Rowan University; the University of Michigan Health and Society Scholars

Program; the Eastern American Studies Association (thank you, Lisa Jarvinen and Charlie Kupfer); the Department of History and Philosophy of Medicine at the University of Kansas Medical Center (thank you, Chris Crenner); the UCLA History of Science Colloquium (thank you, Mary Terrall, Ted Porter, and Bob Frank); Malta's "The Mediterranean Under Quarantine" conference (thank you, John Chircop and Alex Chase-Levenson); and Sydney's "Quarantine: History, Heritage, Place" conference (thank you, Alison Bashford and Lisa Rosner). I am grateful to them all.

Princeton's Shelby Cullom Davis Center for Historical Studies provided a congenial home for research and writing. Special thanks to Keith Wailoo, Alison Isenberg, Phil Nord, Matt Karp, and Center fellows Pam Ballinger, Pierre Force, Atina Grossmann, and Rebecca Nedostup, as well as Alec Dun, Bill Jordan, and the participants in the Princeton History of Science Colloquium.

The members of the Philadelphia Nonfiction Writers Collaborative made the long ordeal of writing this book more bearable and improved my writing. Thank you, Nancy Moses, Margie Patlak, Darl Rastorfer, and Carol Shloss for your company, your collegial support, and your good humor. Audra Wolfe of The Outside Reader spent many hours helping me with query letters, book proposals, and chapter drafts. Michael Willrich, Vincent Cannato, and Jon Zimmerman all volunteered their insights on those same matters, as did Stephen Fried, who went far beyond the call of either duty or friendship. Thank you all! Matt McAdam of Johns Hopkins University Press has been the model of a patient and demanding editor—exactly what this book needed. Jackie Wehmueller read and re-read the entire manuscript when it was much longer and more tangled than it needed and wanted to be. She is the genius behind the reordering and streamlining that made this book, well, readable. Jackie, I can't thank you enough.

Carla Chamberlin, thank you for the innumerable ways in which you have enriched my life during the latter stages of this book's creation. Hard work has never been so thoroughly leavened by joy. This book is dedicated to my sons, Daniel and Nicholas, who during the time I have been working on it have grown from rambunctiously curious schoolkids to passionately committed adults working to build a more sustainable and more just world. My pride in this book pales in comparison to my pride in them.

Notes

Abbreviations

BHAR   Board of Health annual report, *Report of the Board of Health of the City and Port of Philadelphia* (Philadelphia: Board of Health, multiple years)
HSP   Historical Society of Pennsylvania
MPBH   Minutes of the Philadelphia Board of Health, Philadelphia City Archives
NARA   National Archives and Records Administration
RG   Record Group

Introduction

1. *Philadelphia Public Ledger*, February 3, 1838; *North American* (Philadelphia), July 3, 1839; *Philadelphia Inquirer*, January 4, 1876; *Hatboro (PA) Public Spirit*, October 1, 1881.

2. *Hatboro (PA) Public Spirit*, June 9, 1883; resolution of Philadelphia Maritime Exchange, December 18, 1882, and H. G. Sickel to James Beaver, February 19, 1887, Appointments File, box 84, series 41, RG 26, Pennsylvania State Archives, Harrisburg.

3. *Philadelphia Evening Bulletin*, July 17, 1879; *Philadelphia Inquirer*, July 18, 1879; *Philadelphia Times*, July 18, 1879; René La Roche, *Yellow Fever, Considered in Its Historical, Pathological, Etiological, and Therapeutical Relations*, 2 vols. (Philadelphia: Blanchard and Lea, 1855), 1:214–16.

4. *Philadelphia Evening Bulletin*, July 18, 1879.

5. *Philadelphia Record*, July 18, 1879.

6. *Philadelphia Times*, July 24, 1879. On the Chester physicians at the Lazaretto in 1870, see chapter 8. On J. L. Forwood, see Samuel T. Wiley, *Biographical and Historical Cyclopedia of Delaware County, Pennsylvania*, ed. by Winfield Scott Garner, rev. ed. (Richmond, IN: Gresham, 1894), 469–71.

7. *Philadelphia Evening Bulletin*, July 26, 1879.

8. *Philadelphia Evening Bulletin*, August 7, 1879.

9. *Philadelphia Evening Bulletin*, August 8, 1879; *Philadelphia Times*, August 9, 1879.

10. *Philadelphia Times*, August 8, 1879.

11. *Philadelphia Times*, August 8, 1879.

12. *Philadelphia Evening Bulletin*, August 14 and 16, 1879; *Philadelphia Daily Evening Telegraph*, August 15, 1879; *Philadelphia Record*, August 15, 1879.

13. *Philadelphia Evening Bulletin*, August 16 and 19, 1879.

14. *Philadelphia Times*, September 3, 1879; *Philadelphia Inquirer*, September 4, 1879; *Philadelphia Evening Bulletin*, September 4, 5, and 6, 1879.

15. Jeffrey Kluger and Alice Park, "Guardians of the Year: Anthony Fauci and Frontline Health-Care Workers," *Time*, December 11, 2020.

16. John Harley Warner, *The Therapeutic Perspective: Medical Practice, Knowledge, and Identity in America, 1820–1885* (Cambridge, MA: Harvard University Press, 1986), 17–31.

17. James Lewis, "Dr. Krugman's Magic Dogma," *American Thinker*, May 5, 2012, http://www.americanthinker.com/2012/05/dr_krugmans_magic_dogma.html; David Wootton, *Bad Medicine: Doctors Doing Harm Since Hippocrates* (Oxford: Oxford University Press, 2006), 283; Lawrence J. Henderson, paraphrased in H. L. Blumgart, "Caring for the Patient," *New England Journal of Medicine* 270 (1964): 449.

18. Mark Harrison, *Contagion: How Commerce Has Spread Disease* (New Haven, CT: Yale University Press, 2012); Geoff Manaugh and Nicola Twilley, *Until Proven Safe: The History and Future of Quarantine* (New York: Farrar, Straus and Giroux, 2021); Alex Chase-Levenson, *The Yellow Flag: Quarantine and the British Mediterranean World, 1780–1860* (New York: Cambridge University Press, 2020).

CHAPTER ONE: **The Nation's Capital at Rock Bottom, 1793–1798**

1. George Gibbs, ed., *Memoirs of the Administrations of Washington and John Adams*, 2 vols. (New York, 1846), 2:272; Octavius Pickering, *The Life of Timothy Pickering*, 4 vols. (Boston: Little, Brown, 1867–73), 3:315, 414; Bernard C. Steiner, *The Life and Correspondence of James McHenry* (Cleveland: Burrows Brothers, 1907), 321–24.

2. *Cito, longe, tarde* (leave quickly, go far away, and return late) was the Latin motto from the plague epidemics of the fourteenth through eighteenth centuries; Colin Jones, "Languages of Plague in Early Modern France," in *Body and City: Histories of Urban Public Health*, ed. Sally Sheard and Helen Power (London: Routledge, 2017), 45. Both the College of Physicians and the Academy of Medicine, although they disagreed about the nature of the danger, recommended the evacuation of all residents from the affected areas. Thomas Condie and Richard Folwell, *History of the Pestilence Commonly Called Yellow Fever, Which Almost Desolated Philadelphia, in the Months of August, September, and October, 1798* (Philadelphia, 1799), 48–51.

3. Condie and Folwell, *History of the Pestilence*, 55; Allison Plyer, "Facts for Features: Katrina Impact," The Data Center: Independent Analysis for Informed Decisions in Southeast Louisiana, August 26, 2016, http://www.datacenterresearch.org/data-resources/katrina/facts-for-impact/.

4. Simon Finger, *The Contagious City: The Politics of Public Health in Early Philadelphia* (Ithaca, NY: Cornell University Press, 2012), 3–19.

5. Cornelius William Stafford, *The Philadelphia Directory for 1798* (Philadelphia: William W. Woodward, 1798).

6. Stafford, *Philadelphia Directory for 1798*.

7. William Currie, *A Sketch of the Rise and Progress of the Yellow Fever [. . .] in Philadelphia, in the Year 1799* (Philadelphia: Budd and Bartram, 1800), 16; *Philadelphia Gazette*, August 29, 1798; *Claypoole's American Daily Advertiser* (Philadelphia), August 29, 1798.

8. Thomas E. Will, "Liberalism, Republicanism, and Philadelphia's Black Elite in the Early Republic: The Social Thought of Absalom Jones and Richard Allen," *Pennsylvania History* 69, no. 4 (2002): 558–76; Stephen Fried, *Rush: Revolution, Madness, and the Visionary Doctor Who Became a Founding Father* (New York: Crown, 2018); Absalom Jones and Rich-

ard Allen, *A Narrative of the Proceedings of the Black People, during the Late Awful Calamity in Philadelphia* (Philadelphia: William W. Woodward, 1794); Mathew Carey, *A Short Account of the Malignant Fever Lately Prevalent in Philadelphia* (Philadelphia, 1793).

9. Anita DeClue and Billy G. Smith, "Wrestling the 'Pale Faced Messenger': The Diary of Edward Garrigues during the 1798 Philadelphia Yellow Fever Epidemic," *Pennsylvania History* 65 (1998): 243–68; *Philadelphia Gazette*, August 28, September 1 and 7, 1798; *Gazette of the United States* (Philadelphia), August 30, 1798.

10. DeClue and Smith, "Wrestling," 251–64.

11. DeClue and Smith, "Wrestling," 251–64.

12. Condie and Folwell, *History of the Pestilence*, 90–95.

13. Condie and Folwell, *History of the Pestilence*, 55, 108, xxvi (appendix).

14. Gibbs, *Memoirs*, 2:115–16.

15. Eve Kornfeld, "Crisis in the Capital: The Cultural Significance of Philadelphia's Great Yellow Fever Epidemic," *Pennsylvania History* 51, no. 3 (1984): 191–92; Currie, *Sketch*, 130–33; minutes, May 28, August 13 and 24, 1798, MPBH; Benjamin Rush, *Observations upon the Origins of the Malignant Bilious, or Yellow Fever, and upon the Means of Preventing It* (Philadelphia: Thomas Dobson, 1799), 4–5.

16. Bob Arnebeck, *Destroying Angel: Benjamin Rush, Yellow Fever, and the Birth of Modern Medicine* (Thousand Island Park, NY: self-published, 1999), chapter 15, http://bobarnebeck.com/fever1793/chapter15.html.

17. Condie and Folwell, *History of the Pestilence*, 55, 108, xxvi (appendix); Thomas Jefferson to Benjamin Rush, September 12, 1799, in Barbara B. Oberg, ed., *The Papers of Thomas Jefferson*, vol. 31 (Princeton, NJ: Princeton University Press, 2003), 183–84.

18. *Pennsylvania Gazette*, December 12, 1798.

19. *Pennsylvania Gazette*, December 12, 1798.

20. *Pennsylvania Gazette*, December 12, 1798.

21. *Pennsylvania Gazette*, December 12, 1798.

22. *Pennsylvania Gazette*, December 12, 1798.

23. *Pennsylvania Gazette*, December 12, 1798.

CHAPTER TWO: **Righteousness and Desperation, 1799**

1. K. David Patterson, "Yellow Fever Epidemics and Mortality in the United States, 1693–1905," *Social Science and Medicine* 34 (1992): 855–65.

2. State Island was called Province Island until the end of the Revolutionary War. Decades of landfill gradually eliminated all traces of the creeks and channels that separated the island from what is today Southwest Philadelphia and Philadelphia International Airport.

3. College of Physicians of Philadelphia, *Facts and Observations Relative to the Nature and Origin of the Pestilential Fever* (Philadelphia: Thomas Dobson, 1798), 11; minutes, December 4, 1798, MPBH; *Claypoole's American Daily Advertiser* (Philadelphia), April 19, 1799.

4. DeClue and Smith, "Wrestling."

5. Arnebeck, *Destroying Angel*, chapter 16, http://bobarnebeck.com/fever1793/chapter16.html.

6. Edward Garrigues diary, April 29 and June 29, 1799, HSP.

7. Currie, *Sketch*, 5.

8. This description is based on René La Roche's discussion of yellow fever symptoms in his exhaustive 1855 textbook *Yellow Fever*, 1:129–36.

9. Currie, *Sketch*, 5.

10. Currie, *Sketch*, 5–11.

11. Currie, *Sketch*, 9–10.

12. Rush, *Observations*, 21–25.

13. Rush, *Observations*, 3, 4, 28.

14. Minutes, July 2, 1799, MPBH.

15. Currie, *Sketch*, 11–16.

16. Garrigues diary, July 4, 6, and 13, 1799.

17. Currie, *Sketch*, 17–18.

18. Currie, *Sketch*, 19; *Claypoole's American Daily Advertiser* (Philadelphia), June 22, 1799; minutes, June 14, 1799, MPBH.

19. Currie, *Sketch*, 19; *Claypoole's American Daily Advertiser* (Philadelphia), June 22, 1799; minutes, June 14, 1799, MPBH.

20. Currie, *Sketch*, 20–21; Garrigues diary, July 13, 1799.

21. *Claypoole's American Daily Advertiser* (Philadelphia), August 2, 1799; Currie, *Sketch*, 23.

22. Currie, *Sketch*, 23; minutes, August 22, 1799, MPBH; *Universal Gazette* (Philadelphia), August 29, 1799.

23. Garrigues diary, August 18 and September 6, 1799.

24. Garrigues diary, September 12, 1799.

25. Currie, *Sketch*, 25–26; La Roche, *Yellow Fever*, 1:90.

26. *Philadelphia Gazette*, June 20, 1799.

CHAPTER THREE: **A New Lazaretto, 1800–1801**

1. *Claypoole's American Daily Advertiser* (Philadelphia), August 5, 1800.

2. *Claypoole's American Daily Advertiser* (Philadelphia), August 5, 1800; *Philadelphia Gazette and Daily Advertiser*, August 5, 1800; *Gazette of the United States* (Philadelphia), August 20, 1800; manifest of schooner *Phoebe*, August 22, 1800, RG 36, Bureau of Customs, National Archives Mid-Atlantic, Philadelphia; James L. Mooney, ed., *Dictionary of American Fighting Ships*, vol. 3 (Washington, DC: Naval History Division, 1968), 17; Mark Roth, "Surname Ganges Can Be Traced to Warship," *Pittsburgh Post-Gazette*, February 15, 2014; V. Chapman-Smith, "Philadelphia and the Slave Trade: The Ganges Africans," *Pennsylvania Legacies* 5, no. 2 (November 2005): 20; Mark E. Dixon, "Remembering the Ganges," *Main Line Today* (Newtown Square, PA), February 2005.

3. *Claypoole's American Daily Advertiser* (Philadelphia), August 5, 1800; *Philadelphia Gazette and Daily Advertiser*, August 5, 1800; Elizabeth Sandwith Drinker, *The Diary of Elizabeth Drinker*, ed. Elaine Forman Crane, vol. 2 (Boston: Northeastern University Press, 1991), 1327.

4. *Gazette of the United States* (Philadelphia), August 7 and 20, 1800. The story of the emotional reunion was widely reprinted in newspapers throughout the northern states.

5. *Philadelphia Gazette and Daily Advertiser*, August 11, 1800; Edward Needles, *An Historical Memoir of the Pennsylvania Society for Promoting the Abolition of Slavery* (Philadelphia: Merrihew and Thompson, 1848), 46.

6. Chapman-Smith, "Philadelphia and the Slave Trade"; Voyages 36707 and 36992, The Trans-Atlantic Slave Trade Database, Slave Voyages, accessed July 29, 2022, http://www.slavevoyages.org; Lazaretto Hospital Account Book, 1794–1800, 37.11, Philadelphia City Archives.

7. Chapman-Smith, "Philadelphia and the Slave Trade"; series 4, Manumissions, Indentures, and Other Legal Papers, reels 22–23, Pennsylvania Abolition Society Papers, HSP.

8. *Aurora General Advertiser* (Philadelphia), June 11, 1801.

9. *Aurora General Advertiser* (Philadelphia), June 11, 1801.

10. The following summary description of inspection and quarantine procedures is distilled from the Pennsylvania Health Law, excerpted in *Poulson's American Daily Advertiser* (Philadelphia), July 1, 1801, and from discussions and decisions in the MPBH over many years.

11. Lazaretto Hospital Register, collection of the Philadelphia History Museum, now in custody of Drexel University, Philadelphia.

12. Minutes, August 1, 1801, MPBH.

13. This description of typhus symptoms is drawn from several sources: Laurence Turnbull, "Practical Observations on Ship Fever as It Prevailed in Philadelphia and Its Environs, in the Months of June, July, and August, 1847," *Medical Examiner and Record of Medical Science*, September 1, 1847, 528–31; F. W. Sargent, "Report of Cases of Typhus Fever, Observed at the Lazaretto, near Philadelphia," *American Journal of the Medical Sciences*, October 1847, 529–35; Dr. Benedict, discussion of typhus fever at the Blockley Hospital in Philadelphia, College of Physicians of Philadelphia, meeting of June 1, 1847, *Summary of the Transactions of the College of Physicians of Philadelphia* 2 (1846–49): 134–35; Robert D. Lyons, *A Treatise on Fever* (Philadelphia: Blanchard and Lea, 1861), 99–107; George B. Wood, *A Treatise on the Practice of Medicine*, 6th ed., 2 vols. (Philadelphia: Lippincott, 1866), 1:213, 405–6; Hans Zinsser, *Rats, Lice, and History* (Boston: Little, Brown, 1935), 216–17; and Victoria A. Harden, "Typhus, Epidemic," in *Cambridge World History of Human Disease*, ed. Kenneth F. Kiple (Cambridge: Cambridge University Press, 1993), 1080–84.

14. Manifest and passenger list of the brig *Venture Again*, August 3, 1801, *Passenger Lists of Vessels Arriving in the Port of Philadelphia, 1800–1882*, Publication M-425, Bureau of Customs, RG 36, National Archives Mid-Atlantic, Philadelphia.

15. Theodosia Burr Alston to J. Frederick Prevost, October 18, 1801, Theodosia Burr Alston Papers, Library of Congress Manuscript Division, Washington, DC.

16. *Philadelphia Gazette*, October 30, 1801.

17. *Gazette of the United States* (Philadelphia), June 2, 1801.

18. *Gazette of the United States* (Philadelphia), September 19, 1801, and April 5, 1802; *Philadelphia Gazette*, September 21, 1801, and February 6, 1802.

CHAPTER FOUR: **Exodus (Again) and Compromise, 1802–1803**

1. Minutes, July 9, 1802, MPBH; *Philadelphia Gazette*, September 30, 1802; William Currie and Isaac Cathrall, *Facts and Observations Relative to the Origin, Progress, and Nature of the Fever* [. . .] *of Philadelphia* (Philadelphia: William Woodward, 1802), 6–7.

2. Currie and Cathrall, *Facts and Observations*, 8–11, 15; minutes, July 10, 12, 13, 14, and 16, 1802, MPBH.

3. *Philadelphia Gazette*, September 30, 1802; James Robinson, *The Philadelphia Directory, City and County Register, for 1802* (Philadelphia: William Woodward, 1802), 66; minutes, July 16, 1802, MPBH.

4. *Philadelphia Gazette*, August 5, 1802; minutes, August 5, 1802, MPBH.

5. Currie and Cathrall, *Facts and Observations*, 10; Eliza Cope Harrison, ed., *Philadelphia Merchant: The Diary of Thomas P. Cope, 1800–1851* (South Bend, IN: Gateway Editions, 1978), 131; *Gazette of the United States* (Philadelphia), August 9, 1802. New York mayor Edward Livingston wasted no time, announcing on August 7 his city's quarantine and travel ban against vessels and travelers from Philadelphia; *American Citizen* (New York), September 24, 1802; La Roche, *Yellow Fever*, 1:93–94. La Roche's account includes Rush's characterization of the public reaction to the Board of Health's August 5 proclamation.

6. *Philadelphia Gazette*, September 30, 1802; Currie and Cathrall, *Facts and Observations*, 10–17.

7. Minutes, May 19, 29, and June 3, 1802, MPBH.

8. Currie and Cathrall, *Facts and Observations*, 4–6, appendix i–ii. The account of the sailor's illness at the Lazaretto comes from handwritten marginal notes in the copy of the book that is digitized in the Readex database Early American Imprints, Series II: Shaw-Shoemaker, 1801–1819. The marginal notes attribute the information to a conversation with or communication from Dorsey.

9. *Philadelphia Gazette*, September 30, 1802; Currie and Cathrall, *Facts and Observations*, 6–7.

10. Currie and Cathrall, *Facts and Observations*, 9–10.

11. [Charles Caldwell], *Thoughts on the Subject of a Health Establishment for the City of Philadelphia* (Philadelphia, [1802]), 1–2. The pamphlet, which incorporated several newspaper commentaries, was published anonymously, probably shortly after the end of the 1802 epidemic, but Caldwell later claimed authorship.

12. According to the annual Philadelphia city directories, the Health Office migrated over the years from 32 Walnut Street to various locations near Fifth and Chestnut and Sixth and Chestnut Streets, before settling in at the southwest corner of Sixth and George (now Sansom) Streets in the 1840s, where it stayed for the rest of the nineteenth century.

13. *Gazette of the United States* (Philadelphia), August 17, 1805.

14. Charles Caldwell, *Autobiography of Charles Caldwell* (Philadelphia: Lippincott, Grambo, 1855), 288–92; Charles Caldwell, *An Anniversary Oration on the Subject of Quarantines* (Philadelphia: Fry and Kammerer, 1807), 4–6, 8–9, 13, 26; William Shainline Middleton, "Charles Caldwell: A Biographical Sketch," *Annals of Medical History* 3 (1921): 156–78; Thomas L. Maddin, "Remarks of Dr. Maddin," *Southern Practitioner* 25 (1903): 263; Penn and Slavery Project, "Charles Caldwell," accessed August 7, 2022, http://pennandslaveryproject.org/exhibits/show/medschool/southerndoctors/charlescaldwell.

15. Caldwell, *Thoughts on the Subject*, 11–13.

16. Sanford W. Higginbotham, "The Keystone in the Democratic Arch: Pennsylvania Politics, 1800–1816" (PhD diss., University of Pennsylvania, 1952), 60.

CHAPTER FIVE: **A Regime of Vigilance "to Banish from among Us Even the Apprehension of Disease"**

1. Robinson, *Philadelphia Directory*; minutes, April 25, 1803, MPBH.

2. *Gazette of the United States* (Philadelphia), May 6, 1803.

3. *Gazette of the United States* (Philadelphia), May 6, 1803.

4. See, for example, Carolyn Raffensperger and Joel A. Tickner, eds., *Protecting Public Health and the Environment: Implementing the Precautionary Principle* (Washington, DC: Island Press, 1999).

5. *Gazette of the United States* (Philadelphia), May 6, 1803.

6. Minutes, May 5, 1803, MPBH; *Gazette of the United States* (Philadelphia), May 6, 1803.

7. Thomas Paine, *The Crisis* (1776; New York: Peter Eckler, 1918), 69; *The Declaration of Independence* (Washington, DC: National Archives and Records Administration, 1992), 26–28.

8. Patterson, "Yellow Fever Epidemics," 857–58.

9. For example, minutes, May 3 and 5, 1803; and June 2, 1834, MPBH.

10. Minutes, May 19, 1803; May 8, 1804; and May 31, 1816, MPBH.

11. Minutes, May 3, 1802; June 2, 1802; May 28, 1805; and May 27, 1818, MPBH.

12. Minutes, August 13–14, 1802; August 28, 1802; and May 15, 1805, MPBH.

13. *Poulson's American Daily Advertiser (Philadelphia)*, October 1, 1817; minutes, September 24, 1817; October 4, 1817; June 30, 1820; and July 6, 1820, MPBH.

14. Minutes, January 13, 1806; May 29, 1806; and May 27, 1818, MPBH.

15. Minutes, November 22, 1804; November 29, 1804; and September 28, 1819, MPBH.

16. *Poulson's American Daily Advertiser* (Philadelphia), September 13, 1803.

17. *Poulson's American Daily Advertiser (Philadelphia)*, September 13, 1803.

18. La Roche, *Yellow Fever*, 1:94–97.

19. Minutes, June 4, 1803, MPBH.

20. Minutes, August 13, 1804, MPBH.

21. Minutes, August 13, 1804, MPBH.

22. Minutes, September 9 and September 12, 1833, MPBH.

23. Minutes, May 20, May 28, June 4, June 6, June 10, and July 7, 1803, MPBH.

24. For example, minutes, October 2, 1807; and July 26 and September 1, 1808, MPBH.

25. Minutes, April 26, May 2, May 4, May 5, May 10, May 11, May 16, May 18, June 3, June 6, June 21, and July 7, 1803, MPBH.

CHAPTER SIX: **"Expedient" Measures and Rioting Redemptioners, 1804**

1. William Paley, *Principles of Moral and Political Philosophy*, 2 vols. (Boston: N. H. Whitaker, 1830), 2:95–96.

2. James F. Childress et al., "Public Health Ethics: Mapping the Terrain," *Journal of Law, Medicine and Ethics* 30, no. 2 (2002): 173; Ronald Bayer and Amy L. Fairchild, "The Genesis of Public Health Ethics," *Bioethics* 18, no. 6 (2004): 489; Lawrence O. Gostin, *Public Health Law: Power, Duty, Restraint*, 2d ed. (Berkeley: University of California Press, 2008), 68; Peter D. Jacobson and Richard E. Hoffman, "Regulating Public Health: Principles and Applications of Administrative Law," in *Law in Public Health Practice*, ed. Richard A.

Goodman et al. (Oxford: Oxford University Press, 2003), 29–30. I thank Michael Yudell and Jonathan Moreno for very helpful discussions of these issues.

3. Minutes, July 24, 1809, MPBH.

4. Minutes, May 14, 1805, MPBH.

5. Sjaak van der Geest, Susan Reynolds Whyte, and Anita Hardon, "The Anthropology of Pharmaceuticals: A Biographical Approach," *Annual Review of Anthropology* 25 (1996): 168; Susan Reynolds Whyte, Sjaak van der Geest, and Anita Hardon, *Social Lives of Medicines* (Cambridge: Cambridge University Press, 2002), 14–17, 170–71; Charles Rosenberg, "The Therapeutic Revolution: Medicine, Meaning and Social Change in Nineteenth-Century America," *Perspectives in Biology and Medicine* 20 (1977): 485–506; Rosenberg, *Our Present Complaint: American Medicine, Then and Now* (Baltimore, MD: Johns Hopkins University Press, 2007), 9–10; Robert Aronowitz, "From Skid Row to Main Street: The Bowery Series and the Transformation of Prostate Cancer, 1951–1966," *Bulletin of the History of Medicine* 88 (2014): 288–89, 312.

6. Karl Frederick Geiser, *Redemptioners and Indentured Servants in the Colony and Commonwealth of Pennsylvania* (New Haven, CT: Tuttle, Morehouse and Taylor, 1901), 51–52; Sharon V. Salinger, *"To Serve Well and Faithfully": Labor and Indentured Servants in Pennsylvania* (Cambridge: Cambridge University Press, 1987), 97.

7. I focus on Johan Christen in this narrative because documentary evidence survives about his life in the United States after arrival. While there is no direct evidence that he was a redemptioner or indentured servant, we do know that at least one hundred of the *Rebecca's* passengers—mostly Swiss Germans like Christen—were redemptioners. *Poulson's American Daily Advertiser* (Philadelphia), September 10, 1804.

8. Cheesman A. Herrick, *White Servitude in Pennsylvania: Indentured and Redemption Labor in Colony and Commonwealth* (1926; New York: Negro Universities Press, 1969), 184–85; August Ludwig Schlözer, *Briefwechsel* (Göttingen, 1777), quoted in Geiser, *Redemptioners and Indentured Servants*, 18–19.

9. Herrick, *White Servitude in Pennsylvania*; Schlözer, *Briefwechsel*, quoted in Geiser, *Redemptioners and Indentured Servants*, 18–19.

10. Herrick, *White Servitude in Pennsylvania*, 188.

11. Herrick, *White Servitude in Pennsylvania*, 188; Gottlieb Mittelberger, *Gottlieb Mittelberger's Journey to Pennsylvania in the Year 1750 and Return to Germany in the Year 1754*, trans. Carl T. Eben (Philadelphia: John J. McVey, 1898), 20.

12. Herrick, *White Servitude in Pennsylvania*, 188; Mittelberger, *Gottlieb Mittelberger's Journey*, 20; Salinger, *"To Serve Well and Faithfully,"* 93–96.

13. John Christian, *Autobiography of John Christian* (Exeter Township, PA, [1865]), 5–10.

14. Christian, *Autobiography*, 10–11.

15. Christian, *Autobiography*, 11–13.

16. Christian, *Autobiography*, 13–15. This description of typhus symptoms is drawn from several sources: Turnbull, "Practical Observations on Ship Fever," 528–31; Sargent, "Report of Cases of Typhus Fever," 529–35; Dr. Benedict, discussion of typhus fever, June 1, 1847, 134–35; Zinsser, *Rats, Lice and History*, 216–17; and Harden, "Typhus, Epidemic," 1080–84.

17. Farley Grubb, "Morbidity and Mortality on the North Atlantic Passage: Eighteenth-Century German Immigration," *Journal of Interdisciplinary History* 17, no. 3 (1987): 565–

85, and *German Immigration and Servitude in America, 1709–1920* (London: Routledge, 2011), mortality table, 74, depicts the redemption trade as a rational series of voluntary transactions that generally benefited all parties. Sharon V. Salinger, *"To Serve Well and Faithfully"* and "Labor, Markets, and Opportunity: Indentured Servitude in Early America," *Labor History* 38, no. 2-3 (1997): 311–38, argues that conditions were worse and transactions less truly voluntary than the rosy free-market view would suggest.

18. Minutes, August 16, 1804, MPBH.

19. *Poulson's American Daily Advertiser* (Philadelphia), September 10, 1804.

20. Christian, *Autobiography*, 17–19.

21. Christian, *Autobiography*, 17–19.

22. Minutes, September 26, 1804, MPBH.

23. *Aurora General Advertiser* (Philadelphia), October 11, 1804.

24. Minutes, October 12, 1804, MPBH.

25. Samuel H. Williamson, "Seven Ways to Compute the Relative Value of a U.S. Dollar Amount—1774 to Present," *MeasuringWorth*, accessed May 26, 2015, https://www.measuringworth.com/uscompare/.

26. Minutes, December 27, 1804; January 10 and April 25, 1805, MPBH.

CHAPTER SEVEN: **A Mischievous Boy, 1805**

1. *Philadelphia Gazette*, December 9, 1801; minutes, December 24, 1804; and December 23, 1807, MPBH.

2. Ellis P. Oberholtzer, *Philadelphia: A History of the City and Its People*, 4 vols. (Philadelphia: S. J. Clarke, [1912]), 2:112.

3. Among innumerable examples: minutes, October 8 and 12, 1801; May 13, 1802; August 23 and September 18, 1817; and August 7, 1818, MPBH.

4. Minutes, May 28, 1799; and October 16, 1801, MPBH.

5. Minutes, June 29, 1804, MPBH; *Aurora General Advertiser* (Philadelphia), June 30, 1804.

6. *Philadelphia Gazette*, December 9, 1801; minutes, December 24, 1804, and December 23, 1807, MPBH.

7. In August 1818, for example, when word spread "in distant places" that yellow fever was prevalent in Philadelphia, the board immediately published strong denials in the major local newspapers. The following summer, New York's Board of Health wrote to Philadelphia's board asking about similar reports that had come to its attention. When the letter was received, knowing that full disclosure was required if trust between the boards was to be maintained, three members of Philadelphia's board drafted a report on the spot and sent it back. It admitted the existence of six cases of "malignant fever" (which were likely yellow fever) in three adjacent houses just above Market Street Wharf. Three of the patients had died, and the others were recovering. All three houses had been evacuated and disinfected, and known contacts had been taken outside the city. No further cases had occurred, the board added in its reply, and the city was "generally healthy." Somehow, the board's confidential report made it into the New York papers, and calls arose for a quarantine on vessels from Philadelphia. The board felt compelled to issue a statement in the local papers denying the existence of an epidemic. The statement alluded to "a few cases of a malignant character," explained the measures that had been taken in response, and

denounced the "exaggerated alarm, so hastily and prematurely promulgated." Equally importantly, the board pledged always to be forthright in announcing publicly any "cause . . . endangering the lives of the Citizens of Philadelphia, or the Citizens of any other place." A New York ban was averted. Minutes, July 10 and July 22, 1819, MPBH.

8. René La Roche, *Remarks on the Origin and Mode of Progression of Yellow Fever in Philadelphia* (Philadelphia, 1871), 63–64; for "infected district," see, for example, minutes, September 1 and 15, 1820, MPBH.

9. Almshouse information: Almshouse Admissions Book (35.3-4.14), 1801, Board of Guardians of the Poor, Philadelphia City Archives. The following narrative, discussion, and quotations are drawn from the board's public report, published in *Poulson's American Daily Advertiser* (Philadelphia), January 16, 1806, and in the *Aurora General Advertiser* (Philadelphia), January 20, 1806.

10. *Aurora General Advertiser* (Philadelphia), July 31, 1805.

11. "Yellow Fever at Philadelphia in 1805," *Literary Magazine and American Register*, January 1806, 4-7; Charles Caldwell, *An Essay on the Pestilential or Yellow Fever*, published as an appendix to Caldwell's translation of J. L. Alibert, *A Treatise on Malignant Intermittents* (Philadelphia: Fay and Kammerer, 1807), 46–54; La Roche, *Yellow Fever*, 1:97–102.

12. *Poulson's American Daily Advertiser* (Philadelphia), January 16, 1806; *Aurora General Advertiser* (Philadelphia), August 19, 1805.

13. "Yellow Fever at Philadelphia in 1805," 5–6.

14. Caldwell, *Essay on the Pestilential or Yellow Fever*, 57–61; La Roche, *Yellow Fever*, 1:99–100.

CHAPTER EIGHT: **"This Inhuman Traffic," 1817**

1. Grubb, *German Immigration and Servitude*, 343–45.

2. Grubb, *German Immigration and Servitude*, 343–45.

3. Grubb, *German Immigration and Servitude*, 343–45.

4. The following narrative of the *Hope*'s ill-fated journey is based on "The Journey of the Ship *Hope*," a firsthand account written a year after the fact by Adrian Rudolf Märk in Pittsburgh and published in the *Swiss Messenger* newspaper in Aarau, Switzerland: no. 50 (December 10, 1818): 393–94, and no. 51 (December 17, 1818): 401–5, translated by Alfred Hilfiker and reproduced at R. A. Gase's website, accessed May 29, 2015, https://www.gase.nl/shiphope.htm.

5. Grubb, *German Immigration and Servitude*, 344–45.

6. *Grotjan's Philadelphia Public Sale Report*, August 18, 1817; "Extract of a Letter from the Lazaretto," *New York National Advocate*, August 11, 1817.

7. Märk, "Journey of the Ship *Hope*"; minutes, August 11, 1817, MPBH; *Philadelphia True American*, quoted in *Ladies' Weekly Museum* (New York), August 23, 1817.

8. Andrea Barrett, *Ship Fever* (New York: Norton, 1996), 180–81.

9. "Extract of a Letter from the Lazaretto." (Lehman's reference to the abolition of "the slave trade" refers to the Act Prohibiting the Importation of Slaves passed by Congress in 1807.) The letter is unsigned, but passages such as "I immediately remanded the healthy passengers on board the *Johanna*" could only have been written by the Lazaretto physician. *Philadelphia True American*, quoted in *Ladies' Weekly Museum* (New York), August 23, 1817; *New-York Evening Post*, December 11, 1817.

10. *Poulson's American Daily Advertiser* (Philadelphia), August 12, 1817; *Relf's Philadelphia Gazette*, August 12 and 15, 1817; minutes, August 11 and 12, 1817, MPBH.

11. Minutes, August 8 and 13, 1817, MPBH.

12. Minutes, August 18, September 3 and 5, 1817, MPBH.

13. Minutes, August 7, 8, 9, 11, 12, 13, 16, and 18, 1817, MPBH.

14. Minutes, August 11 and 16, 1817, MPBH.

15. Ronald A. Gase, "Family Tree of the American Gase," accessed June 2, 2015, http://www.gase.nl/Internettree/index.htm.

16. John E. Hilficker, "Brief Summary of the Family of Jacob Hilfiker/Hilficker/Hilfiger," accessed June 2, 2015, http://www.hilficker.addr.com/hilficker/hilficker_genealogy.htm; John Hilficker, personal communication, May 28, 2015.

17. Märk, "Journey of the Ship *Hope*."

18. Minutes, August 14, 19, 20, and 21; September 1, 5, 8, 11, 12, 17, and 18; and November 21, 1817, MPBH.

19. *New-York Evening Post*, December 11, 1817.

20. *New-York Evening Post*, December 11, 1817.

21. *New-York Evening Post*, December 11, 1817.

22. *New-York Evening Post*, December 11, 1817.

23. *Relf's Philadelphia Gazette*, May 13, 1818; Märk, "Journey of the Ship *Hope*."

24. Minutes, October 4, 7, and 11; and December 23, 1817, MPBH.

25. Farley Grubb, "The End of European Immigrant Servitude in the United States: An Economic Analysis of Market Collapse, 1772–1835," *Journal of Economic History* 54, no. 4 (1994): 815–16, and *German Immigration and Servitude*, 358–9; James Boyd, "The Rhine Exodus of 1816/1817 within the Developing German Atlantic World," *Historical Journal* 59. no. 1 (2016): 99–123; Friedrich Kapp, *Immigration and the Commissioners of Emigration of the State of New York* (New York: Douglas Taylor, 1870), 23–24; Donald MacKay, *Flight from Famine: The Coming of the Irish to Canada* (Toronto: McClelland and Stewart, 1990), 198–99.

CHAPTER NINE: **Fencing in Yellow Fever, 1820**

1. Lehman made his strong rejection of the contagiousness of yellow fever clear in his letter to Nicolas Chervin, May 24, 1821, Nicolas Chervin Papers, National Library of Medicine, Bethesda, Maryland.

2. Minutes, July 3, 1820, MPBH; *Poulson's American Daily Advertiser* (Philadelphia), July 4, 1820; *Franklin (PA) Gazette*, July 7 and 12, 1820; Samuel Jackson, *An Account of the Yellow or Malignant Fever, as It Occurred in the City of Philadelphia in 1820* (Philadelphia: M. Carey and Sons, 1821), 33–34, 36–37.

3. Minutes, July 26, 1820, MPBH; Jackson, *Account of the Yellow or Malignant Fever*, 16, 34–35.

4. Minutes, July 27, 1820, MPBH; Jackson, *Account of the Yellow or Malignant Fever*, 35–36, 113–14.

5. Minutes, July 29, 1820, MPBH; Jackson, *Account of the Yellow or Malignant Fever*, 18–19.

6. Jackson, *Account of the Yellow or Malignant Fever*, 19.

7. Minutes, July 19, 20, 21, 22, 24, and 25; and August 5 and 9, 1820, MPBH; *Franklin (PA) Gazette*, August 11, 1820.

8. Jackson, *Account of the Yellow or Malignant Fever*, 19–20.

9. Jackson, *Account of the Yellow or Malignant Fever*, 20.

10. Jackson, *Account of the Yellow or Malignant Fever*, 20–21.

11. Jackson, *Account of the Yellow or Malignant Fever*, 21.

12. Jackson, *Account of the Yellow or Malignant Fever*, 22.

13. Jackson, *Account of the Yellow or Malignant Fever*, 22–24; *Franklin (PA) Gazette*, August 18, 1820.

14. Minutes, September 2 and 3, 1820, MPBH.

15. Minutes, September 4, 1820, MPBH.

16. Minutes, September 4, 1820, MPBH; *Philadelphia Democratic Press*, September 5, 1820; *Franklin (PA) Gazette*, September 8, 1820.

17. Minutes, September 5 and 6, 1820, MPBH; *Poulson's American Daily Advertiser* (Philadelphia), September 6, 1820.

18. *Franklin (PA) Gazette*, September 8, 1820.

19. Minutes, July 31, August 4 and 11, and September 3, 7, and 8, 1820, MPBH.

20. Minutes, September 7 and 8, 1820, MPBH.

21. Minutes, September 7, 9, 11, and 12, 1820, MPBH.

22. Minutes, September 15, 16, 17, 20, and 21, 1820, MPBH.

23. Minutes, September 11, 1820, MPBH.

24. Minutes, September 21–23 and 27, 1820, MPBH; *Franklin (PA) Gazette*, September 23, 1820.

25. Minutes, October 5, 7, and 10, 1820, MPBH; Jackson, *Account of the Yellow or Malignant Fever*, 24.

26. Jackson, *Account of the Yellow or Malignant Fever*, 25.

CHAPTER TEN: **"Detained on Account of Her Hides"**

1. Thomas Harrison to William Boone, August 24, 1821, doc. 1995, box 7, Jeremiah Boone Papers (coll. 66), HSP.

2. Thomas Harrison to William Boone, July 23, 1821, doc. 1989, Boone Papers.

3. Harrison to Boone, July 23, 1821, doc. 1988, Boone Papers.

4. Harrison to Boone, July 28 and July 30, 1821, docs. 1990–91, Boone Papers.

5. Manfred J. Waserman and Virginia Kay Mayfield, "Nicolas Chervin's Yellow Fever Survey, 1820–1822," *Journal of the History of Medicine and Allied Sciences* 26, no. 1 (1971): 40–51; Nicolas Chervin, *Pétition adressée à la Chambre des Députés* (Paris: J. B. Baillière, 1833).

6. The replies are in the Nicolas Chervin Papers held by the History Medicine Division of the National Library of Medicine in Bethesda, Maryland. The quoted passages come from Thomas Mitchell's letter of May 12, 1821, William Currie's letter of June 1, 1821, and Samuel Emlen Jr.'s letter of May 11, 1821.

7. Waserman and Mayfield, "Nicolas Chervin's Yellow Fever Survey," 51.

8. William H. Ukers, *All About Coffee* (New York: Tea and Coffee Trade Journal Company, 1922), 129–30; *The Philadelphia Directory and Register for 1821* (Philadelphia: McCarty and Davis, 1821).

9. Minutes, September 4–20, 1820, MPBH.

10. As seen through the filter of the Board of Health minutes. With very few exceptions, the original Lazaretto physicians' letters to the board do not survive. The Board of Health minutes survive in an almost uninterrupted series since 1794.

11. A cargo insurance company in the twenty-first century describes the odor of rotting green coffee beans as musty, rotten, rancid, and repellent. "Coffee," Transport Information Service, accessed August 2, 2022, http://www.tis-gdv.de/tis_e/ware/genuss/kaffee/kaffee.htm.

12. Benjamin Rush, *An Account of the Bilious Remitting Yellow Fever, as It Appeared in the City of Philadelphia in 1793* (Philadelphia: Thomas Dobson, 1794), 12–13, 20.

13. Minutes, August 3 and 6, 1798, MPBH. At the time, the quarantine was located at the old Lazaretto or Marine Hospital on State Island, at the confluence of the Schuylkill and Delaware Rivers.

14. *Philadelphia Gazette and Daily Advertiser*, July 1, 1801.

15. Minutes, May 3, 17, 18, 19, and 24, 1803, MPBH.

16. Minutes, May 7, 8, and 23, 1804; June 2 and 21, 1804; July 5, 1804; June 27, 1809; and July 1, 1818, MPBH; *Oxford English Dictionary*, online edition, s.v. "triage (*n.*)," accessed August 2, 2022, http://www.oed.com/view/Entry/205658.

17. *Oxford English Dictionary*, online edition, "damaged (*adj.*, b)," accessed August 2, 2022, http://www.oed.com/view/Entry/47009; "sound (*adj.*, I.3.a)," accessed August 2, 2022, http://www.oed.com/view/Entry/185128; and "sweet (*adj.*, A.3.a)," accessed August 2, 2022, http://www.oed.com/view/Entry/195665; minutes, May 24, 1803 and May 12, 1804, MPBH.

18. Minutes, July 11, 1803; July 6, 1831; and September 21, 1838, MPBH.

19. A. N. Bell, "On the Cause, Malignancy, and Persistence of Yellow Fever Aboard Ship" (1864), *Trans. Epidemiol. Soc. London* 2 (1867): 225; John Gamgee, *Yellow Fever: A Nautical Disease* (New York: Appleton, 1879), 27. On hides, putrefaction, and tanning in the nineteenth century, see "Leather, and the Process of Tanning," *Working Man's Friend and Family Instructor* 3, no. 61 (1852): 134–35; and *One Hundred Years' Progress of the United States* (Hartford: L. Stebbins, 1871), 316–21.

20. Francis B. Thurber, *Coffee: From Plantation to Cup*, 6th ed. (New York: American Grocer, 1884), 18.

21. Thurber, *Coffee*, 19.

22. Such lists appeared routinely in local quarantine laws and regulations, and in manuals published to assist merchants and mariners in navigating through the thicket of global commerce. For example, I. Stikeman, *Steel's Shipmaster's Assistant and Owner's Manual*, 20th ed. (London: Longman, Rees, Orme, Brown, Green, and Longman, 1832), 304–6; and "Papers Relating to Quarantine Laws," in House of Commons (Great Britain), *Accounts and Papers, January–June 1860*, vol. 22, *Shipping* (London: Eyre and Spottiswoode, 1860). Philadelphia's Board of Health also occasionally issued its own list of dangerous cargo. This one dates from 1817:

Cotton
Coffee
Cocoa in bags
Hides or Tallow in Hides
Rags

Turkey carpets
Camel's hair
Turkey wool
Yarns of hair or wool
Clothing, beds, and bedding from the West Indies or Mediterranean

Minutes, June 10, 1817, MPBH.

23. A. J. Valente, *Rag Paper Manufacture in the United States, 1801–1900* (Jefferson, NC: McFarland, 2010); John Bowring, *Report on the Statistics of Tuscany, Lucca, the Pontifical, and the Lombardo-Venetian States* (London: Clowes and Sons, 1837), 21–28; *Annual Report of the Supervising Surgeon-General of the Marine-Hospital Service of the United States for the Fiscal Year 1893*, vol. 2 (Washington, DC: Government Printing Office, 1895), 317.

24. Carl Zimring, "Dirty Work: How Hygiene and Xenophobia Marginalized the American Waste Trades, 1870–1930," *Environmental History* 9, no. 1 (2004): 80–101; Henry Mayhew, *London Labour and the London Poor* (1861; New York: Dover, 1968), 2:136–42; Henry Thomas Buckle, *Introduction to the History of Civilization in England*, rev. ed. (London: Routledge, 1904), 818–19; Alain Faure, "Classe malpropre, classe dangereuse? Quelques remarques à propos des chiffonniers parisiens aux XIXe siècle et leurs cités," *Recherches* 29 (1978): 79–102; Barrie Ratcliffe, "Perception and Realities of the Urban Margin: The Rag Pickers of Paris in the First Half of the Nineteenth Century," *Can. J. Hist./Annales canadiennes d'histoire* 27, no. 2 (1992): 198–233; Catherine J. Kudlick, *Cholera in Post-Revolutionary Paris: A Cultural History* (Berkeley: University of California Press, 1996), 177–83.

25. Minutes, August 10, 1867, MPBH.

26. Minutes, June 27 and July 14 and 16, 1804, MPBH.

27. Minutes, June 24, 1809, MPBH. That importation did not necessarily imply contagion in the nineteenth century applies not only to yellow fever but to other diseases as well. The boundaries of disease categories were more fluid before about 1880 than afterward, and many official discussions of quarantine were not explicitly disease specific.

28. Thomas D. Mitchell, "Notes from Lecture on Yellow Fever," *Transylvania Med. J.* 12 (1839): 164–76, quotation on 170.

29. David Hosack, "Observations on the Laws of Contagion" and "Observations on the Nature and Treatment of Yellow Fever," in *Essays on Various Subjects of Medical Science*, 3 vols. (New York: J. Seymour, 1824–1830), 1:253–61 and 3:419–41.

30. Caldwell, *Anniversary Oration*, 4–6, 8–9, 13, 26.

31. Charles Caldwell, *Thoughts on Quarantine and Other Sanitary Systems* (Boston: Marsh, Capen and Lyon, 1834), quoted in *Boston Medical and Surgical Journal* 11 (1834): 277–78.

32. Caldwell, *Thoughts on Quarantine*. The same recommendation appears in his 1807 *Anniversary Oration*, 26.

33. For example, James Copland, *A Dictionary of Practical Medicine* (New York: Harper, 1848), 6:279; and David L. Huntington, "Quarantine: Its Efficacy and Necessity" (MD thesis, University of Pennsylvania, 1857).

34. *Oxford English Dictionary*, online edition, "infection (n.)," accessed August 2, 2022, http://www.oed.com/view/Entry/95273 and "infect (v.)," accessed August 2, 2022, http://www.oed.com/view/Entry/95266.

35. Bacteriologists advocating disinfection in the late nineteenth century often referred to the long pedigree of this practice while taking pains to emphasize its newly scientific justification and efficacy. See, for example, Samuel Rideal, *Disinfection and Disinfectants* (London: Charles Griffin, 1895), 2–3.

36. *New-York Gazette*, September 14, 1821; Alexander F. Vaché, *Letters on Yellow Fever, Cholera and Quarantine* (New York: McSpedon and Baker, 1852), 34.

37. John Duffy, "Nineteenth Century Public Health in New York and New Orleans: A Comparison," *Louisiana History* 15 (1974), 325–37; "Report of a Special Committee of the House of Assembly of the State of New York on the Present Quarantine Laws." *New York Journal of Medicine* 7 (1846): 221–22, 232–33; *New York Daily Advertiser*, July 13, 1805; *The Revised Statutes of the State of New-York*, 3 vols. (Albany, NY: Packard and Van Benthuysen, 1829), 1:430–31; Vaché, *Letters on Yellow Fever*, 7, 29; New York Chamber of Commerce, *Report of Select Committee on Quarantine* (New York: D. Van Nostrand, 1859), 27–30; *Annual Report of the Metropolitan Board of Health, 1866* (New York: C. S. Westcott, 1867), 385. The midcentury quarantine conventions and the many published guides for mariners to worldwide maritime laws and customs show similar general regulations on the books at the large American seaports, with variations in the list of cargo items deemed "liable to infection." For example, Joseph Blunt, *The Shipmaster's Assistant, and Commercial Digest: Containing Information Useful to Merchants, Owners, and Masters of Ships*, 2d ed. (New York: E. and G. W. Blunt, 1837), 279–313. In New York in 1837, the following articles were subject to stricter rules than other cargo: rags, hides, skins, cotton, and "all other articles likely to imbibe or retain infection." Blunt, *Shipmaster's Assistant*, 290.

38. Chase-Levenson, *Yellow Flag*, 14; Peter Baldwin, *Contagion and the State in Europe, 1830–1930* (Cambridge: Cambridge University Press, 1999), 135, 150–51, 203–4. Beginning in 1851, the major European and Mediterranean powers gathered for a series of International Sanitary Conferences with the goal of formulating a uniform international quarantine and sanitary policy that would limit the spread of plague, yellow fever, and cholera. The proceedings of the first conference in Paris reviewed the practices that had prevailed over the previous decades. *Procès-verbaux de la Conférence sanitaire internationale* (Paris: Imprimerie nationale, 1852): sessions of September 16 and October 16, 18, and 21, 1851. The course of the debate in subsequent conferences can be seen in *Procès-verbaux de la conférence sanitaire internationale* (Constantinople: Imprimerie centrale, 1866), session of September 26, 1866; and *Procès-verbaux de la conférence sanitaire internationale* (Vienna: Imprimerie impériale et royale, 1874), 429–30.

39. This pathogenic influence was often referred to as *infection*, which overlaps with but is not synonymous with *miasma*, a word that refers to a disease-causing principle emanating from decaying organic matter. In historical scholarship, *miasma* or *miasmatism* has generally referred to strictly *local* sources of disease (including marshes, corpses, garbage, human waste); see Frank M. Snowden, *Naples in the Time of Cholera, 1884–1911* (Cambridge: Cambridge University Press, 1995), 67; and Dorothy Porter, *Health, Civilization, and the State: A History of Public Health from Ancient to Modern Times* (London: Routledge, 1999), 80. Many nineteenth-century observers believed that infection, under certain circumstances, could be transported over great distances. Extended discussions of the medical meanings and cultural resonance of *infection* can be found in Owsei Temkin, "An

Historical Analysis of the Concept of Infection," in *The Double Face of Janus and Other Essays in the History of Medicine* (Baltimore, MD: Johns Hopkins University Press, 1977), 456–73; and David S. Barnes, *The Great Stink of Paris and the Nineteenth-Century Struggle against Filth and Germs* (Baltimore, MD: Johns Hopkins University Press, 2006), 241–43.

CHAPTER ELEVEN: **"Brought to Our Shores by the Cupidity of Others,"** 1847

1. Christian, *Autobiography*, 17–19; Märk, "Journey of the Ship *Hope*."

2. Passenger manifest, ship *Swatara*, Philadelphia, September 18, 1847, Pennsylvania, U.S., Arriving Passenger and Crew Lists, 1798–1962 accessed March 25, 2015, Ancestry.com Library Edition. I have inferred the family relationships based on the ages listed on the manifest, where the five Coulters are listed as a single family unit. I found no evidence regarding the wife/mother of James, Mary, and Alexander; my speculation about her death is based only on the high mortality rates of the Irish famine and of this voyage of the *Swatara*.

3. John MacGregor, *The Progress of America, from the Discovery by Columbus to the Year 1846*, 2 vols. (London: Whittaker, 1847), 2:996; search results for "owned by Stephen Baldwin," Immigrant Ships Transcribers Guild, accessed June 5, 2015, https://immigrantships .net; *Philadelphia Press*, December 29, 1859.

4. Christine Kinealy and Gerard Mac Atasney, *The Hidden Famine: Poverty, Hunger and Sectarianism in Belfast, 1840–50* (London: Pluto Press, 2000), 86–88; "The Emigrant Ship 'Swatara': Melancholy Condition of the Passengers," *Belfast News-Letter*, April 6, 1847, Irish Emigration Database, last updated 2012, http://www.dippam.ac.uk/ied/records/45046.

5. Stephen E. De Vere to T. F. Elliot, in *Evidence before the Select Committee of the House of Lords on Colonisation from Ireland, 1847*, quoted in Edwin C. Guillet, *The Great Migration: The Atlantic Crossing by Sailing-Ship Since 1770*, 2d ed. (1937; Toronto: University of Toronto Press, 1963), 96.

6. John H. Griscom, in *Report of a Special Committee on the Subject of the Quarantine Laws at the Port of New York* (1846), quoted in Cecil Woodham-Smith, *The Great Hunger: Ireland, 1845–1849* (New York: Harper and Row, 1962), 254.

7. "News of the Ship *Swatara*," *Belfast Commercial Chronicle*, May 8, 1847, Irish Emigration Database, accessed August 2, 2022, https://www.dippam.ac.uk/ied/records/43430.

8. Roger K. French, "Scurvy," in *Cambridge World History of Human Disease*, ed. Kenneth F. Kiple (Cambridge: Cambridge University Press, 1993), 1000–1005; the description of Andrew Coulter's scurvy symptoms is drawn from Robley Dunglison, *The Practice of Medicine*, 2 vols. (Philadelphia: Lea and Blanchard, 1842), 2:691–2. Typhus symptoms are drawn from several sources: Turnbull, "Practical Observations on Ship Fever," 528–31; Sargent, "Report of Cases of Typhus Fever," 529–35; Zinsser, *Rats, Lice and History*, 216–17; and Harden, "Typhus, Epidemic," 1080–84.

9. Andrew's and James's diagnoses are found in the 1847 listings of the Lazaretto Hospital Register, Philadelphia History Museum. The sequence I give here for scurvy and typhus is speculative, and I inferred the sequence of the two brothers' illnesses from the order of their release dates from the Lazaretto hospital.

10. Barrett, *Ship Fever*, 183–84.

11. William A. Spray, "Irish Famine Emigrants and the Passage Trade to North America," in *Fleeing the Famine: North America and Irish Refugees, 1845–1851*, ed. Margaret M.

Mulrooney (Westport, CT: Praeger, 2003), 3–20; Woodham-Smith, *Great Hunger*, 216–17; Herman Melville, *Redburn: His First Voyage* (1849; New York: Modern Library, 2002), 279.

12. Kerby A. Miller, *Emigrants and Exiles: Ireland and the Irish Exodus to North America* (Oxford: Oxford University Press, 1985), 292. Some of these figures may include passengers who died in quarantine or shortly after arrival.

13. Pamela S. Nadell, "United States Steerage Legislation: The Protection of the Emigrants En Route to America," *Immigrants and Minorities* 5, no. 1 (1986): 62–72; "Steerage Act," in *Immigration and Multiculturalism: Essential Primary Sources*, ed. K. Lee Lerner, Brenda Wilmoth Lerner, and Adrienne Wilmoth Lerner (Detroit, MI: Gale, 2006), 23–25.

14. Melville, *Redburn*, 337–39.

15. "Extract of a Letter from the Lazaretto."

16. Nadell, "United States Steerage Legislation," 62–72.

17. Michael Feldberg, *The Philadelphia Riots of 1844: A Study of Ethnic Conflict* (Westport, CT: Greenwood Press, 1975); Kenneth W. Milano, *The Philadelphia Nativist Riots: Irish Kensington Erupts* (Charleston, SC: History Press, 2013).

18. The newspapers reported 230 arrivals, but the official passenger manifest listed 227. *Philadelphia Inquirer*, September 20, 1847; *Philadelphia Public Ledger*, September 20, 1847; *Washington (DC) Daily Union*, September 21, 1847; *Swatara* passenger manifest, Philadelphia, September 18, 1847. Because of the three interruptions in the ship's journey, it is impossible to know how many of the original passengers died during the journey. Some may have been left in a hospital or other facility at one of the ports of call and survived. Others may have boarded to take the place of passengers who had died or been left behind. If the newspaper-reported figure of twenty births is accurate, and if all of the original 296 passengers either died en route or arrived alive in Philadelphia, then there were eighty-nine deaths, or 30 percent of the original number of passengers.

19. For example, the consecutive advertisements for the Lloyds' and for Baldwin's goods: *North American* (Philadelphia), June 9, 1847 (just a few days before the *North Star's* arrival at the Lazaretto); minutes, August 30, 1847, MPBH.

20. Minutes, August 30, 1847, MPBH.

21. Variations on these themes can be found in the following works, among others: Alan M. Kraut, *Silent Travelers: Germs, Genes, and the "Immigrant Menace"* (Baltimore, MD: Johns Hopkins University Press, 1995); Howard Markel, *Quarantine! East European Jewish Immigrants and the New York City Epidemics of 1892* (Baltimore, MD: Johns Hopkins University Press, 1997); Judith Walzer Leavitt, *Typhoid Mary: Captive to the Public's Health* (Boston: Beacon Press, 1996); Susan Craddock, *City of Plagues: Disease, Poverty, and Deviance in San Francisco* (Minneapolis: University of Minnesota Press, 2000), 300; Nayan Shah, *Contagious Divides: Epidemics and Race in San Francisco's Chinatown*, vol. 7 (Berkeley: University of California Press, 2001), 384; Marilyn Chase, *The Barbary Plague: The Black Death in Victorian San Francisco* (New York: Random House, 2003), 276; Guenter B. Risse, *Plague, Fear, and Politics in San Francisco's Chinatown* (Baltimore, MD: Johns Hopkins University Press, 2012). Edward T. Morman, "Guarding Against Alien Impurities: The Philadelphia Lazaretto, 1854–1893," *Pennsylvania Magazine of History and Biography* 108, no. 2 (1984): 131–52, acknowledges that quarantine targeted vessels and cargo as well as passengers, but implies that distrust or stereotyping of foreigners shaped quarantine policy in Philadelphia throughout those years.

22. On the Great Famine, see Christine Kinealy, *The Great Irish Famine: Impact, Ideology, and Rebellion* (New York: Palgrave, 2002).

CHAPTER TWELVE: **The Care Cure**

1. Eduardo Licéaga, "Typhus Fever," in *Twentieth-Century Practice: An International Encyclopedia of Modern Medical Science*, ed. Thomas L. Stedman, 20 vols. (New York: William Wood, 1898), 15:311.

2. John Harley Warner, *The Therapeutic Perspective: Medical Practice, Knowledge, and Identity in America, 1820–1885* (Cambridge, MA: Harvard University Press, 1986), 58–60, 86, 92–93; K. Codell Carter, *The Decline of Therapeutic Bloodletting and the Collapse of Traditional Medicine* (New Brunswick, NJ: Transaction, 2012), 20–22.

3. Samuel Jackson gives examples of such observation and adjustment in *Account of the Yellow or Malignant Fever*, 67.

4. Charles E. Rosenberg, "The Therapeutic Revolution: Medicine, Meaning, and Social Change in Nineteeenth-Century America," *Perspectives in Biology and Medicine* 20 (1977): 485–506; Warner, *Therapeutic Perspective*, 92–93, 133; Carter, *Decline of Therapeutic Bloodletting*, 21–22.

5. Audrey Davis and Toby Appel, *Bloodletting Instruments in the National Museum of History and Technology* (Washington, DC: Smithsonian Institution Press, 1979).

6. Benjamin Rush to John R. B. Rodgers, October 3, 1793, in L. H. Butterfield, ed., *Letters of Benjamin Rush*, 2 vols. (Philadelphia: American Philosophical Society, 1951), 2:695; Warner, *Therapeutic Perspective*, 135.

7. Davis and Appel, *Bloodletting Instruments*, 5; Dr. Hope, "Inflammation of the Brain," in *A System of Practical Medicine*, ed. Alexander Tweedie and W. W. Gerhard, 2d American ed., 3 vols. (Philadelphia: Lea and Blanchard, 1842), 1:515.

8. Davis and Appel, *Bloodletting Instruments*, 17–25.

9. Davis and Appel, *Bloodletting Instruments*, 34–36.

10. Wood and Bache, *Dispensatory*, 377–81, 796–97.

11. Richard Swiderski, *Calomel in America: Mercurial Panacea, War, Song, and Ghosts* (Boca Raton, FL: BrownWalker Press, 2009), 33–34; Dunglison, *Medical Lexicon*, 162; Wood and Bache, *Dispensatory*, 359–61, 388.

12. Jackson, *Account of the Yellow or Malignant Fever*, 18, 65–67.

13. Lazaretto hospital register, 1847–1893, collection of the Philadelphia History Museum (in custody of Drexel University).

14. Abel Tennant, *The Vegetable Materia Medica and Practice of Medicine* (Batavia, NY: D. D. Waite, 1837), 361; Stephen W. Williams, "Report on the Indigenous Medical Botany of Massachusetts," *Transactions of the American Medical Association* 2 (1849): 909.

15. Joshua Y. Jones, "Typhus Fever" (medical thesis, University of Pennsylvania, 1829).

16. F. W. Sargent was one of the physicians called on by the Board of Health to fill in for Joshua Jones in June 1847 while Jones was ill—reportedly with typhus. Jones recovered and resumed his duties at the Lazaretto after about a month. Minutes, May 26 and 29, June 30, and July 5, 1847; and January 6, 1849, MPBH; College of Physicians of Philadelphia, meeting of June 1, 1847, *Summary of the Transactions of the College of Physicians of Philadelphia* 2 (1846–49): 134. It is theoretically possible but highly unlikely that Sargent or

others imposed a completely different treatment protocol while Jones was ill, and that Jones then reasserted an aggressive depletive regimen when he recovered. The treatments described by Sargent match those used for typhus at other Philadelphia hospitals around the same time, and neither the Board of Health nor norms of professional courtesy would likely have countenanced radically divergent treatments under the circumstances.

17. Sargent, "Report of Cases of Typhus Fever," 535; George B. Wood and Franklin Bache, *The Dispensatory of the United States of America*, 4th ed. (Philadelphia: Grigg and Elliot, 1839), 360–61, 380, 422; Robley Dunglison, *Medical Lexicon: A Dictionary of Medical Science*, 9th ed. (Philadelphia: Blanchard and Lea, 1852), 730.

18. William Frederick Norwood, *Medical Education in the United States before the Civil War* (Philadelphia: University of Pennsylvania Press, 1944), 405–6; Steven Stowe, *Doctoring the South: Southern Physicians and Everyday Medicine in the Mid-Nineteenth Century* (Chapel Hill: University of North Carolina Press, 2004), 69–71.

19. Warner, *Therapeutic Perspective*, 175–79.

20. Warner, *Therapeutic Perspective*, 166–67; Carter, *Decline of Therapeutic Bloodletting*, 90–91.

21. W. W. Gerhard, "On the Typhus Fever Which Occurred at Philadelphia in the Spring and Summer of 1836," *American Journal of the Medical Sciences* 19 (1837): 288–321 and 20 (1837): 289–322; unsigned editorial, "W. W. Gerhard, Typhoid vs. Typhus Fever," *Journal of the American Medical Association* 181, no. 2 (1962): 154–55.

22. Gerhard, "On the Typhus Fever"; "W. W. Gerhard, Typhoid vs. Typhus Fever."

23. Gerhard, "On the Typhus Fever," 20:310–21.

24. Gerhard, "On the Typhus Fever," 20:310–21.

25. Warner, *Therapeutic Perspective*, 17–31.

26. Lewis, "Dr. Krugman's Magic Dogma"; David Wootton, *Bad Medicine: Doctors Doing Harm since Hippocrates* (Oxford: Oxford University Press, 2006), 283; Lawrence J. Henderson, paraphrased in Blumgart, "Caring for the Patient," 449.

27. Iowa State University Center for Food Security and Public Health, "Typhus Fever—*Rickettsia prowazekii*," last updated February 2017, http://www.cfsph.iastate.edu /Factsheets/pdfs/typhus_fever.pdf. The World Health Organization also reports a case-fatality rate of "up to 40% in the absence of specific treatment." World Health Organization, "Typhus Fever (Epidemic Louse-Borne Typhus)," April 23, 2020, http://www.who .int/ith/diseases/typhusfever/en/. Case-fatality rates cited here for nineteenth-century yellow fever epidemics are for white patients; 95 percent of the yellow fever patients treated at the Lazaretto between 1847 and 1893 were listed as white. Lauren E. Blake and Mariano A. Garcia-Blanco, "Human Genetic Variation and Yellow Fever Mortality during 19th-Century U.S. Epidemics," *mBio* 5, no. 3 (2014): e01253-14; T. P. Monath, "Yellow Fever Vaccine," *Expert Review of Vaccines* 4, no. 4 (2005): 553–74.

28. All data about the number of patients and average length of stay are calculated from the Lazaretto hospital register, collection of the Philadelphia History Museum (in custody of Drexel University). On the continual requests for more staff and supplies, see, for example, minutes, June 5, 14, 16, 17, 19, 21, 22, 25, and 30; July 14, 16, 17, and 23; August 6 and 7; and September 13 and 15, 1847, MPBH.

29. T. J. P. Stokes, June 1853 notes, Lazaretto Hospital Register.

30. Gerhard, "On the Typhus Fever," 20:320.

31. Gerhard, "On the Typhus Fever," 20:321; Sargent, "Report of Cases of Typhus Fever," 535; minutes, May 26; June 3, 16, and 30; July 10, 12, 16, and 28; August 3, 5, 11, and 12, 1847, MPBH.

32. Centers for Disease Control and Prevention, "2014–2016 Ebola Outbreak in West Africa," accessed August 3, 2022, http://www.cdc.gov/vhf/ebola/history/2014-2016-outbreak /index.html.

33. Matthew Wynia, "Why Confusion Still Surrounds the Ebola Risk," *Denver Post*, November 16, 2014.

34. The most widely read heralds of the "emerging diseases" scare were Richard Preston, *The Hot Zone* (New York: Random House, 1994); and Laurie Garrett, *The Coming Plague: Newly Emerging Diseases in a World Out of Balance* (New York: Farrar, Straus and Giroux, 1994). The most insightful analysis of the "outbreak narrative" that these works helped to popularize is Priscilla Wald, *Contagious: Cultures, Carriers, and the Outbreak Narrative* (Durham, NC: Duke University Press, 2008).

35. Centers for Disease Control and Prevention, "2014–2016 Ebola Outbreak in West Africa."; CDC, "Ebola (Ebola Virus Disease): Case Counts," last reviewed February 19, 2020, http://www.cdc.gov/vhf/ebola/outbreaks/2014-west-africa/case-counts.html; BBC News, "Ebola: Mapping the Outbreak," June 19, 2015, http://www.bbc.com/news/world -africa-28755033; Anemona Hartocollis, "Craig Spencer, New York Doctor with Ebola, Will Leave Bellevue Hospital," *New York Times*, November 10, 2014; Denise Grady, "Better Staffing Seen as Crucial to Ebola Treatment in Africa," *New York Times*, October 31, 2014; Paul Farmer, "Diary," *London Review of Books*, October 23, 2014, 38–39.

CHAPTER THIRTEEN: **"Gross and Criminal Negligence" at the Lazaretto, 1853**

1. The following description of the inspection of the bark *Mandarin* is based on information from the following sources: *Philadelphia Public Ledger*, July 14 and July 29, 1853; Wilson Jewell, "The Fever Prevailing in the Vicinity of South Street Wharf," *Summary of the Transactions of the College of Physicians of Philadelphia*, vol. 2 (Philadelphia: J.B. Lippincott,1856), 60; and the procedures prescribed by the Health Law of Pennsylvania: *The Laws of Pennsylvania in Relation to the Board of Health and the Health Laws of the City and County of Philadelphia* (Philadelphia: Crissy and Markley, 1848), 98–101.

2. This chapter includes some reconstructed dialogue based on the legally proscribed procedure for questioning arriving captains at the Lazaretto.

3. *Philadelphia Public Ledger*, July 14 and 29, 1853; minutes, July 27, 1853, MPBH; Jewell, "Fever Prevailing," 60.

4. Minutes, May 25, 1854, MPBH.

5. Jewell, "Fever Prevailing," 54, 60.

6. René La Roche, "Remarks on the Origin of the Yellow Fever Which Prevailed in Philadelphia, in 1853" (presented to College of Physicians of Philadelphia, April 5, 1854), *Summary of the Transactions of the College of Physicians of Philadelphia*, n.s., 2 (1853–56): 231–32.

7. *Philadelphia Public Ledger*, March 6, 1850.

8. The following description is based on the classic symptoms of severe yellow fever cases. La Roche, *Yellow Fever*, 1:129–36; T. P. Monath, "Yellow Fever: An Update," *Lancet*

Infectious Diseases 1, no. 1 (2001): 11–20; Donald B. Cooper and Kenneth F. Kiple, "Yellow Fever," in *The Cambridge World History of Human Disease*, ed. Kenneth F. Kiple (Cambridge: Cambridge University Press, 1993), 1100–1107.

9. Jewell, "Fever Prevailing," 54–58.

10. Jewell, "Fever Prevailing," 56–57, 91.

11. Jewell, "Fever Prevailing," 55, 68–71, 91; minutes, July 25, 26, 27, and 28, 1853, MPBH.

12. Jewell, "Fever Prevailing," 71–73.

13. Jewell, "Fever Prevailing," 91, 123–25; *New York Times*, September 20, 1853; Lazaretto Hospital Register, 1847–1893, collection of the Philadelphia History Museum (in custody of Drexel University).

14. Jewell, "Fever Prevailing," 60, 91, 118–20, 123–25.

15. Jewell, "Fever Prevailing," 61–62, 117–18.

16. Frederick P. Henry, ed., *Standard History of the Medical Profession of Philadelphia* (Chicago: Goodspeed Brothers, 1897), 306; *Transactions of the College of Physicians of Philadelphia*, 3rd s., 9 (1887): cclxx; William T. Taylor, "Wilson Jewell, M.D., 1800–1867," *Transactions of the Medical Society of the State of Pennsylvania* 13 (1880): 368–74; minutes, June 15 and September 20, 1848; and January 17, 20, and 24, and April 4, 1849, MPBH; Jewell, "Fever Prevailing."

17. *Philadelphia Public Ledger*, July 27, 28, and 29, 1853.

18. *Philadelphia Public Ledger*, July 29, 1853.

19. *Philadelphia Public Ledger*, July 30, 1853.

20. *Philadelphia Public Ledger*, August 2, 1853.

21. *Philadelphia Public Ledger*, August 8, 1853.

22. *Philadelphia Public Ledger*, September 6, 1853.

23. *North American and United States Gazette* (Philadelphia), April 4, 1854; *Philadelphia Bulletin*, April 3 and 4, 1854; *Philadelphia Public Ledger*, April 4, 1854; *Commonwealth v. Stokes and Van Dusen*, Court of Quarter Sessions, April 3–5, 1854, RG 21, Court of Quarter Sessions, Philadelphia City Archives.

24. *Philadelphia Public Ledger*, April 4 and 5, 1854.

25. Jewell, "Fever Prevailing," 54, 65.

26. *Philadelphia Public Ledger*, August 8, 1853.

27. *North American and United States Gazette* (Philadelphia), April 5 and 6, 1854; *Philadelphia Bulletin*, April 5, 1854; *Philadelphia Public Ledger*, April 6, 1854; minutes, April 12 and May 25, 1854, MPBH.

28. T. J. P. Stokes to James Buchanan, June 12 and August 28, 1855, in James Buchanan Papers (collection 91), HSP; *Philadelphia Public Ledger*, February 19, 1857.

29. *Philadelphia Public Ledger*, September 6, 1853.

30. Wilson Jewell, welcoming address to the first National Quarantine Convention (later renamed National Quarantine and Sanitary Convention), Philadelphia, May 13, 1857, in *Minutes of the Proceedings of the Quarantine Convention* (Philadelphia: Crissy and Markley, 1857), 4–6.

31. Jewell, *Historical Sketches of Quarantine*, address delivered to the Philadelphia County Medical Society, January 28, 1857 (Philadelphia: T. K. and P. G. Collins, 1857), 26–30.

32. *Minutes of the Proceedings of the Quarantine Convention*, 3–11, 20–23.

33. *Minutes of the Proceedings of the Quarantine Convention*, 36–37.

34. *Proceedings and Debates of the Third National Quarantine and Sanitary Convention* (New York: Edmund Jones, 1859) 24, 29–33, 36–7, 56, 64, 315.

35. *Proceedings and Debates of the Third National Quarantine*, 71–72, 76–77.

36. See, for example, Kari S. McLeod, "Our Sense of Snow: The Myth of John Snow in Medical Geography," *Social Science and Medicine* 50, no. 7/8 (2000): 923–35.

37. *Minutes of the Proceedings of the Second Annual Meeting of the Quarantine and Sanitary Convention* (Baltimore: John D. Toy, 1858); *Proceedings and Debates of the Third National Quarantine*, 40–44; *Proceedings and Debates of the Fourth National Quarantine and Sanitary Convention* (Boston: Rand and Avery, 1860), 171, 186–87.

38. Mazyck P. Ravenel, "The American Public Health Association, Past, Present, Future," *American Journal of Public Health* 11, no. 12 (1921): 1031.

CHAPTER FOURTEEN: The Darkest Hour, 1870

1. *Philadelphia Inquirer*, August 12, 1870.

2. *Philadelphia Public Ledger*, August 11, 1870; *Philadelphia Inquirer*, August 12, 1870.

3. Drew Gilpin Faust, *This Republic of Suffering: Death and the American Civil War* (New York: Knopf, 2008), 267.

4. *Philadelphia Inquirer*, June 30, 1870, 21. The following accounts of the 1870 epidemic are pieced together from Goodman's, Taylor's, and La Roche's reports to the Board of Health, and from the tables of cases presented in the BHAR 1870, 39–65; La Roche, *Remarks on the Origin and Mode of Progression*, 20–26.

5. BHAR 1870, 61; *Philadelphia Morning Post*, August 12, 1870.

6. Minutes, October 12, 1801, July 3, 1806, and July 11, 1808, MPBH.

7. On the disarray among the surviving staff: *Delaware County (PA) American*, September 14, 1870.

8. *Philadelphia Inquirer*, August 9, 1870.

9. BHAR 1870, 39–65.

10. Henry Graham Ashmead, *History of Delaware County, Pennsylvania* (Philadelphia: L. H. Everts, 1884), 398–401; Wiley, *Biographical and Historical Cyclopedia*, 119.

11. *Philadelphia Inquirer*, April 1, 1861.

12. *Delaware County American*, August 17, 1870.

13. *Philadelphia Inquirer*, September 26, 1870.

14. BHAR 1870, 61; La Roche, *Remarks on the Origin and Mode of Progression*, 25.

15. George F. Lehman (Lazaretto physician) to Nicolas Chervin, May 24, 1821, box 3, Nicolas Chervin Papers; Patricia D'Antonio, *American Nursing: A History of Knowledge, Authority, and the Meaning of Work* (Baltimore, MD: Johns Hopkins University Press, 2010), 3–4; Susan Reverby, *Ordered to Care: The Dilemma of American Nursing, 1850–1945* (Cambridge: Cambridge University Press, 1987), 30; Charles Rosenberg, *The Care of Strangers: The Rise of America's Hospital System* (New York: Basic Books, 1987), 213–14.

16. *Delaware County (PA) American*, September 14, 1870.

17. US Census, 1850, Allegheny County, PA, City of Pittsburgh, 1st Ward; US Census, 1870, Philadelphia County, PA, 18th District, 7th Ward; *Gopsill's Philadelphia City Directory for 1869* (Philadelphia, 1869); *Philadelphia Sunday Dispatch*, September 11, 1870; G. T. Rid-

lon, *History of the Ancient Ryedales* (Manchester, NH, 1884), 182; Michael R. Murphy, "The Mayors of Pittsburgh," Brookline Connection, last updated January 28, 2021, http://www.brooklineconnection.com/history/Facts/PghMayors.html.

18. BHAR 1870, 46–47; La Roche, *Remarks on the Origin and Mode of Progression*, 24–25.

19. *Philadelphia Sunday Dispatch*, September 11, 1870; BHAR 1870, 46–47.

20. *Philadelphia Sunday Dispatch*, September 11, 1870.

21. BHAR 1870, 61; *Philadelphia Morning Post*, August 12, 1870.

22. The three accounts that follow are based on the evidence presented in BHAR 1870, 39–65; and La Roche, *Remarks on the Origin and Mode of Progression*, 20–26.

23. Currie, *Sketch*, 71 (emphasis added).

24. Currie, *Sketch*, 72–73.

25. Currie, *Sketch*, 71.

26. Board of Health committee to Secretary of Treasury Richard Rush, January 13, 1827; and Charles Penrose, Thomas D. Groves, and William Bethell to William Jones (Customs Collector of the Port of Philadelphia), March 27, 1827, RG 36, Office of the Collector of Customs, Letters and Circulars Received, 1798–1912, vol. 3 (1827–32), NARA Mid-Atlantic.

27. Reports of Dr. H. Earnest Goodman and Dr. J. Howard Taylor, BHAR 1870, 48, 64.

28. Jewell, "Fever Prevailing," 54–62.

29. Port physician's report and "Appendix: Table of Yellow Fever Cases Contracted in Swanson Street Locality," BHAR 1870, 52, 55.

30. La Roche, *Yellow Fever*.

31. La Roche, *Remarks on the Origin and Mode of Progression*, 3–5.

32. La Roche, *Remarks on the Origin and Mode of Progression*, 18, 22–23; report of Dr. Goodman, BHAR 1870, 41.

33. BHAR 1870, 42–44, 60–61; La Roche, *Remarks on the Origin and Mode of Progression*, 4–5, 24, 28–50.

34. La Roche, *Remarks on the Origin and Mode of Progression*, 64–70.

CHAPTER FIFTEEN: **Quarantine, a Political Minefield**

1. Finger, *Contagious City*, 142–45.

2. *Relf's Philadelphia Gazette*, July 3, 1806; *Aurora General Advertiser* (Philadelphia), July 11 and 12, 1806; minutes, July 11, 1808, MPBH; James Hedley Peeling, "Governor McKean and the Pennsylvania Jacobins (1799–1808)," *Pennsylvania Magazine of History and Biography* 54 (1930): 343–52.

3. Philip Shriver Klein, *Pennsylvania Politics, 1817–1832: A Game without Rules* (Philadelphia: Historical Society of Pennsylvania, 1940), 77–84; Philip S. Klein and Ari Hoogenboom, *A History of Pennsylvania* (New York: McGraw-Hill, 1973), 118–19.

4. *Weekly Aurora* (Philadelphia), March 31, 1817; *Berks and Schuylkill Journal* (Reading, PA), March 29, 1817. Slightly different versions of the Sutherland letter were published in various newspapers. On the political background of the Sutherland scandal and the 1817 campaign, see Klein and Hoogenboom, *History of Pennsylvania*, 118–19; and Klein, *Pennsylvania Politics*, 79–96.

5. *Weekly Aurora* (Philadelphia), March 31, 1817.

6. *Weekly Aurora* (Philadelphia), March 24 and 31, 1817; *Berks and Schuylkill Journal* (Reading, PA), March 29, 1817; *National Register* (Washington, DC), April 5, 1817; Thomas Brothers, *The United States of North America as They Are* (London: Longman, Orme, Brown, Green, and Longmans, 1840), 136–39; William L. Mackenzie, *The Lives and Opinions of Benjamin Franklin Butler and Jesse Hoyt* (Boston: Cook, 1845), 182; J. Thomas Scharf and Thompson Westcott, *History of Philadelphia, 1609–1884*, 3 vols. (Philadelphia: L. H. Everts, 1884), 1:588.

7. *Berks and Schuylkill Journal* (Reading, PA), May 13, 1826.

8. "Sutherland, Joel Barlow (1792–1861)," *Biographical Directory of the U.S. Congress*, accessed August 2, 2022, http://bioguide.congress.gov/scripts/biodisplay.pl?index=S001083; Mackenzie *Lives and Opinions*, 182.

9. Appointments File, box 84, series 41, RG 26, Pennsylvania State Archives, Harrisburg.

10. H. G. Sickel to James Beaver, February 19, 1887, in Appointments File, box 84, series 41, RG 26, Pennsylvania State Archives.

11. Appointments File, box 84, series 41, RG 26, Pennsylvania State Archives.

12. Appointments File, box 84, series 41, RG 26, Pennsylvania State Archives.

13. *Hatboro (PA) Public Spirit*, June 9 and August 25, 1883.

14. Samuel T. Wiley, ed., *Biographical and Portrait Cyclopedia of Montgomery County, Pennsylvania* (Philadelphia: Biographical Publishing, 1895), 394; Steven Peitzman, *A New and Untried Course: Woman's Medical College and Medical College of Pennsylvania, 1850–1998* (New Brunswick, NJ: Rutgers University Press, 2000), 32–33.

15. Wiley, *Biographical and Portrait Cyclopedia*, 394; Peitzman, *New and Untried Course*, 32–33.

16. *Hatboro (PA) Public Spirit*, June 7 and September 20, 1879; and June 5, 1880. Northern scorn and condescension toward the South pervaded national policy discussions throughout the decades of superficial postwar reconciliation and national reunification. See especially Natalie Ring, *The Problem South: Region, Empire, and the New Liberal State, 1880–1930* (Athens: University of Georgia Press, 2012).

17. *Hatboro (PA) Public Spirit*, July 3, 1880; Eric Foner, *Reconstruction: America's Unfinished Revolution, 1863–1877*, updated ed. (New York: Harper Perennial, 2014), 307–8.

18. *Hatboro (PA) Public Spirit*, July 3, 1880. ("Fag-end" meant a cigarette butt or, figuratively, residue or dregs.)

19. W. W. H. Davis, *History of the 104th Pennsylvania Regiment* (Philadelphia, 1866; Beford, MA: Applewood Books, n.d.), 317–18; Alice J. Gayley, "104th Regiment Pennsylvania Volunteers," accessed August 3, 2022, http://www.pa-roots.com/pacw/infantry/104th/104thorg.htm, excerpting Samuel P. Bates, *History of Pennsylvania Volunteers, 1861–65*, 5 vols. (Harrisburg, PA: B. Singerly, 1868–1871).

20. In a letter to Major-General J. G. Foster, commanding officer of all US forces in South Carolina, his Confederate counterpart Major-General Samuel Jones indicated his intention to release Robinson "as soon as it can be done," because Foster had assured him that Robinson had not been out "reconnoitering" when he was captured. Jones's letter was written on August 2, 1864, however, less than a month after Robinson's capture, and Colonel Davis of the 104th notes that Robinson was released after "about three months" as a prisoner. Samuel Jones to J. G. Foster, August 2, 1864, in "Letters on the Treatment and

Exchange of Prisoners," *Southern Historical Society Papers* 3 (1877): 81; Davis, *History of the 104th*, 318; *Hatboro (PA) Public Spirit*, September 14, 1933.

21. Davis, *History of the 104th*, 21, 318, 331–33.

22. This included, among other innovations, a steam-powered tug that allowed inspections of arriving vessels to take place without the ships even slowing down, much less coming to anchor, at the Lazaretto. *Philadelphia Inquirer*, January 4, 1876; *Philadelphia Evening Bulletin*, June 18, 1879; "Life on the 'Visitor': How the Quarantine Officials Visit the Foreign Ships that Pass Up the Delaware," *Hatboro (PA) Public Spirit*, May 22 and July 10, 1880; and October 1, 1881.

23. Thomas A. Lewis, "When Washington, D.C. Came Close to Being Conquered by the Confederacy," *Smithsonian*, July 1988, https://www.smithsonianmag.com/history/when-washington-dc-came-close-to-being-conquered-by-the-confederacy-180951994/.

24. "Life on the 'Visitor'"; *Hatboro (PA) Public Spirit*, June 23, 1883.

25. "Life on the 'Visitor.'"

26. *Hatboro (PA) Public Spirit*, October 4, 1879; and July 1 and 8, 1882.

27. *Hatboro (PA) Public Spirit*, June 7, 1879.

28. *Hatboro (PA) Public Spirit*, July 24, 1880.

29. *Hatboro (PA) Public Spirit*, October 9, 1880. Twenty-first-century readers may find irony in Robinson's mention of the mosquito, but Robinson could not have connected that insect with yellow fever. It wasn't until the following year that Cuban physician Carlos Finlay first suggested that *Aedes aegypti* played a role in the disease's transmission, and only after the experiments conducted by the US military commission led by Walter Reed in 1900 was the mosquito hypothesis widely accepted. Carlos Finlay, "The Mosquito Hypothetically Considered as an Agent in the Transmission of Yellow Fever Poison," trans. Rudolph Matas, *New Orleans Medical and Surgical Journal* 9 (1882): 601–16; François Delaporte, *The History of Yellow Fever: An Essay on the Birth of Tropical Medicine* [*Histoire de la fièvre jaune*], trans. Arthur Goldhammer (Cambridge, MA: MIT Press, 1991); Mariola Espinosa, *Epidemic Invasions: Yellow Fever and the Limits of Cuban Independence, 1878–1930* (Chicago: University of Chicago Press, 2009), 56–63.

30. *Hatboro (PA) Public Spirit*, June 17, 1882.

31. George B. Wood, *A Treatise on Therapeutics, and Pharmacology or Materia Medica*, 2 vols. (Philadelphia: Lippincott, 1856), 2:267–68.

32. Warner, *Therapeutic Perspective*, 175–79; Alfred Stillé, *The Origins, Nature, Symptoms and Treatment of Yellow Fever* (Philadelphia: Samuel M. Miller, [1879]), 19. See chapter 12 for a discussion of heroic depletion.

33. Stillé, *Origins, Nature, Symptoms*, 19–20; Warner, *Therapeutic Perspective*, 149–53; *Philadelphia Times*, July 18, 1879.

34. *Hatboro (PA) Public Spirit*, July 28, 1883.

35. *Hatboro (PA) Public Spirit*, July 28, 1883.

36. *Hatboro (PA) Public Spirit*, July 28, 1883; Lazaretto Hospital Register, 1847–1893, collection of the Philadelphia History Museum (in custody of Drexel University).

37. William Osler, valedictory address to the University of Pennsylvania Faculty of Medicine, May 1, 1889, reprinted in Osler, *Aequanimitas, with Other Addresses to Medical Students, Nurses, and Practitioners of Medicine* (Philadelphia: P. Blakiston's Son, 1904), 4.

38. *Harrisburg Daily Patriot,* May 17, 1887; *Philadelphia Inquirer,* May 27 and 28, 1887. After his Lazaretto service, during which he clashed repeatedly with the steward, Brusstar distinguished himself primarily by providing advertising testimonials for Horsford's Acid Phosphate (a patent remedy for "nervous troubles") and by being targeted by the state Board of Health for polluting the Schuylkill River through improper dumping or draining at his property in Birdsboro. *Christian Work: Illustrated Family Newspaper* 61 (1896): 444; *Sixteenth Annual Report of the State Board of Health and Vital Statistics of the Commonwealth of Pennsylvania* ([Harrisburg, PA]: Wm. Stanley Ray, 1901), 279.

39. Epitaph of William T. Robinson, Hatboro Cemetery, Hatboro, Pennsylvania.

40. *Hatboro (PA) Public Spirit,* June 9 and July 28, 1883.

41. I borrow the phrase "the double face of Janus" from Owsei Temkin's book of collected essays, *The Double Face of Janus and Other Essays in the History of Medicine* (1977; Baltimore, MD: Johns Hopkins University Press, 2006).

CHAPTER SIXTEEN: **The Final Days, 1888–1895**

1. "Delaware County Population and Census," Old Chester, PA, last updated October 18, 2005, http://www.oldchesterpa.com/population_census.htm.

2. Minutes, August 9 and 12, 1884, and August 18, 1885, MPBH.

3. Minutes, February 7 and June 6, 1888, MPBH.

4. *Philadelphia Inquirer,* June 13, 1888. To re-create the atmosphere of the raucous meeting, I have converted the newspaper's indirect quotation to a direct quotation beginning "Dr. Brusstar is not fit."

5. *Philadelphia Inquirer,* July 6, 1888.

6. *Philadelphia Inquirer,* July 12, 1888.

7. *Philadelphia Inquirer,* July 12, 1888.

8. *Philadelphia Inquirer,* July 21, 1888.

9. *Philadelphia Inquirer,* August 23, 24, 25, and 31, 1888.

10. "Ward R. Bliss," Pennsylvania House of Representatives, Historical Biographies, accessed August 4, 2022, http://www.legis.state.pa.us/cfdocs/legis/BiosHistory/MemBio .cfm?ID=2782&body=H; Wiley, *Biographical and Historical Cyclopedia,* 469–71.

11. *Philadelphia Inquirer,* May 29, 1889.

12. Among the dozens of newspaper articles repeating variations of the allegations and rebuttals between 1891 and 1893: *Philadelphia Press,* undated clipping (early 1891), in Board of Health scrapbook, 76.38, Philadelphia City Archives; *Philadelphia Inquirer,* December 28, 1890; and February 9 and 22, 1891.

13. The following sources are all in the Board of Health scrapbook: Board of Health resolution, January 29, 1891; Board of Health "Memorial" to the state legislature, February 3, 1891; *Philadelphia Press,* undated clipping (early 1891); clipping from *Philadelphia Call,* March 17, 1891.

14. Board of Health scrapbook: protest against Bliss bill by coalition of business interests, February 13, 1891; clippings from *Philadelphia Inquirer,* January 31, 1891; and *Public Ledger,* March 9, 1891.

15. *Philadelphia Inquirer,* February 22, 1891; *Philadelphia Call,* March 7, 1891.

16. *Philadelphia Press,* undated clipping (early 1891), in Board of Health scrapbook.

17. *Philadelphia Times,* April 16, 1891.

18. *Philadelphia Inquirer*, April 14, 1891.

19. *Chester (PA) Times*, March 17, 1891.

20. *Philadelphia Press*, May 6, 1891.

21. Many newspaper clippings in the Board of Health scrapbook offer various accounts of these developments. For example: *Philadelphia Times*, May 14, 1891; *Philadelphia Call*, May 14, 1891; *Delaware County (PA) Advocate*, May 16, 1891; *Philadelphia Public Ledger*, May 21, 1891; *Delaware County (PA) American*, June 3, 1891.

22. Spread of cholera in 1892: Richard J. Evans, *Death in Hamburg: Society and Politics in the Cholera Years, 1830–1910* (London: Penguin, 1990), 279–80.

23. *Philadelphia Inquirer*, July 10, 1892; minutes, July 6, 8, 9, and 12, 1892, MPBH.

24. *Philadelphia Inquirer*, August 2 and 9, 1892; Evans, *Death in Hamburg*, 280–84.

25. Charles Bright, *Submarine Telegraphs: Their History, Contruction, and Working* (London: C. Lockwood, 1898), 99–105.

26. *Philadelphia Inquirer*, August 26 and 27, 1892; minutes, August 29, 1892, MPBH.

27. Kraut, *Silent Travelers*, 59–60; Markel *Quarantine!*, 73; *Philadelphia Inquirer*, August 29 and 31, 1892.

28. *Philadelphia Inquirer*, August 30, 1892.

29. Minutes, August 30 and September 1 and 2, 1892, MPBH.

30. *Philadelphia Inquirer*, September 2, 1892.

31. *Philadelphia Inquirer*, September 2 and 3, 1892; minutes, September 2, 1892, MPBH.

32. *Philadelphia Inquirer*, September 4, 1892; minutes, September 3, 1892, MPBH.

33. *Philadelphia Inquirer*, September 6, 1892.

34. Minutes, October 3 and 13, and November 28, 1892, MPBH.

35. Minutes, August 29, September 2, 8, 12, 16, and 20, and October 27, 1892, MPBH.

36. Evans, *Death in Hamburg*; Markel, *Quarantine!*, 130.

37. Minutes, September 2, 1892, MPBH; *Philadelphia Inquirer*, December 28, 1892.

38. Joseph J. Kinyoun to T. Mitchell Prudden, September 8, 1892; William H. Welch to Prudden, September 13, 1892; and Prudden, Stephen Smith, Abraham Jacobi, Edward G. Janeway, Alfred L. Loomis, Richard H. Derby, and Allan McLane Hamilton to Alexander E. Orr (chairman, Quarantine Committee, Chamber of Commerce of the State of New York), October 19, 1892. All three letters are in MS 1051, series 1, box 1, T. Mitchell Prudden Papers, Yale University Library Manuscripts and Archives, New Haven, Connecticut.

39. Markel, *Quarantine!*, 173–78; *Philadelphia Bulletin*, March 21, 1893.

40. Various newspaper clippings, April and May 1893, in Board of Health scrapbook.

41. *Philadelphia Inquirer*, May 7, 1893.

42. *Philadelphia Press*, April 22, 1893, in Board of Health scrapbook.

43. *Philadelphia Press*, April 22, 1893.

44. *Philadelphia Press*, May 30 and June 1, 1893, in Board of Health scrapbook; minutes, June 1, 1893, MPBH; *Harrisburg (PA) Patriot*, June 2, 1893.

45. *Philadelphia Inquirer*, June 6, 1893; *Philadelphia Public Ledger*, June 7, 1893, in Board of Health scrapbook.

46. Minutes, June 15, 1893, MPBH; *Hatboro (PA) Public Spirit*, June 17, 1893.

47. William Faulkner, *Requiem for a Nun* (1950; New York: Vintage Books, 2011), 73; Albert Camus, *The Plague*, trans. Stuart Gilbert (1947; New York: Vintage Books, 1991), 308.

CHAPTER SEVENTEEN: **Afterlives**

1. *Philadelphia Inquirer*, May 15, 1898.

2. *Philadelphia Inquirer*, January 14, 1900.

3. *Philadelphia Inquirer*, January 14, 1900; James H. Dormon, "Shaping the Popular Image of Post-Reconstruction American Blacks: The 'Coon Song' Phenomenon of the Gilded Age," *American Quarterly* 40 (1988): 450–71; Lynn Abbott and Doug Seroff, *Ragged but Right: Black Traveling Shows, "Coon Songs," and the Dark Pathway to Blues and Jazz* (Jackson: University Press of Mississippi, 2007), 11–80.

4. *Philadelphia Inquirer*, September 8, 1915; "Penn People: Robert Edward Glendinning, 1867–1936," University of Pennsylvania Archives, accessed August 4, 2022, https://archives.upenn.edu/exhibits/penn-people/biography/robert-edward-glendinning/.

5. *Philadelphia Inquirer*, February 4 and 27, and March 1 and 8, 1916; Frank Kingston Smith and James P. Harrington, *Aviation and Pennsylvania* (Philadelphia: Franklin Institute Press, 1981), 30–40; William F. Trimble, *High Frontier: A History of Aeronautics in Pennsylvania* (Pittsburgh: University of Pittsburgh Press, 1982), 91–93.

6. Walt Ellis, "An Outline of the History of the Philadelphia Seaplane Base and the Mills Family of Essington, PA," Essington Seaplane Base at Philadelphia, August 2, 2022, http://www.phillyseaplanebase.com/logbook/.

7. Todd Mason, "A Preservation Battle over Immigrant Site," *Philadelphia Inquirer*, June 21, 2006.

8. Elana Gordon, "Preservation of the Lazaretto, America's Oldest Surviving Quarantine Center, Finally Gets Underway," WHYY radio, October 28, 2016 https://whyy.org/articles/preservation-of-the-lazaretto-americas-oldest-surviving-quarantine-center-finally-gets-underway/.

9. The Lazaretto: America's Oldest Quarantine Station, home page, accessed June 27, 2022, http://www.Lazaretto.site.

10. City of Philadelphia, "Social Distancing, Isolation, and Quarantine during COVID-19 Coronavirus," March 31, 2020, https://www.phila.gov/2020-03-31-social-distancing-isolation-and-quarantine-during-covid-19-coronavirus/.

Afterword

1. The following description is based on the classic symptoms of severe yellow fever cases. La Roche, *Yellow Fever*, 1:129–36; Monath, "Yellow Fever: An Update"; Cooper and Kiple, "Yellow Fever," 1100–1107.

2. Harden, "Typhus, Epidemic," 1080–84.

3. Anne Hardy, "Urban Famine or Urban Crisis? Typhus in the Victorian City," *Medical History* 32, no. 4 (1988): 401–25; K. David Patterson, "Typhus and Its Control in Russia, 1870–1940," *Medical History* 37, no. 4 (1993): 361–81; Margaret Humphreys, "A Stranger to Our Camps: Typhus in American History," *Bulletin of the History of Medicine* 80, no. 2 (2006): 269–90.

4. Humphreys, "Stranger to Our Camps."

5. Margaret Humphreys, *Yellow Fever and the South* (Baltimore, MD: Johns Hopkins University Press, 1999), 4–5; J. R. McNeill, *Mosquito Empires: Ecology and War in the Greater Caribbean, 1620–1914* (New York: Cambridge University Press, 2010), 40–52.

6. McNeill, *Mosquito Empires*, 43; Joseph L. Melnick, "Yellow Fever," *McGraw-Hill Encyclopedia of Science and Technology*, 8th ed., 20 vols. (New York: McGraw-Hill, 1997), 19:684.

7. A sampling: Richard H. Shryock, *The Development of Modern Medicine* (Philadelphia: University of Pennsylvania Press, 1936), 215; David Musto, "Quarantine and the Problem of AIDS," *Milbank Quarterly* 64 (1986): 104, 108, 113, 115; Myron J. Echenberg, *Plague Ports: The Global Urban Impact of Bubonic Plague, 1894–1901* (New York: NYU Press, 2007), 142; World Health Organization, *The World Health Report 2007: A Safer Future: Global Public Health Security in the 21st Century* (Geneva: World Health Organization, 2007), 2, 7; Charles E. Rosenberg, "Commentary: Epidemiology in Context," *International Journal of Epidemiology* 38, no. 1 (2009): 28–30.

8. Patterson, "Yellow Fever Epidemics," 855–65; Humphreys, *Yellow Fever and the South*. Humphreys argues that the shorter quarantine detentions accompanied by thorough disinfection that became more common in southern ports in the 1880s "offered the prospect of a truly effective quarantine" and "probably did a fair job of killing mosquitoes" (180). Thomas Apel, "The Rise and Fall of Yellow Fever in Philadelphia, 1793–1805," in *Nature's Entrepôt: Philadelphia's Urban Sphere and Its Environmental Thresholds*, ed. Brian C. Black and Michael J. Chiarappa (Pittsburgh: University of Pittsburgh Press, 2012), 55–72, attributes the retreat of yellow fever from Philadelphia to several factors, including quarantine, which "isolated victims, making it more difficult for the *Aedes aegypti* mosquitoes to travel between an infected person and a healthy one" (57). He gives the lion's share of the credit, however, to the new water supply provided by the Center Square Water Works (which, like the Tinicum Lazaretto, opened in 1801), which "eliminat[ed] the necessity of keeping standing water in people's yards" (70).

9. *Proceedings and Debates from the Third National Quarantine and Sanitary Convention* (New York: Edmund Jone, 1859), 71–72, 76–77.

10. Patterson, "Typhus and Its Control in Russia."

11. van der Geest, Whyte, and Hardon, "Anthropology of Pharmaceuticals," 168; Whyte, van der Geest, and Hardon, *Social Lives of Medicines*, 14–17, 170–71; Rosenberg, "Therapeutic Revolution," 485–506; Rosenberg, *Our Present Complaint*, 9–10; Aronowitz, "From Skid Row to Main Street," 288–89, 312.

12. Peter Glaskowsky, "Bruce Schneier's New View on Security Theater," *CNET*, April 9, 2008, http://www.cnet.com/news/bruce-schneiers-new-view-on-security-theater/; Charles C. Mann, "Smoke Screening," *Vanity Fair* (web exclusive), December 20, 2011, http://www.vanityfair.com/culture/features/2011/12/tsa-insanity-201112;

13. Childress et al., "Public Health Ethics," 173; Bayer and Fairchild, "Genesis of Public Health Ethics," 489; Gostin, *Public Health Law*, 68; Jacobson and Hoffman, "Regulating Public Health," 29–30. I thank Michael Yudell and Jonathan Moreno for very helpful discussions of these issues.

14. Tyler Gay, Sam Hammer, and Erin Ruel, "Examining the Relationship between Institutionalized Racism and COVID-19," *City and Community* 19, no. 3 (2020): 523–30; Lucy Prior, "Allostatic Load and Exposure Histories of Disadvantage," *International Journal of Environmental Research and Public Health* 18, no. 14 (2021): 7222; Rebekah Rollston and Sandro Galea, "COVID-19 and the Social Determinants of Health," *American Journal of Health Promotion* 34, no. 6 (2020): 687–89; Sandro Galea, *The Contagion Next Time* (New York: Oxford University Press, 2022).

Index

Page numbers ending with *f* refer to figures.

yellow fever (*cont.*)
    168; extrinsic incubation period and, 245; in
    Jamaica, 3, 172, 183, 188; Lazaretto's overall
    success at treating, 7, 143–44, 208; Lower
    Mississippi Valley epidemic (1878) of, 212;
    medical treatments for, 135, 137, 139, 205–6;
    mortality rates from, 17; mosquitoes and, 7,
    17, 182, 243–45; partisan politics and, 26;
    Philadelphia epidemic (1793) of, 17–18, 21,
    25, 114–15, 137, 229; Philadelphia epidemic
    (1797) of, 20–21, 25, 191; Philadelphia
    epidemic (1798) of, 13–14, 16–22, 25, 33, 115;
    Philadelphia epidemic (1799) of, 21, 26–31,
    39, 45; Philadelphia epidemic (1800) of, 36;
    Philadelphia epidemic (1801) of, 43–44;
    Philadelphia epidemic (1802) of, 45–49, 51;
    Philadelphia epidemic (1803) of, 60–62;
    Philadelphia epidemic (1805) of, 84–86;
    Philadelphia epidemic (1820) of, 99–108,
    112, 113, 139; Philadelphia epidemic (1853)

of, 154–58, 159f, 160–64, 171, 187; Philadelphia epidemic (1870) of, 171–90; Philadelphia's decade (1790s) of outbreaks of, 8,
13, 20–21, 39, 86, 229; scientific theories
during eighteenth and nineteenth century
regarding, 7, 19–21, 26, 29, 47, 50–52, 54,
81, 85, 111–15, 117–21, 158, 168, 182–90,
244–46; seasonal patterns regarding, 7, 20,
28, 32–33, 46, 59, 246, 247; *Shasta* quarantine (1879) and, 2–6, 196, 210–11; Spain
outbreaks (1804) and, 59; supportive care
and, 179–81, 206–7; symptoms of, 17,
27–28, 43, 100, 102, 114–15, 207, 243
*Yellow Fever, Considered in Its Historical,
    Pathological, Etiological, and Therapeutical
    Relations* (La Roche), 175, 187
Young, Elizabeth, 83–84, 86
Young, Peter, 82–86

zymotic diseases, 188